Benzodiazepines
Today and Tomorrow

Benzodiazepines Today and Tomorrow

Proceedings of the 1st International Symposium on Benzodiazepines in Rio de Janeiro
28–30 September 1979

Edited by

R.G. PRIEST
Professor of Psychiatry, St. Mary's Hospital Medical School, University of London, England

U. VIANNA FILHO
Professor of Psychiatry, Psychiatry Institute
President of Brazilian Psychiatry Association
Rio de Janeiro, Brazil

R. AMREIN
F. Hoffmann–La Roche & Co. Ltd.,
Basle, Switzerland

M. SKRETA
F. Hoffmann-La Roche & Co. Ltd.,
Basle, Switzerland

MTP PRESS LIMITED
International Medical Publishers

All names of products in this book are legally protected as Trade Marks.

Published by
MTP Press Limited
Falcon House
Lancaster, England

Softcover reprint of the hardcover 1st edition 1980

First published 1980

British Library Cataloguing in Publication Data

International Symposium on Benzodiazepines,
1st, Rio de Janeiro, 1979
Benzodiazepines today and tomorrow.
1. Benzodiazepines – Congresses
I. Title II. Priest, Robert G.
615'.7882 RM666.B42

ISBN 978-94-011-7240-0 ISBN 978-94-011-7238-7 (eBook)
DOI 10.1007/978-94-011-7238-7

REDWOOD BURN LIMITED
Trowbridge and Esher.

Contents

List of Contributors and Participants

M. A. ALBUQUERQUE
Dept° Psiquiatria
Pontifícia Universidade Católica
90000 Porto Alegre, RS
BRAZIL

J. L. ALHO FILHO
Rua Sabará 401 apt° 102
01239 São Paulo, SP
BRAZIL

R. AMREIN
Dept. of Clinical Investigation and Development
F. Hoffmann–La Roche & Co. Ltd.
CH 4002 Basle
SWITZERLAND

E. AZZI
Dept° Psiquiatria e Psicologia Médica
Fac. Ciências Médicas
Rua Dr. Cesário Motta Jr. 112
01221 São Paulo, SP
BRAZIL

O. BASTOS
Dept.° de Psiquiatria
Centro de Ciências da Saúde
Univ. Federal de Pernambuco
50000 Recife, PE
BRAZIL

V. BOTELHO Herrera
Casilla de Correo 2207
La Paz
BOLIVIA

J. P. BOULENGER
c/o Produits Roche S.A.
52, Boulevard du Parc
92241 Neuilly-sur-Seine
FRANCE

F. J. BRAGA DE ALMEIDA
Dept° de Psiquiatria e Psicologia Médica
Fac. Ciências Médicas/UNICAMP
Rua José Theodoro Lima 44
13100 Campinas, SP
BRAZIL

T. R. BROWNE
Dept. of Neurology
Boston University Medical Center
80 East Concord Street
Boston, Mass. 02118
USA

J. R. BUENO
Assoc. Bras. Psiquiatria
Rua Paulino Fernandes 78
22270 Rio de Janeiro, RJ
BRAZIL

E. D. BUSNELLO
Rua Luciana de Abreu 210 apt° 602
90000 Porto Alegre, RS
BRAZIL

A. CORREIA
SQS 111, bloco D, apt° 504
70377 Brasília, DF
BRAZIL

J. A. COSTA E SILVA
Rua Getúlio das Neves 22
22461 Rio de Janeiro, RJ
BRAZIL

J. L. CROISY
Centre Hospitalier Spécialisé
67170 Brumath
FRANCE

W. G. CROUTHAMEL
Dept. of Pharmacokinetics and Biopharmaceutics
Hoffmann–La Roche Inc.
Nutley, NJ 07110
USA

J. H. DIÁZ
Edificio del Banco de América
3ero piso
Panama Ciudad
PANAMA

A. J. M. DE PAULA
Rua Araguaia 48
36100 Juiz de Fora, MG
BRAZIL

M. DISTEFANI
Rua Nove de Julho 830 apt° 26
14800 Araraquara, SP
BRAZIL

A. C. ESPONDA
CIAT – Centro de Informaciones y Asesoramiento Toxicológico
Hospital de Clínicas
Montevideo
URUGUAY

N. de Moura FÉ
Rua Joaquim Lima 436
60000 Fortaleza, CE
BRAZIL

R. G. FELDMAN
Dept. of Neurology
Boston University Medical Center
80 East Concord Street
Boston, Mass. 02118
USA

M. P. de Toledo FERRAZ
Rua Borges Lagoa 394
04038 São Paulo, SP
BRAZIL

V. GENTIL FILHO
Dept° de Farmacologia
Inst. de Ciências Biomédicas/USP
Cidade Universitária
05568 São Paulo, SP
BRAZIL

C. H. de GOUVEIA
Roche Farmacêutica Química Ltda.
Apartado 2549
1113 Lisboa
PORTUGAL

J. R. GRABOWSKI
Av. Silva Jardim 921 apt° 32
80000 Curitiba, PR
BRAZIL

W. E. HAEFELY
Pharmaceutical Research Dept.
F. Hoffmann–La Roche & Co. Ltd.
CH 4002 Basle
SWITZERLAND

H. HIGUERO Juliao
Dept° de Psiquiatría
Universidad de Panama
Panama Ciudad
PANAMA

G. M. JACOBIDES
Neofitou Vamva 5
Athens 138
GREECE

F. JESSURUM
c/o Hoffmann–La Roche B.V.
Nijverheidsweg 38
3641 RR Mijdrecht
NETHERLANDS

M. R. JORGE
Rua Joinville 651 – Ibirapuera
São Paulo, SP
BRAZIL

S. C. KAIM
Biometric Research Institute, Inc.
1010 Wisconsin Ave. N.W.
Washington, DC 20007
USA

S. A. KAPLAN
Dept. of Pharmacokinetics and Biopharmaceutics
Hoffmann–La Roche Inc.
Nutley, NJ 07110
USA

I. G. KARNIOL
Dept° de Psiquiatria e Psicologia Médica
Fac. Ciências Médicas/UNICAMP
Rua José Theodoro Lima 44
13100 Campinas, SP
BRAZIL

D. KELLY
The Priory Hospital
Priory Lane, Roehampton
London SW15 5JJ
ENGLAND

A. van der KUY
c/o Hoffmann–La Roche B.V.
Nijverheidsweg 38
3641 RR Mijdrecht
NETHERLANDS

D. LADEWIG
Psychiatrische Universitätsklinik
Wilhelm Klein-Strasse 27
CH 4025 Basle
SWITZERLAND

Y. D. LAPIERRE
197 Cumberland Street
Ottawa, Ontario K1N 7H4
CANADA

B. LEISHMAN
Dept. of Clinical Investigation and Development
F. Hoffmann–La Roche & Co. Ltd.
CH 4002 Basle
SWITZERLAND

J. LEMOS
Dept° de Psiquiatria
Centro de Ciências da Saúde
Univ. Federal de Pernambuco
50000 Recife, PE
BRAZIL

L. M. LESSA
Parque Lucaia, rua D, qd.E, lote 3
Rio Vermelho
40000 Salvador, BA
BRAZIL

M. LEVY Jr.
Rua Caraúna 148
05449 São Paulo, SP
BRAZIL

M. P. LISON
Rua Visconde de Inhaúma 1566
14100 Ribeirão Preto, SP
BRAZIL

J. L. LOPES
Rua Visconde de Caravelas 111
22271 Rio de Janeiro, RJ
BRAZIL

G. LORETO
Rua Virgínia Loreto 88
50000 Recife, PE
BRAZIL

J. C. MADALENA
Casa de Saúde Dr. Eiras
Rua Assunção 2
22251 Rio de Janeiro, RJ
BRAZIL

P. MARIZ
Coordenadoria de Saúde Mental
Praça Oswaldo Cruz, s/n
50000 Recife, PE
BRAZIL

M. C. C. A. MARTINS
Dept° de Psiquiatria
Centro de Ciências da Saúde
Univ. Federal de Pernambuco
50000 Recife, PE
BRAZIL

E. G. MATOS
Dept° de Psiquiatria e Psicologia Médica
Fac. Ciências Médicas/UNICAMP
Rua José Theodoro Lima 44
13100 Campinas, SP
BRAZIL

D. McCLURE
St. Mary's Hospital
3830 Lacombe Ave., room 3207
Montréal, Québec H3T 1M5
CANADA

R. MONTENEGRO
Instituto Equatoriano de Securidad Social
Quito
EQUADOR

M. J. F. MOREIRA
Dept° de Psiquiatria e Psicologia Médica
Fac. Ciências Médicas/UNICAMP
Rua José Theodoro Lima 44
13100 Campinas, SP
BRAZIL

M. S. MOREIRA
Clínica Psiquiátrica da Escola de Medicina e Cirurgia
Rio de Janeiro, FEFIERJ, RJ
BRAZIL

E. M. OLIVEIRA NETO
Rua Clodomiro Amazonas 443
04537 São Paulo, SP
BRAZIL

I. F. PAIM
SQS 114, bloco H, apt° 102
70377 Brasília, DF
BRAZIL

J. PAPROCKI
GPC – Grupo de Estudos em Psicofarmacologia Clínica
Rua Dom Lúcio Antunes 360
30000 Belo Horizonte, MG
BRAZIL

L. PEPPLINKHUIZEN
c/o Hoffmann–La Roche B.V.
Nijverheidsweg 38
3641 RR Mijdrecht
NETHERLANDS

P. E. PICANÇO
Rua Dr. José Lourenço 1645
60000 Fortaleza, CE
BRAZIL

A. E. PIEDRABUENA
Dept° de Psiquatria e Psicologia Médica
Fac. Ciências Médicas/UNICAMP
Rua José Theodoro Lima 44
13100 Campinas, SP
BRAZIL

W. PÖLDINGER
Kantonale Psychiatrische Klinik A
CH 9500 Wil/St. Gallen
SWITZERLAND

M. POINEAU
Produits Roche S.A.
52, Boulevard du Parc
92241 Neuilly-sur-Seine
FRANCE

J. U. POSTMA
c/o Hoffmann–La Roche B.V.
Nijverheidsweg 38
3641 RR Mijdrecht
NETHERLANDS

R. G. PRIEST
St. Mary's Hospital
Dept. of Psychiatry
Harrow Road
London W9 3RL
ENGLAND

L. RAMIREZ Ruiz
Centro Nacional de Farmacobiología
Ministerio de Sanidad y Securidad Social
Majadahonda
Madrid
SPAIN

J. M. van ROSSUM
c/o Hoffmann–La Roche B.V.
Nijverheidsweg 38
3641 RR Mijdrecht
NETHERLANDS

Á. RUBIM DE PINHO
Largo da Vitória 2 apt° 101
40000 Salvador, BA
BRAZIL

N. de Souza SAMPAIO
Escola de Medicina e Saúde Pública
Rua Frei Henrique 8
40000 Salvador, BA
BRAZIL

M. A. S. L. SANTOS
Dept° de Psiquiatria
Centro de Ciências da Saúde
Univ. Federal de Pernambuco
50000 Recife, PE
BRAZIL

J. A. SCHIPPER
c/o Hoffmann–La Roche B.V.
Nijverheidsweg 38
3641 RR Mijdrecht
NETHERLANDS

E. SCHWARZ
Psychiatrische Universitätsklinik
Wilhelm Klein-Strasse 27
CH 4025 Basle
SWITZERLAND

S. D. SEIBEL
Rua Pará 65 conj. 24
01238 São Paulo, SP
BRAZIL

K. R. SETYONEGORO
Mental Health Dept.
Ministry of Health
Prapatan 10
Jakarta
INDONESIA

I. SHIRAKAWA
Rua Dr. Rafael de Barros 238
04003 São Paulo, SP
BRAZIL

M. SKRETA
Dept. of Clinical Investigation
and Development
F. Hoffmann–La Roche & Co. Ltd.
CH 4002 Basle
SWITZERLAND

G. SOLARI Canessa
Unidad de Salud Mental
Ministerio de Salud
Monjitas 689, 4° piso
Santiago
CHILE

J. de SOUZA CAMPOS
Sanatório N.S. Aparecida
Rua Dona Mariana 182
22280 Rio de Janeiro, RJ
BRAZIL

J. G. SPECIALI
c/o M. P. Lison
Rua Visconde de Inhaúma 1566
14100 Ribeirão Preto, SP
BRAZIL

L. H. STERNBACH
Research Division
Hoffmann–La Roche Inc.
Nutley, NJ 07110
USA

H. TAVARES FILHO
Rua Maranhão 1566
30000 Belo Horizonte, MG
BRAZIL

R. TAVERAS Lucas
Dept° de Neuropsiquiatría
Hospital Psiquiátrico
Santo Domingo
DOMINICAN REP.

C. H. TOBLER
Av. Luis A. de Herrera 2431
Montevideo
URUGUAY

A. VIANNA FILHO
Rua Andre Wendhausen 113
88000 Florianópolis, SC
BRAZIL

U. VIANNA FILHO
Associação Brasileira de Psiquiatria
Rua Paulino Fernandes 78
22270 Rio de Janeiro, RJ
BRAZIL

W. A. VILELA
Dept° de Psiquiatria e Psicologia
Médica
Fac. Ciências Médicas/UNICAMP
Rua José Theodoro Lima 44
13100 Campinas, SP
BRAZIL

L. H. M. van WILGENBURG
Hoffmann–La Roche B.V.
Nijverheidsweg 38
3641 RR Mijdrecht
NETHERLANDS

A. ZAGLUL
Dept° de Psiquiatría
Universidad de Santo Domingo
DOMINICAN REP.

The 1st International Symposium on Benzodiazepines in Rio de Janeiro
was organized by the
'Associação Brazileira de Psiquiatria'
under the chairmanship of its president
Prof. U. Vianna Filho.

Particular mention should be made of the very valuable scientific contribution of the guest of honour,
Prof. Dr. Leo Sternbach,
pioneer in the research concerned with the development of the benzodiazepine drugs.

Editing Office and Translations:

Edith van de Benque, Rio de Janeiro
Marc Berkowitz, Rio de Janeiro
Jürg Burckhardt, Basle
Sergio Campos Mello, Rio de Janeiro
Elisabeth Hart, Rio de Janeiro
Barbara Leishman, Basle
Sonja Mani, Basle
Claudia Miranda, Rio de Janeiro
Sergio Montuori, Rio de Janeiro
Milan Skreta, Basle
Hans Weidner, Basle

Address of Editing Office:

Dr Milan Skreta,
F. Hoffmann–La Roche & Co. Ltd.,
Basle, Switzerland

Acknowledgement

For critical reading of some of the contributions and their helpful advice with regard to the publication of these proceedings, we would like to thank Dr Roland Dubuis (F. Hoffmann–La Roche, Basle) and Dr Phillip H. Bookman (Hoffmann–La Roche, Nutley).

1

Introduction

U. Vianna Filho

In his historical evolution, man has been able to dominate nature by means of his technological achievements, his knowledge and his inventiveness, attaining an increasing control over the world and its organization. As a result, his power over his fellow men has also increased, giving him more and more responsibility which leads, of necessity, to one existential problem: is the contemporary man, with all his power and knowledge, really happy?

Technological progress has brought him several rights and desires: health, better insight into the future and greater control over his own destiny, but despite all this he still suffers from insecurity and from all the new problems that he has to face, which fact accounts for his imperfections and limitations that inevitably generate anxiety.

Anxiety, therefore, constitutes one of the main characteristics of modern man. It can be foreseen today that, in the near future, the entire population of any large city will suffer from anxiety and behave in a 'neurotic' way.

Man is seeking relief from pain, suffering and, naturally, also anxiety. Thus all possible efforts are being made to find a solution for this anxiety. The search for substances that are able to eliminate anxiety is one of the constant concerns of modern science, and, in this context, one of the turning points, as we will see in this volume, has been the discovery of the chemical agents known as the benzodiazepines.

Their use has become so widespread that they are probably the most largely prescribed drugs in the world, their importance for the relief of anxiety being possibly equivalent to that of aspirin for physical pain.

Their utilization has been constantly increasing and may even lead to abuse and misuse. No drug can be free from side-effects and problems of dependence may occur with some of them. For this reason, the greatest care should be taken in order to avoid misapplications by doctors and patients.

A few words now about our view of the future and the forthcoming chemical developments with their consequences for therapeutics: On the basis of present human and technological resources, it is fair to expect that the quest for the ideal drug, that is, the most effective and side-effect free, will continue to be the goal of psychopharmacology in future years.

In the pursuit of this aim, we can expect the synthesis of new anxiolytic agents in the near future for the benefit of all mankind.

2

The Benzodiazepines Today and Tomorrow

R. G. Priest

Emotional distress is widespread. It respects neither class, colour nor nationality. It is common in all countries and the full extent of its prevalence is only gradually being recognized by the medical profession. Sometimes radical curative remedies are available, sometimes not. Frequently the distress is self-limiting, and all that the patient requests is some relief from the mental anguish while it lasts. Sometimes the treatment of the underlying psychological disorder is slow to come to fruition, and the sufferer requires some amelioration of his symptoms meanwhile.

The benzodiazepines are very effective at melting away the arctic terror of *anxiety*. They have replaced the older, traditional, toxic and notoriously addictive remedies for the treatment of *insomnia*. These two effects are of transcendental importance. Anxiety and insomnia are likely to occur as features of almost any acute personal distress[1, 2]. It is a tremendous boon to the medical profession to have active weapons in the fight against misery that are not only effective but are relatively safe when abused by despairing and desperate patients.

The benzodiazepines have numerous other uses. They are effective in the control of seizures. They reduce pathological excesses of muscular tension. They normalize the disordered autonomic nervous system. They are valued by the anaesthetist. There is scarcely a branch of medicine that has not been affected by their arrival.

The ballot paper of the medical profession is the prescription form. Physicians have given an overwhelming vote in favour of the benzodiazepines. Such a revolution in medical practice demands, and has produced, a cautionary reaction. The widespread use of benzodiazepines has given rise to intense controversy. Is it right that so many people should be taking minor tranquillizers? Is their wholesale prescription an indictment of the medical profession, a risky mistake in judgement? Or on the other hand is this wide availability a conspicuous social benefit?

It is time to review the advantages and the costs of the use of this class of drug. Previous conferences have examined in meticulous detail the pharmacological effects of benzodiazepines[3]. We now have the opportunity to take a broad look at the place of these drugs in medicine. What are their dangers, either in ordinary use or when misused? What advances would we like to witness in the drug treatment of anxiety, insomnia, epilepsy and muscle spasm? In what other conditions do we envisage enlisting the use of these and related drugs? What improvements would the clinician be keen to see in the effectiveness, selectivity or pharmacokinetics of benzodiazepines? The First International Symposium in Brazil addressed itself to these important issues. The benefit of the experience of practising clinicians in a country of 100 million people was synthesized with the expertise of an international array of invited speakers. The papers and the ensuing discussions are presented in the following pages. There will be few physicians who will read them without learning something new that is of value to his patients. What is more, the doctor who can share the visions seen by the participants and authors will be ready for the advances that are bound to come in the lifetime of most of us present.

References

1. Bedford, A., Foulds, G. A. and Sheffield, B. F. (1976). A new proposal disturbance scale (DSSI/sAD). *Br. J. Soc. Clin. Psychol.*, **15**, 387
2. Foulds, G. A. (1965). *Personality and Personal Illness* (London: Tavistock Publications)
3. Priest, R. G., Pletscher, A. and Ward, J. (eds.) (1979). *Sleep Research.* (Lancaster: MTP Press)

3

The Benzodiazepine Story

L. H. Sternbach

In this chapter, I would like to discuss the discovery and development of the centrally acting 1,4-benzodiazepines which started with the synthesis and pharmacological evaluation of a compound which is the active ingredient of Librium and is now known by the generic name chlordiazepoxide.

In the mid-fifties, almost a quarter of a century ago, when a new class of therapeutic agents, the tranquillizers, were shown to have considerable clinical value, Roche decided to initiate a programme concerned with the search for products of this type. The pharmacological tests for the screening of sedatives and tranquillizers were well in hand, and the chemists were asked to produce a new compound which would be superior to the then existing tranquillizers.

The chemist faced with a problem of this kind has various approaches at his disposal. He can start in a rather sophisticated manner with a biochemical working hypothesis, with other intelligent speculations, or select a more prosaic approach.

Our knowledge of the processes occurring in the brain was rather limited, and we could not conceive of an intelligent working hypothesis. We decided therefore to take the low road and to attack this problem in a purely empirical manner. Since our main interest was synthetic chemistry, we planned to select an approach which would be most attractive, challenging and satisfying for the bench chemist. In order to increase our chances of success, we considered it most practical to look for a group of compounds which would enable us to synthesize a large number of new representatives within a relatively short time. This class of compounds would be expected to fulfil the criteria indicated below:

(1) Be relatively unexplored,
(2) Be readily accessible,
(3) Give the possibility of a multitude of variations and transformations,
(4) Offer some chemically challenging problems and
(5) 'Look' as if it could lead to biologically active products.

A group of heterocycles I had worked with in the early thirties during my dyestuff chemistry years at the Cracow University[1,2] seemed to be ideally suited and now looked particularly attractive and promising to me. These were the easily crystallized benzheptoxdiazines shown in Figure 3.1 which were readily accessible by a simple sequence of reactions. We were sure that the accessibility of these compounds and the usual excellent co-operation of our Pharmacology Department under the direction of Dr Lowell Randall would considerably increase our chances of finding a biologically active product.

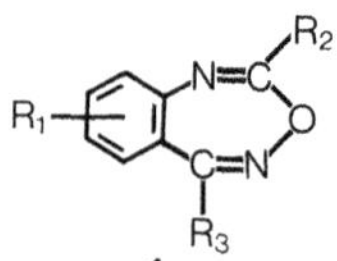

1

Figure 3.1

We thought it most promising to prepare new types of benzheptoxdiazines into which a basic substituent could be introduced, since it is known to the medicinal chemist that basic side chains often impart biological properties. Thus, we synthesized a number of products of type **2** and transformed them by treatment with secondary amines into products of type **3** (see Figure 3.2). The products were formed in good yield, crystallized well, formed nice water-soluble salts, but unfortunately did not possess any interesting biological properties.

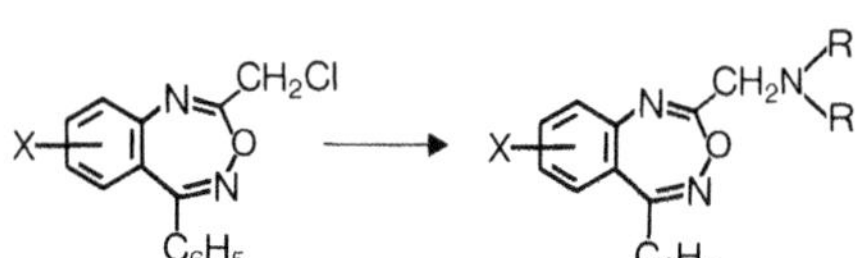

2 3

Figure 3.2

However, during these studies, we made the interesting discovery that these compounds known as heptoxdiazines were not heptoxdiazines at all, but were in fact the quinazoline 3-oxides[11] **4** and **5** (see Figure 3.3).

Shortly after this discovery, we had, to our regret, to stop our work in the quinazoline field since other problems seemed to be more important and required our full attention. This intensive work in new areas of research

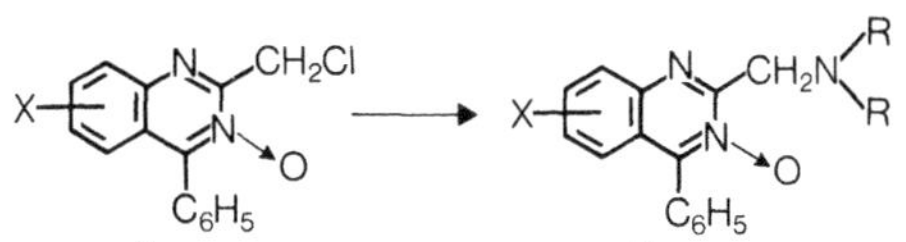

4 5

Figure 3.3

resulted finally in April 1957 in an almost unbearable situation. The laboratory benches were covered with dishes, flasks and beakers containing various more or less crystalline samples and mother liquors. The bench work area had shrunk to almost zero, and a major house cleaning was in order.

During this clean-up operation, my co-worker, Mr Earl Reeder, drew my attention to a few hundred milligrams of two products, a nicely crystalline base and its hydrochloride. The base had been prepared in 1955 by treatment of the quinazoline *N*-oxide (**6**) with methylamine; its hydrochloride shortly afterwards (Figure 3.4). The products were not submitted for pharmacological testing at that time because of our involvement with other problems. Since the compounds were pure and had the expected composition, we submitted in 1957 the water-soluble salt for pharmacological evaluation. We were quite prepared for a negative result and considered this the end of our work with quinazoline 3-oxides. We thought, however, that the material on hand would then be complete enough to yield a chemically interesting publication. Little did we know that this experiment would start a program which would keep us busy for many years.

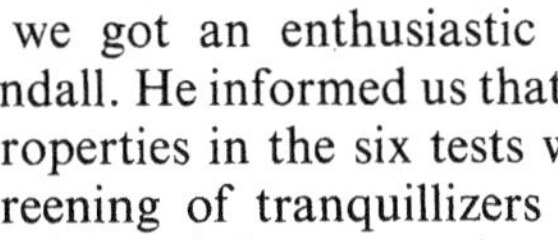

6

Figure 3.4

Within a few days we got an enthusiastic telephone call from our pharmacologist, Dr Randall. He informed us that this compound possessed unusually interesting properties in the six tests which were generally used for the preliminary screening of tranquillizers and sedatives. Table 3.1 shows the screening results and the comparison of the properties of this new compound with those of meprobamate, chlorpromazine and phenobarbital[3,4,12,14].

I am sure that these tests will be familiar to many[13]. I would, however, like to mention again that the first test indicates muscle relaxation and sedation in mice, the second a taming effect in mice, the third, muscle

Table 3.1 Pharmacological properties of 'new compound', meprobamate, chlorpromazine and phenobarbital

				Anticonvulsant tests		
					Electroshock	
Compound	*Incl. screen*	*Foot shock*	*Cat*	*Pentylenetetrazole*	*Max.*	*Min.*
New compound	100	40	2	18	92	150
Meprobamate	250	250	100	150	200	167
Chlorpromazine	17	20	2.5	42	150	600
Phenobarbital	120	80	10	75	18	90

relaxation in the cat. The last three tests in mice show anticonvulsant and sedative properties. The numbers in this and all other tables represent the dose (in mg/kg) of the orally administered drug which were needed to achieve the desired effect. Therefore, high figures indicate low activity, and low figures high activity. The table shows that the new compound was much more effective than meprobamate in each of our six preliminary tests. Compared with chlorpromazine, it was weaker in the first two tests, but was of equal strength as a muscle relaxant in the cat and had a more pronounced anticonvulsant activity in the mouse. As the last line shows, our new compound was in most tests even superior to phenobarbital. It is also worth noticing that unlike chlorpromazine and reserpine it had no effect at all on the autonomic nervous system. The product had a pronounced taming effect on monkeys. Particularly encouraging was the low toxicity (620 mg/kg in mice) which, as was found later, is typical for compounds of this group.

While the compound underwent a whole gamut of sophisticated pharmacological tests by Dr Randall and his staff, we in our laboratory were concerned with the chemistry of this unusual compound. We had reservations about its structure from the very beginning since the u.v. and i.r. spectra were completely different from those of the starting material **6** or those of other related quinazoline 3-oxides. Our studies showed, indeed, that the compound was not the quinazoline *N*-oxide **7** but the product of an unusual ring enlargement to the benzodiazepine derivative **8**; instead of the six-membered pyrimidine-ring the compound contained a seven-membered diazepine ring (Figure 3.5).

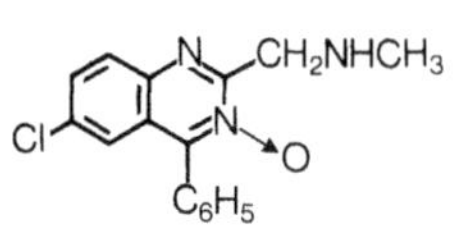

7

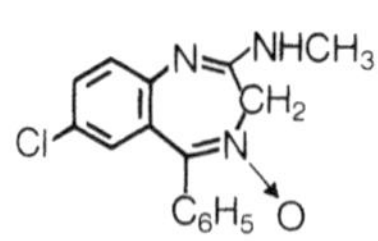

8

Figure 3.5

We elucidated the reaction mechanism[8] and synthesized a number of related compounds[16] as indicated in Figure 3.6.

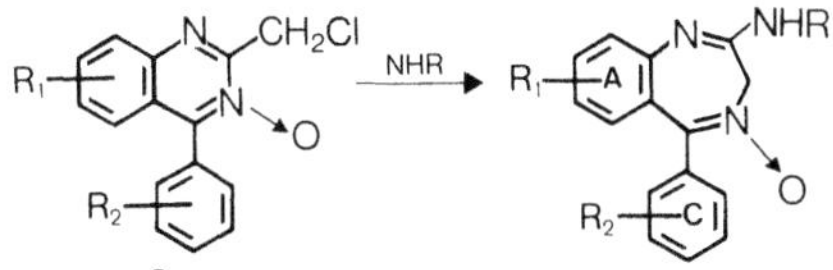

R = H, alkyl, alkenyl etc.
R_1 and R_2 = halogen, alkyl, CF_3 etc. in different positions of rings A and C

Figure 3.6

This enabled us to file a broad patent application in May 1958 claiming 2-amino-1,4-benzodiazepine 4-oxides bearing various substituents in the benzo- and phenyl rings. Because of the novelty of these products, the patent[7] was granted without any difficulties whatsoever, and appeared in July 1959.

All of these benzodiazepine derivatives possessed similar biological properties but neither of them was superior to, or significantly different from, the first product **8**. We therefore selected this first compound for closer investigation.

Long-term toxicity studies gave excellent results, also the clinical investigation looked very promising. The interest of the clinical investigators grew at such a rate that within a relatively short time around 16000 patients had been treated with this drug. The NDA application was submitted, and thanks to the then positive attitude of the FDA, the approval was obtained in record time. The drug was introduced under the trade name Librium in 1960, 2½ years after the pharmacological studies had started. The generic name which was later generally accepted was chlordiazepoxide.

At about the same time also the effect on wild animals was studied, at the San Diego Zoo and in our laboratories. Dr Leonard Hines initiated these studies. While Librium was prepared for introduction, we became interested in a form which would lend itself for the preparation of a pharmaceutically acceptable elixir or syrup for paediatric or geriatric use. This was necessary since chlordiazepoxide hydrochloride, the water-soluble clinically used salt, was extremely bitter: an unsurprising fact, since it is generally known to every medicinal chemist that any useful drug is either bitter, hygroscopic or unstable. Since this compound was rather valuable, it possessed all three properties.

In our search for a tasteless form we found that neither the base nor a salt could be used for these purposes; we discovered, however, on that occasion that the hydrochloride was not quite stable in aqueous solution. It hydrolyzed to the lactam *N*-oxide **11**[15], which to our pleasant surprise possessed the same pharmacological properties as chlordiazepoxide (Figure 3.7).

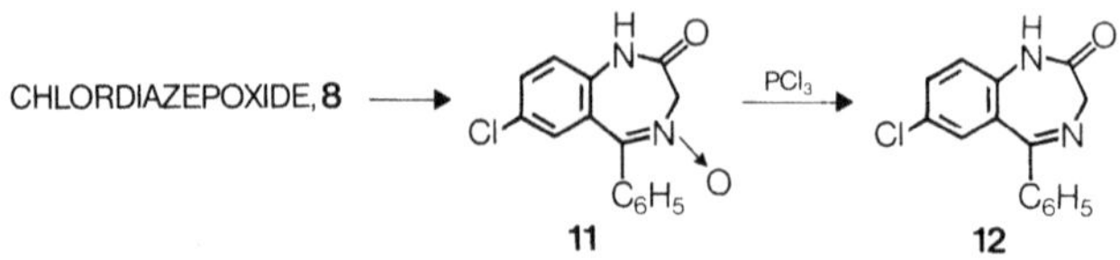

Figure 3.7

Also, the removal of the *N*-oxide oxygen did not diminish its activity, as can be seen in Table 3.2. Thus, it turned out that some of the unique features which seemed so characteristic for chlordiazepoxide were not at all needed for its pharmacological activity. The *N*-oxide function and particularly the basic substituent, which was the cornerstone of our initial working hypothesis, proved to be only unnecessary adornments.

Table 3.2 Pharmacological properties of compounds 8, 11 and 12

Compound	*Incl. screen*	*Foot shock*	*Cat*	*Metrazol*	*Max.*	*Min.*
8	100	40	2	18	92	150
11	75	40	1	6	52	400
12	75	20	1	6	25	61

The only features which were common to these biologically active compounds were the 1,4-benzodiazepine ring system bearing a chlorine in the 7-position and the phenyl group in the 5-position. Based on this knowledge, we started the intensive study of this type of compounds. We were particularly interested in the rather simple benzodiazepinones of type **12**, and developed methods[6,10] for their synthesis. The first two methods which were used most extensively are shown below.

As can be seen (Figure 3.8), in both cases, *o*-aminoketones (**13**) in which R is a hydrogen or an alkyl are used as starting materials. Treatment of the appropriately substituted aminobenzophenone with a haloacetyl halide (Method A) yielded a compound of type **14** which, on treatment with ammonia, gave the benzodiazepinone **15** via an amino derivative **16**. This product cyclizes readily on heating and in many cases spontaneously. Another extensively used method (B) consisted in the treatment of an aminobenzophenone with an amino acid ester salt in a solvent, preferably pyridine, leading directly from **13** to **15**. The first multi-step method (A) generally gave better overall yields, up to 70–80% of very pure products. The second method (B), on the other hand, facilitated the synthesis of

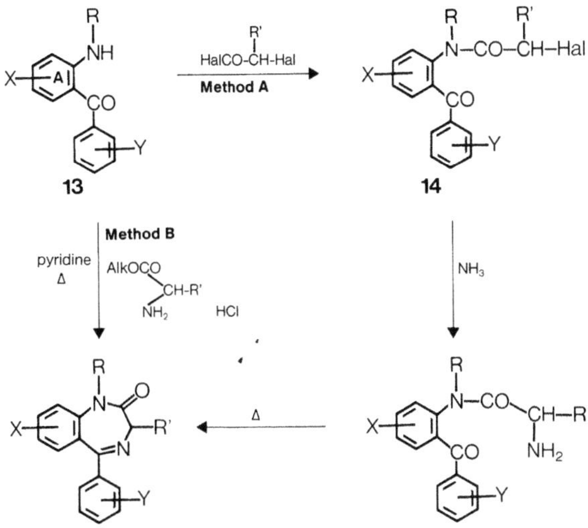

Figure 3.8

benzodiazepinones bearing substituents at position 3, since many α-amino acids bearing additional substituents on the α-carbon are commercially available.

The first transformation of the benzodiazepinones so obtained was the alkylation at position 1 (when R in compound **15** was hydrogen). Since this reaction could be readily carried out by treatment with a base and an alkylating agent, a considerable number of such products was synthesized and pharmacologically tested[14]. These substitution products were on hand when the clinical evaluation of Librium approached its completion. The excellent results encouraged us, even before the introduction of Librium, to look for a 'superior' compound with broader clinical utility. The comparison with the compounds which were at that time available showed that all of them had very similar spectra of activity in our six primary tests; the products varied essentially only in their potency. Since it is difficult, based on animal data, to predict the clinical effect in man of centrally acting drugs, we selected the most potent compound[5], holding that this increased potency would be accompanied by, *a priori*, unpredictable differences in its clinical action. This compound was the 1-methyl derivative **17** (Figure 3.9) and Table 3.3 shows the comparison of its pharmacological activity with that of chlordiazepoxide.

The pharmacology and the toxicity of this compound were studied in depth and gave only favourable data. Clinical studies were started, extended and, after good results were obtained, the introduction was planned. The product was given the generic name diazepam and it was introduced near

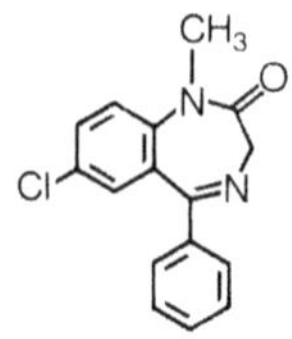

17

DIAZEPAM (VALIUM®)

Figure 3.9

Table 3.3 Comparison of the pharmacological activity of chlordiazepoxide with that of diazepam

Compound	*Incl. screen*	*Foot shock*	*Cat*	*Pentylenetetrazole*	*Max.*	*Min.*
Chlordiazepoxide **8**	100	40	2	18	92	150
Diazepam **17**	30	10	0.2	1.4	6.4	64

the end of 1963 under the trademark Valium. It had indeed a broader spectrum of activity than Librium; particularly the muscle relaxant properties are more pronounced. The toxicity was extremely low.

The intensive study of benzodiazepine derivatives was continued. Within a few years well over 3000 1,4-benzo- and heterodiazepines were in our hands. This involved the preparation, identification, and pharmacological investigation of about 4000 intermediates and byproducts.

The large number of benzodiazepinones made it possible to study the structure–activity relationships[13] in this series of compounds, and led to the data which are summarized in Figure 3.10.

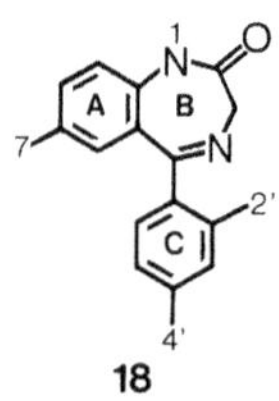

18

Figure 3.10 Effects of substituents on the biological activity of benzodiazepinone.

Ring A: position 7: increased by electron-withdrawing groups, e.g. Cl, NO_2, CF_3. Decreased by electron-releasing groups like CH_3, OCH_3. Substituents in any other position than 7 decrease the activity.

Ring B: position 1: increased by a methyl group. Decreased by larger substituents.

Ring C: increased by halogens in 2′-position (Cl, F). Very strongly decreased by a substituent in 4′-position.

It became apparent at the very beginning of our studies that the substitution pattern played an important role, particularly the substituent at the 7-position (ring A). We studied over 80 substituents at 7 and at other positions in ring A and found, with a few exceptions, good agreement with our initial findings. The effect of hundreds of substituents at the 1-position was explored. The position of substituents in ring C also showed a profound effect on the pharmacological activity. The available data resulted finally in the synthesis of compound **19**[9] which combined all the features known to impart high activity: the CH_3 group at 1, the nitro group at 7 and a fluorine at 2′ (Figure 3.11). It is, as expected, one of the pharmacologically[13] most potent benzodiazepinones, illustrating well the additive or potentiating properties of pharmacophoric groups in the benzodiazepine series (Table 3.4). It was introduced in Switzerland and other countries in 1975 as a potent hypnotic acting in 1–2 mg doses.

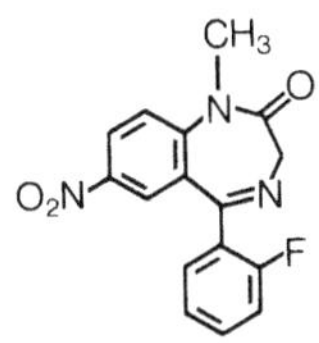

19

Flunitrazepam (Rohypnol®)

Figure 3.11

Table 3.4 Comparison of the pharmacological activity of diazepam with that of flunitrazepam

Compound	*Incl. screen*	*Foot shock*	*Cat*	*Met.*	*Max.*	*Min.*
Diazepam	30	10	0.2	1.4	6.4	64
Flunitrazepam	1	0.8	0.02	0.12	12	354

A host of 1,4-benzodiazepine derivatives has been introduced in the course of the years, indicative of the clinical value of these compounds. At this time there are 23 representatives of this class of compounds available to the clinician. Most of them are anxiolytics, some are hypnotics and one product is specifically used in epilepsy.

Figure 3.12 shows the 8 products marketed in the United States, also under various other trade names in other countries. All of them, with one exception, possess as the main pharmacophoric group a chlorine in the 7-position.

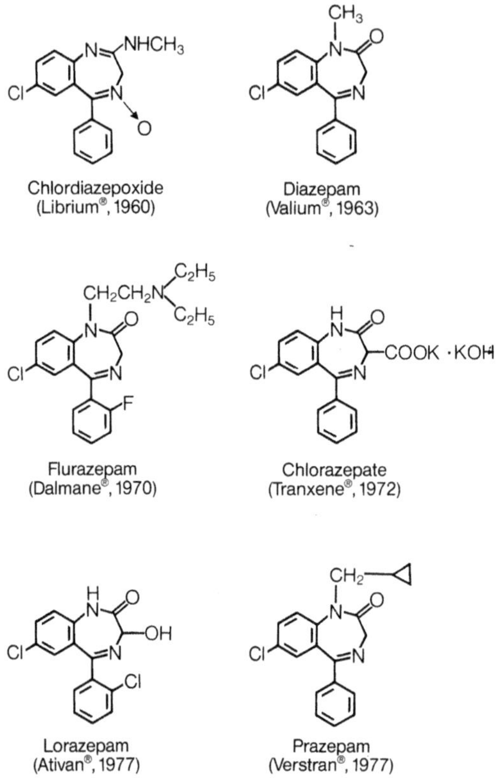

Figure 3.12 Benzodiazepines marketed in the United States

In addition to the generic names, Figures 3.12 and 3.13 show the introduction dates and one of the trade names. Figure 3.13 shows 15 additional products available in other countries under various trade names.

The main pharmacophoric group in 7 is in most cases a chlorine atom; three of the compounds have nitrogroups in 7. Compounds with heteronuclei attached to the B ring have also been introduced as can be seen in the oxazolo derivatives and particularly in the very potent triazolobenzodiazepines.

One related compound is also included. It formally resembles 1,4-benzodiazepines and has similar clinical properties. It is the 1,5-benzodiazepine clobazam.

Intensive research in the benzodiazepine field is still continuing and is concerned with the search for compounds possessing a different spectrum of activity. Another objective is the elucidation of the mode of action of these drugs, particularly at the molecular level. It can be expected that

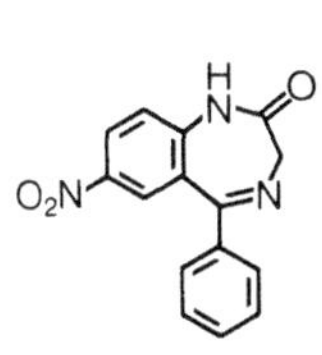
Nitrazepam
(Mogadon®, 1965)

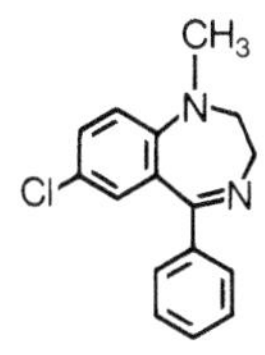
Medazepam
(Nobrium®, 1968)

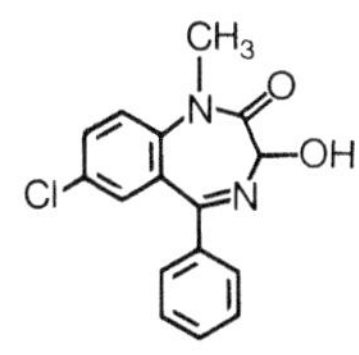
Temazepam
(Levanxol®, 1970)

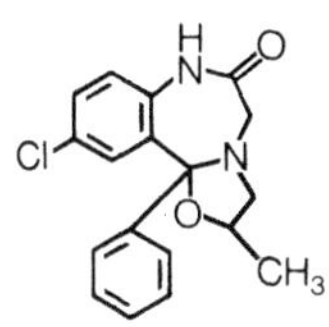
Oxazolam
(Serenal®, 1971)

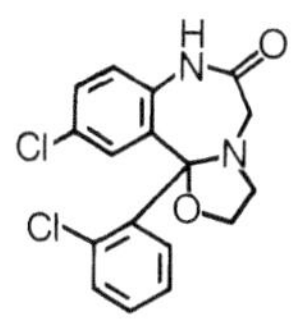
Cloxazolam
(Sepazon®, 1974)

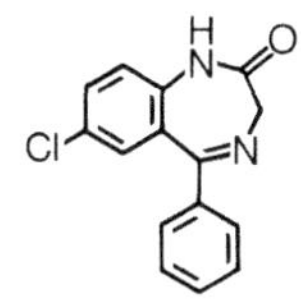
Desmethyldiazepam
(Madar®, 1973)

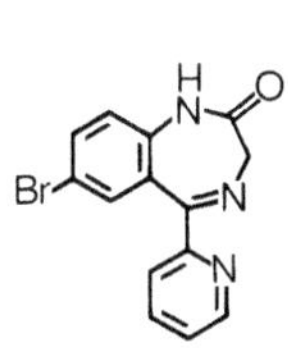
Bromazepam
(Lexotanil®, 1974)

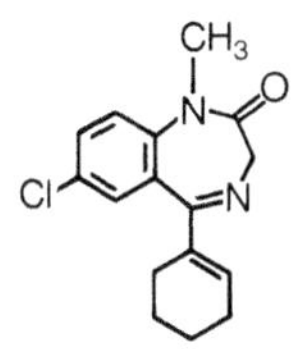
Tetrazepam
(Myolastan®, 1974)

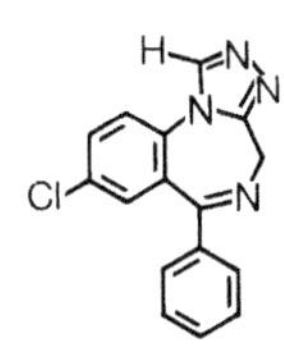
Estazolam
(Eurodin®, 1975)

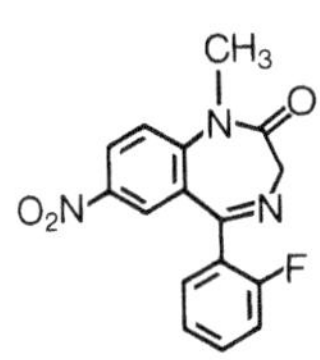
Flunitrazepam
(Rohypnol®, 1975)

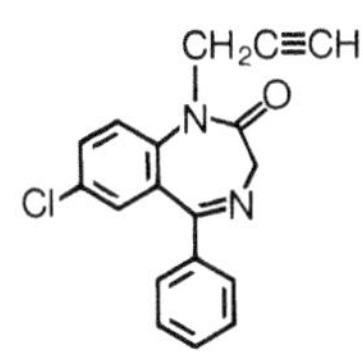
Pinazepam
(Domar®, 1975)

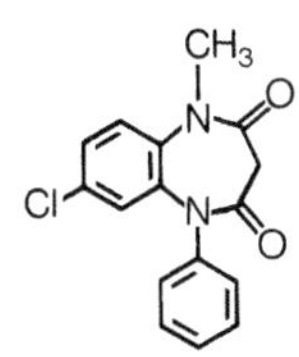
Clobazam
(Urbanyl®, 1975)

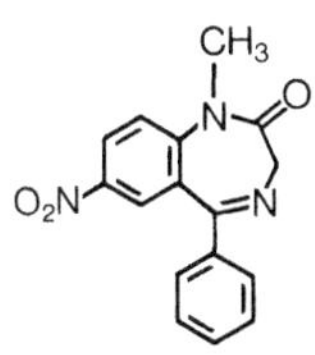
Nimetazepam
(Elimin®, 1977)

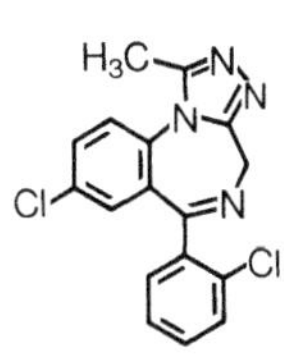
Triazolam
(Halcion®, 1977)

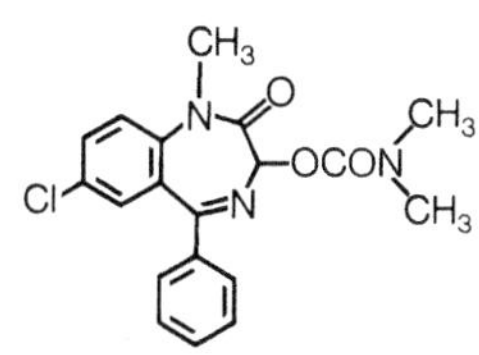
Camazepam
(Albego®, 1977)

Figure 3.13 Benzodiazepines marketed in countries other than the United States these efforts will finally lead to a better understanding of the effect of these compounds on the central nervous system.

References

1. Dziewoński, K. and Sternbach, L. (1933). Ueber die Einwirkung von Benzoylchlorid auf α-Naphthylamin. *Bull. Intern. Acad. Polonaise, Classe Sci. Math. Nat. Sér. A*, 416; *Chem. Abstr.*, **28**, 2717 (1934)
2. Dziewoński, K. and Sternbach, L. (1935). Weitere Studien über Reaktionen zwischen Benzoylchlorid und aromatischen Aminen und über ihre Produkte, Verbindungen der Chinazolinreihe. *Bull. Intern. Acad. Polonaise, Classe Sci. Math. Nat. Sér.* A, 333; *Chem. Abstr.*, **30**, 2971 (1936)
3. Randall, L. O. (1960). Pharmacology of methaminodiazepoxide. In *Dis. Nerv. System*, **XXI**, Sec. 2. Suppl. pp. 7–10
4. Randall, L. O. (1961). Pharmacology of chlordiazepoxide (Librium). In *Dis. Nerv. System*, **XXII**, Sec. 2, Suppl. pp. 7–15
5. Randall, L. O., Heise, G. A., Schallek, W., Bagdon, R. E., Banziger, R. F., Boris, A., Moe, R. A. and Abrams, W. B. (1961). Pharmacological and clinical studies on Valium®. A new psychotherapeutic agent of the benzodiazepine class. *Curr. Ther. Res.*, **3**, 405
6. Stempel, A. and Landgraf, F. W. (1962). Quinazolines and 1,4-benzodiazepines. IX. 2-Carbobenzoxyglycylamidobenzophenones and their conversion to 1,4-benzodiazepinones. *J. Org. Chem.*, **27**, 4675
7. Sternbach, L. H. (1959). US Patent 2,893,992, July 7
8. Sternbach, L. H. (1971). 1,4-Benzodiazepine. Chemie und Betrachtungen zur Beziehung zwischen Struktur und Wirkung. *Angew. Chem.*, **83**, 70
9. Sternbach, L. H., Fryer, R. I., Keller, O., Metlesics, W., Sach, G. and Steiger, N. (1963). Quinazolines and 1,4-benzodiazepines. X. Nitro-substituted 5-phenyl-1,4-benzodiazepine derivatives. *J. Med. Chem.*, **6**, 261
10. Sternbach, L. H., Fryer, R. I., Metlesics, W., Reeder, E., Sach, G., Saucy, G. and Stempel, A. (1962). Quinazolines and 1,4-benzodiazepines. VI. Halo-, methyl- and methoxy- substituted 1,3-dihydro-5-phenyl-*2H*-1,4-benzodiazepin-2-ones. *J. Org. Chem.*, **27**, 3788
11. Sternbach, L. H., Kaiser, S. and Reeder, E. (1960). Quinazoline 3-oxide structure of compounds previously described in the literature as 3,1,4-benzoxadiazepines. *J. Am. Chem. Soc.*, **82**, 475; and unpublished results (E. Reeder and L. H. Sternbach)
12. Sternbach, L. H. and Randall, L. O. (1966). Some aspects of structure–activity relationship in psychotropic agents of the 1,4-benzodiazepine series. In *CNS Drugs*, pp. 53–69, Symposium Regional Research Laboratory, Hyderabad, India (New Delhi: Council of Scientific and Industrial Research)
13. Sternbach, L. H., Randall, L. O., Banziger, R. and Lehr, H. (1968). Structure–activity relationships in the 1,4-benzodiazepine series. In A. Burger (ed.). *Drugs affecting the Central Nervous System*, **2**, pp. 237–264. (New York: Marcel Dekker Inc.)
14. Sternbach, L. H., Randall, L. O. and Gustafson, S. R. (1964). 1,4-benzodiazepines (chlordiazepoxide and related compounds). In M. Gordon (ed.). *Psychopharmacological Agents*, **1**, pp. 137–224. (New York: Academic Press)
15. Sternbach, L. H. and Reeder, E. (1961). Quinazolines and 1,4-benzo-

diazepines. IV. Transformations of 7-chloro-2-methylamino-5-phenyl-*3H*-1,4-benzodiazepine 4-oxide. *J. Org. Chem.*, **26,** 4936

16. Sternbach, L. H., Reeder, E., Keller, O. and Metlesics, W. (1961). Quinazolines and 1,4-benzodiazepines. III. Substituted 2-amino-5-phenyl-*3H*-1,4-benzodiazepine 4-oxides. *J. Org. Chem.*, **26,** 4488; and additional unpublished results

4

Biological Basis of the Therapeutic Effects of Benzodiazepines

W. E. Haefely

The aim of this chapter is to summarize in a very condensed form our present knowledge of the biological basis of the therapeutic effects of benzodiazepines, i.e. of the changes on a molecular, cellular and brain structural level that underlie the neuropsychotropic effects of these drugs[8,9,10,14]. Although considerable efforts to understand the mechanism of action of these drugs were made in many laboratories since the first representative of this chemical class, chlordiazepoxide, was introduced in therapy twenty years ago, it is only in the past five years that a considerable breakthrough has been achieved. The reason for this was the discovery in the early seventies of the neurotransmitters involved in the function of synaptic inhibition.

The first part is a brief review of the main pharmacological effects of benzodiazepines in the experimental animal which are relevant for their therapeutic use in man. The second part presents the evidence for the view that most, if not all, pharmacological and therapeutic effects of these drugs are due to a selective influence on inhibitory synaptic mechanisms in which γ-aminobutyric acid (GABA) is involved as neurotransmitter. The third part deals with a molecular aspect of the actions of benzodiazepines, namely with the benzodiazepine receptors, those molecules of neuronal membranes with which benzodiazepines interact in a highly specific manner to initiate their pharmacological effects.

The main pharmacological effects of benzodiazepines

In Table 4.1 the main characteristic effects of benzodiazepines in the experimental animal are indicated on the left. On the right-hand side are listed the main therapeutic indications that result from the pharmacological activity.

Table 4.1 Characteristic pharmacological effects of benzodiazepines in the animal and their relations to therapeutic use

Pharmacology	*Indications*
Antipunishment and anti-frustration activity, behavioural disinhibition	anxiety, anxious depression
Arousal reduction, anti-aggressive activity, sleep facilitation	hyperemotional states, insomnia
Anticonvulsant action	various forms of epileptic activity
Damping of central pathways connecting afferents from the periphery and emotions with efferents of the autonomic nervous and endocrine system	psychosomatic disorders (cardiovascular, gastro-intestinal, hormonal)
Central muscle relaxation	somatic and psychogenic muscle spasms, tetanus
Potentiation of the activity of centrally depressant agents, anterograde amnesia	surgical anaesthesia

The most characteristic action of benzodiazepines is a normalization of behavioural responses that are suppressed by punishment or absence of reward[8, 13, 31]. It is important to note that this effect, which may be termed in a more general manner 'behavioural disinhibition', does not consist in a depression of behaviour, but in a distinct increase of behavioural responses. Figure 4.1A shows a rat in a Skinner box pressing a lever in order to obtain food. The animal may be trained to emit a certain number of lever presses for which it is then rewarded by a pellet of food (Figure 4.1B). Rats trained in such a schedule of operant behaviour emit a very constant number of lever press responses over several hours of experimentation. When periods are introduced, during this constant working for food, in which each reward with food is coupled with a punishment in the form of an electric foot shock, the animals almost completely cease to lever press (Figure 4.2A). The animal is said to be in a 'conflict' situation, in which the desire of food is competing with the fear of painful punishment. The latter prevails and the animal produces only a few, if any, hesitant lever presses. Under the effect of benzodiazepines the behavioural responses suppressed by punishment reappear (Figure 4.2B) and, depending on the dose, the animal may behave as if no painful shocks were being coupled with the reward. Similar results are obtained with barbiturates (Figure 4.2C),

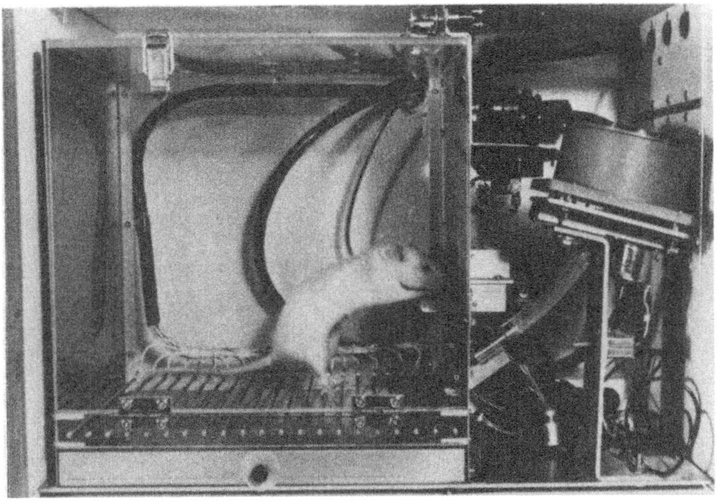

A

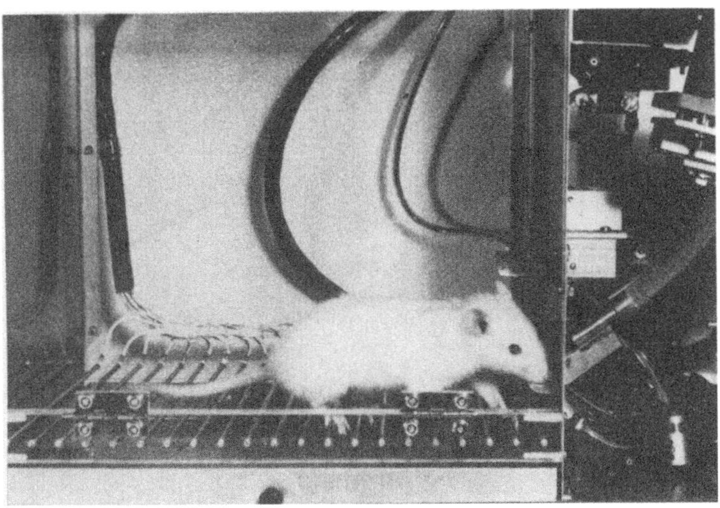

B

Figure 4.1 Example of the experimental procedures used to assess the anxiolytic potential of drugs in animals. Rats are trained in a schedule-controlled behaviour test ('conflict test'). **A.** The animal is pressing a lever placed on one wall of a Skinner box in order to obtain food. **B.** The animal is rewarded for lever pressing by a food pellet offered by an autonomic delivery system

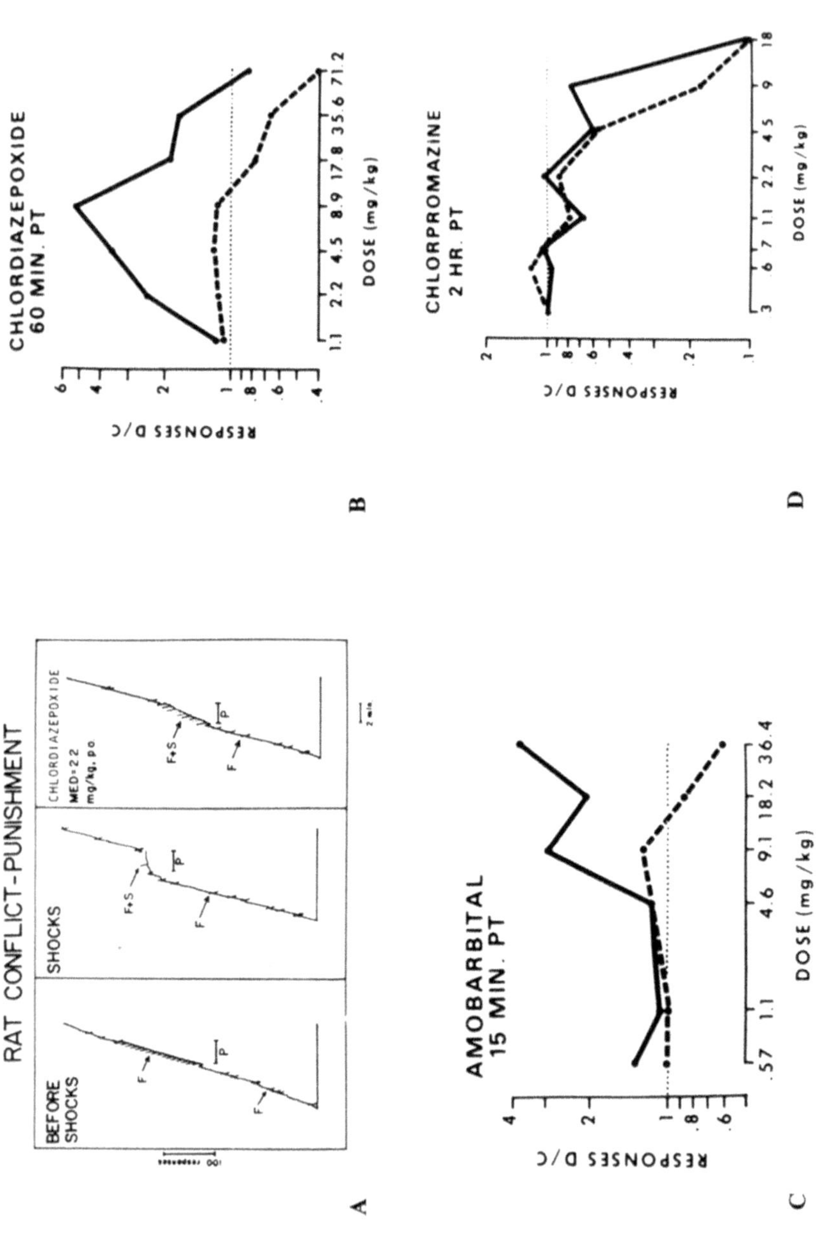

RAT CONFLICT-PUNISHMENT
BEFORE SHOCKS
SHOCKS
CHLORDIAZEPOXIDE
MED=22 mg/kg, po
CHLORDIAZEPOXIDE 60 MIN. PT
AMOBARBITAL 15 MIN. PT
CHLORPROMAZINE 2 HR. PT
DOSE (mg/kg)
RESPONSES D/C
A
B
C
D

although the dose range at which the action is restricted to punished responses is smaller than with benzodiazepines. Neuroleptics, even in small doses, do not produce a selective increase of punished responses (Figure 4.2D); they block punished and non-punished responses in parallel. Instead of coupling reward with punishment, reducing or eliminating reward[36] may be used to depress the operant behaviour of an animal that has been trained to lever press for food. Also in this condition of non-reward, benzodiazepines increase behavioural responses; whereas the increase of punishment-depressed behaviour by benzodiazepines is generally considered to be due to a reduction of fear, their increase of non-rewarded behaviour may indicate an anti-frustration activity. Simpler animal models than the operant tests just described are often used to detect anti-anxiety activity of drugs. Animals placed in a novel environment initially show little exploratory behaviour, obviously because the unfamiliar situation induces fear. This fear of novelty is also reduced by benzodiazepines[34], which increase exploratory activity. A number of

---

Figure 4.2 Effects of chlordiazepoxide, amobarbitone and chlorpromazine in a 'conflict' procedure in rats.

A. Segments of a cumulative record illustrating the response pattern of a rat during a component (P) of punished FR (fixed ratio) 10 (every tenth lever press is simultaneously rewarded with a food pellet and punished by an electric foot shock) and two non-punished VI (variable interval) 30 s components (food reward occurs at variable intervals, in the mean of 30 s duration). Each lever press deflects the pen writer upwards on the slowly revolving kymograph; the slope of the oblique line, therefore, indicates the rate at which the lever is pressed. Food rewards are indicated by small deflections of the pen writer (F). When food reward is not coupled with foot shock during the FR 10 component (before shocks), the animals emit a rather constant number of lever pressing responses. When, during the P phase, each reward is coupled with punishment (shocks), the animal virtually ceases to work for food. After treatment with chlordiazepoxide (Librium) the rat emits a greater number of lever pressing responses during the P phase than when untreated; it, therefore, gets food and shock (F + S) more frequently than in the absence of the drug. The effect of a drug dose is expressed as the ratio of response rate after drug treatment to pre-drug control rate (D/C) for both the 'punished' and the 'non-punished' segments of the experimental session.

B. Dose–response curve for chlordiazepoxide. The ratios D/C during 'punished' segments (full line) and during 'non-punished' segments (broken line) are plotted on the ordinate against the dose on the abscissa. The effect on punished and on non-punished responses was measured at the peak of action of chlordiazepoxide (60 min after administration).

C. Dose–response curve for amobarbitone (15 min after administration).

D. Dose–response curve for chlorpromazine (measurements made 2 hours after administration). Taken from Cook and Davidson[6], used by kind permission of Raven Press other tests based on punishment and novelty have been described[3] and are used to detect anti-anxiety activity. In all these tests, benzodiazepines can be clearly differentiated from most other psychotropic drugs. Antipsychotics, antidepressants and stimulants are unable to increase depressed behaviour in these tests, whereas barbiturates and alcohol, but only in a very narrow dose range, show some similarity to the benzodiazepines. The relative potencies of various benzodiazepines in animal tests of anxiety and frustrations correlate usually rather well with their therapeutic doses in anxiety and anxious depressed states in man.

Benzodiazepines produce various effects which are often summed up as 'sedation', an ill-defined term. What the term in animal experiments implies is, in fact, a reduced arousal to physiological and, in particular, to excessive stimuli. This reduced arousal can be assessed by careful observation and by complicated electrophysiological techniques, such as EEG and evoked potential analysis. A reduction of spontaneously occurring or induced aggressive behaviour is observed with benzodiazepines in some, but not in all animals. Arousal reduction is probably responsible to a large extent for the increase of sleep amount and the reduction of sleep latency in animals. A facilitation of sleep is usually not easily detectable in the laboratory animal under physiological conditions. However, if sleep is disturbed by any of numerous possible ways, the effect of these drugs can be easily seen. As an example (Figure 4.3) the effect of flunitrazepam on a cat with chronic EEG electrodes is shown, whose sleep is almost abolished by a small dose of morphine, which in this species increases arousal. In a dose as small as 0.01 mg/kg, flunitrazepam completely abolished the effect of morphine and re-installed a normal sleep behaviour. The arousal-reducing action of benzodiazepines in the animal corresponds to their effect on human hyperemotional behaviour and insomnia, especially when the latter is due to excessive stimuli or psychogenic factors.

The anticonvulsant actions of benzodiazepines are easily detected in animal experiments[14]. These drugs block convulsions and epileptiform EEG activity induced by chemical agents. These convulsants may interfere with GABAergic mechanisms either by inhibiting the synthesis of GABA (e.g. isoniazid) or by blocking the effects of GABA (e.g. bicuculline and picrotoxin); they may block glycine receptors, such as strychnine, or induce paroxysmal neuronal activity in a yet not fully understood way (e.g. pentetrazole, penicillin, local anaesthesics). Localized epileptic foci can be induced with local application of inhibitors of the neuronal membrane sodium pump (e.g. ouabain) or local irritants (e.g. cobalt). Benzodiazepines also block seizures induced by withdrawal in animals made physically dependent on barbiturates or alcohol. They are also active in suppressing seizures induced by hyperbaric oxygen, electroshock, the so-called kindling (focal epilepsies developing after repeated electric stimulation) and by photic stimulation in photosensitive *Papio papio* monkeys. In accordance with the pronounced anticonvulsant activity in numerous

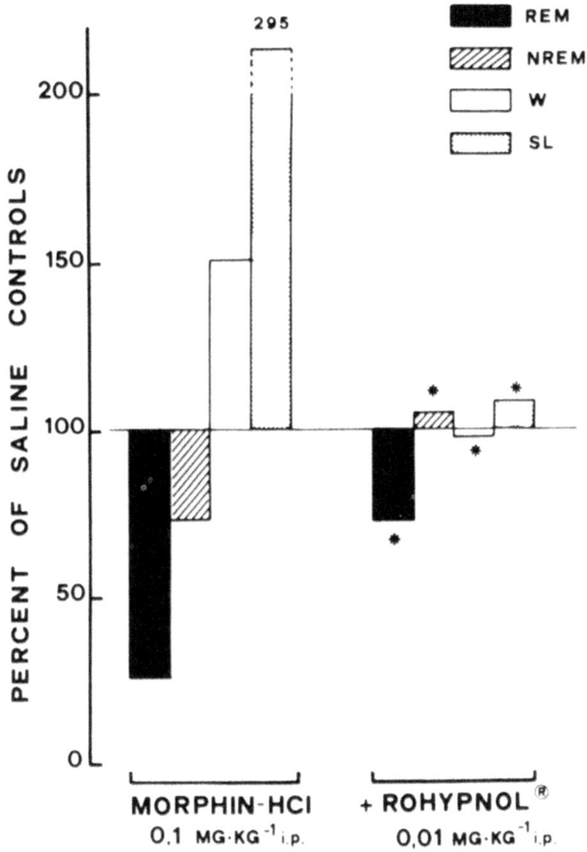

Figure 4.3 Interaction between the effects of morphine and flunitrazepam (Rohypnol) on the sleep–wakefulness cycle of cats. Shown is the effect of a small dose of morphine (0.1 mg/kg i.p.) on REM and non-REM sleep (NREM), as well as on wakefulness (W) and sleep latency (SL). The reduction of both phases of sleep and the increase of wakefulness and sleep latency by morphine is completely antagonized by flunitrazepam 0.01 mg/kg[29]

models of animals seizures, benzodiazepines are useful drugs in various forms of human epilepsy.

Although benzodiazepines in therapeutic doses are completely devoid of a direct action on peripheral autonomic functions, they potently reduce autonomic (cardiovascular, gastro-intestinal) responses to the direct electrical stimulation of the hypothalamus and other brain structures, and autonomic reflexes induced by various peripheral stimuli. As an example, benzodiazepines reduce the increase of plasma noradrenaline and, more markedly, of plasma adrenaline in response to a few moderately painful electric shocks to the feet (Figure 4.4). The damping effect of benzodiazepines on the central substrates of sympathetic, parasympathetic and hormonal activity is the basis of their therapeutic use in psychosomatic cardiovascular, gastro-intestinal, urogenital and endocrinological disorders.

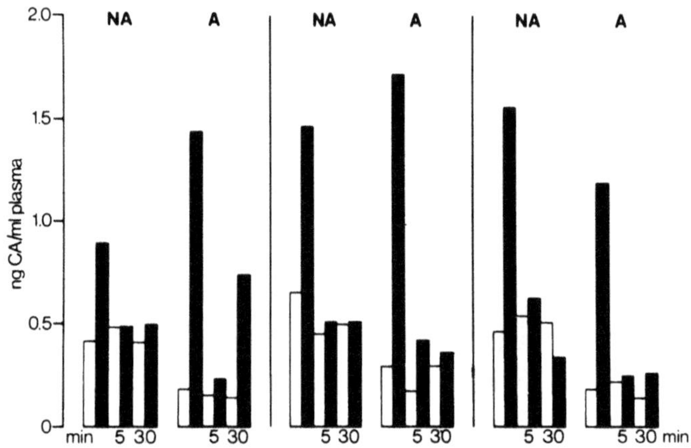

Figure 4.4 The effect of midazolam on the increase of plasma noradrenaline (NA) and adrenaline (A) levels in 3 different rats induced by 6 consecutive unescapable electric foot shocks applied at intervals of 10s. The rats had indwelling intravenous catheters for the withdrawal of blood. The first two columns under NA and A represent the catecholamine levels before (open columns) and after exposure to the footshock stress (filled columns) in the absence of any drug. The following pairs of open and filled columns indicate the pre- and post-stress values of plasma catecholamines 5 and 30 minutes, respectively, after midazolam 10mg/kg i.v.[7]

The therapeutic efficacy of benzodiazepines in states of increased muscle tone of somatic as well as psychogenic aetiology is reflected by their muscle relaxant activity in animals with normal muscle tone and with muscular rigidity (e.g. decerebrate rigidity) and by their depressant effect on supraspinal and spinal reflexes involved in the control of muscle tone.

Benzodiazepines potentiate the effects of various central depressant agents and, in high intravenous doses, produce anterograde amnesia[33,35]. These actions are very useful for the induction and maintenance of surgical anaesthesia. With the availability of the short-acting and water-soluble midazolam, benzodiazepines will increasingly replace barbiturates in anaesthesiology.

Synaptic actions of benzodiazepines

In order to understand the effects of benzodiazepines on the level of synaptic transmission, a few words on inhibitory synapses in the central nervous system are necessary.

The GABAergic inhibitory synapses

The amino acid γ-aminobutyric acid (GABA) is now recognized as the most important inhibitory transmitter in the mammalian central nervous system[19, 28]. Two types of GABAergic inhibition exist which differ in the arrangement of neuronal elements and the functional consequences of their activation (Figure 4.5).

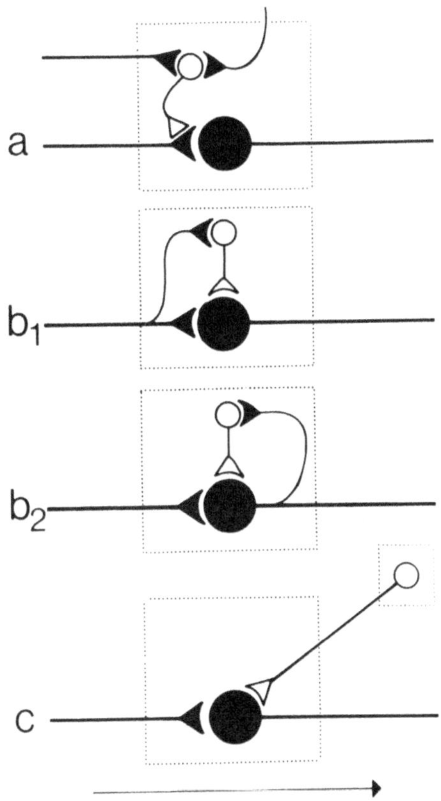

Figure 4.5 Schematic diagrams of presynaptic (a) and postsynaptic inhibitory circuits (b and c). In a (presynaptic inhibition), b_1 (collateral inhibition) and b_2 (recurrent inhibition) GABAergic interneurons are involved; in c postsynaptic inhibition produced by a projecting GABAergic principal neuron is shown. Excitatory neurons are depicted in black, GABAergic neurons in white

So-called postsynaptic inhibition is mediated by axosomatic or axodendritic synapses. The GABAergic neuron may be a projection neuron connecting two different structures, e.g. the caudate nucleus with the substantia nigra, or an interneuron. This interneuron may be activated by a recurrent collateral of the very neuron on which it exerts an inhibitory influence, or by a collateral of afferent neurons which excite the neuron innervated by the GABAergic interneuron. The former circuit occurs very frequently throughout the central nervous system and is called 'recurrent inhibition'. GABA released at the axosomatic or axodendritic synapses acts on a specific GABA receptor in the subsynaptic membrane, which is coupled with a chloride channel. Activation of the GABA receptor opens the chloride channel and allows chloride anions to flow down their concentration gradient from the extracellular fluid into the cell interior. This chloride influx makes the cell interior more negative than it already is at rest and, hence, leads to a hyperpolarization of the cell. This hyperpolarization makes it more difficult for the excitatory synapses to depolarize the neuron beyond the critical level for the generation of an action potential; this type of synaptic inhibition renders the cell less sensitive to all incoming excitatory influences. The operation of the recurrent inhibitory circuit is quite obviously to prevent principal neurons from being overexcited and firing at a high frequency.

So-called presynaptic inhibition operates via an axo-axonal synapse. A GABAergic inhibitory interneuron, which may be excited by a variety of pathways, makes contact with the nerve ending of an excitatory neuron. GABA which is released at this synapse produces a decrease of the amount of excitatory transmitter which is released in response to an action potential. An essential difference of presynaptic inhibition as compared with postsynaptic inhibition is that the former reduces selectively some distinct excitatory inputs to a neuron without affecting the sensitivity of this neuron to other excitatory inputs. Presynaptic inhibition has so far been detected only on the endings of primary afferents of spinal or cranial nerves.

Enhancement of GABAergic synaptic inhibition by benzodiazepines

At all GABAergic synapses studied so far, benzodiazepines have been found to have a facilitating action. Different methods were used to demonstrate this effect, but there is no space to give details here.

Spinal cord

The first indication for a specific interaction of benzodiazepines with inhibitory synaptic transmission was provided by Schmidt and collaborators[30] in 1967 in the cat spinal cord. These neurophysiologists observed that diazepam enhanced presynaptic inhibition, but not postsynaptic inhibition, in the spinal cord disconnected from the brain. At the time of this study it was not yet known that GABA acted as the transmitter at the presynaptic inhibitory synapse. When the role of GABA became increasingly clear in the early seventies, we wanted to re-examine the effects of diazepam on the spinal cord in the light of these recent findings. The pathways for presynaptic and postsynaptic inhibition in the spinal cord are schematically indicated in Figure 4.6. Presynaptic inhibition can be assessed in several ways. The simplest is to elicit and record a monosynaptic reflex by stimulating an afferent muscle nerve and recording the reflex response

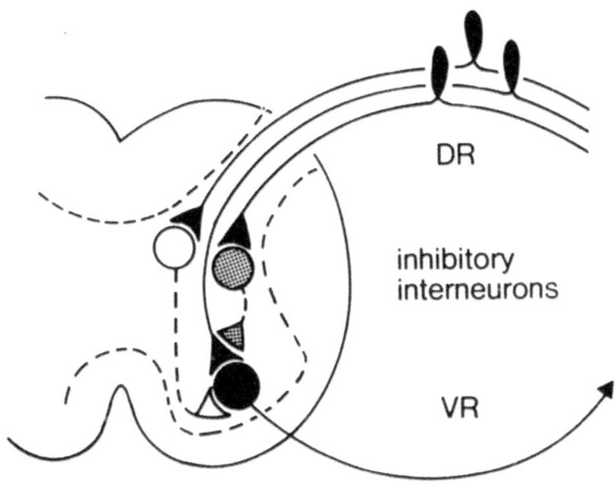

Figure 4.6 Schematic diagram of the monosynaptic excitatory, the postsynaptic inhibitory, and the presynaptic inhibitory pathways on spinal motoneurons. For the sake of simplicity only one interneuron (the GABAergic neuron indicated in white and cross-hatched, respectively) is shown in the inhibitory pathways, whereas in reality there is at least another (excitatory) interneuron. Excitatory neurons are depicted in black. DR = dorsal root, VR = ventral root

of corresponding motoneurons in a ventral root. When the monosynaptic reflex is elicited shortly after a conditioning stimulus in a cutaneous nerve, which activates the presynaptic inhibitory circuit, its amplitude is reduced for up to 500 ms. This inhibition curve is dose-dependently augmented by diazepam, i.e. under the influence of diazepam, the presynaptic inhibition of the monosynaptic reflex is more marked and lasts longer (Figure 4.7).

We were able to show that the effect of benzodiazepines depended on the presence of normal amounts of GABA in the spinal cord[26]. When we inhibited the biosynthesis of GABA, e.g. with thiosemicarbazide, which by itself greatly reduced or abolished presynaptic inhibition, benzodiazepines were no longer able to result in a more marked inhibition. However, when presynaptic inhibition was blocked by a GABA antagonist, e.g. the convulsant bicuculline, then benzodiazepines were able to reinforce the effectiveness of presynaptic inhibition. We were not able, however, on the basis of these experiments on the spinal cord, to decide whether the benzodiazepines interacted selectively with some mechanisms characteristic for presynaptic inhibition or selectively with the GABA transmitter system, because in the spinal cord postsynaptic inhibition appears to operate mainly through glycine. We therefore turned to another structure to study this question.

Dorsal column nuclei

In the dorsal column nuclei of the medulla (the nuclei of Goll and Burdach), the relay neurons projecting to the thalamus are subject to both presynaptic

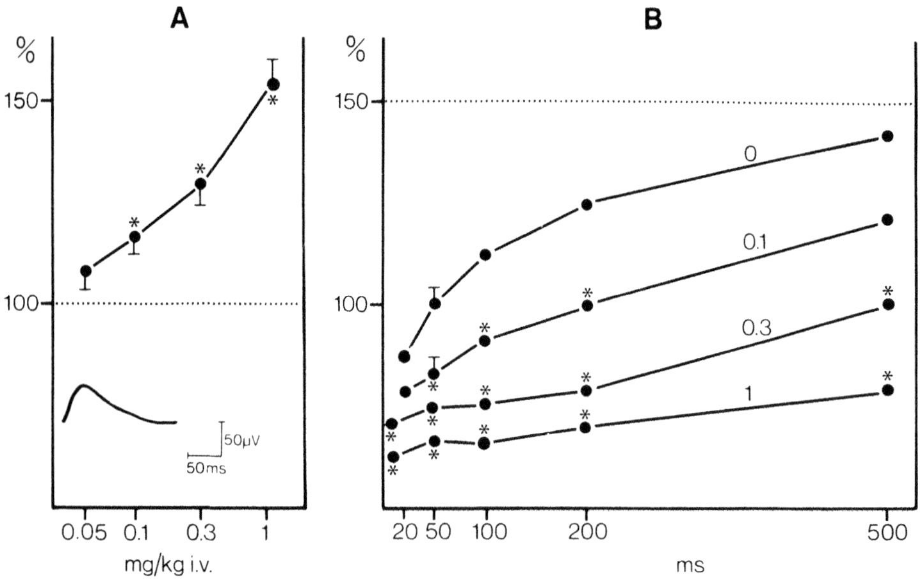

Figure 4.7 Effect of diazepam on the dorsal root potential (DRP area) (A) and on presynaptic inhibition of monosynaptic ventral root reflex responses (B) in spinal cats. Dorsal root potentials were elicited by single stimuli to the nerves to the gastrocnemius and biceps femoris muscles or to the sural nerve. The inset in A shows a typical dorsal root potential. In B the amplitude of the test monosynaptic ventral root reflex response (evoked by single shocks in the nerve to the gastrocnemius muscle) at different times after a conditioning inhibitory volley in the nerve to the biceps femoris muscle is expressed as a percentage of the control reflex response in the absence of a preceding conditioning volley. The values are the means of 6 animals. Values significantly different from pre-drug values are indicated by asterisks. Modified from Polc *et al.*[26]

and postsynaptic inhibition, and in both types of inhibition GABA is the neurotransmitter (Figure 4.8). We found in our laboratories[25] that in the cuneate nucleus benzodiazepines enhanced both presynaptic and postsynaptic inhibition. This very strongly suggested that benzodiazepines interacted specifically with GABAergic transmission independent of whether the type of inhibition was presynaptic or postsynaptic. Studies of the benzodiazepine actions in other brain structures fully confirmed this view.

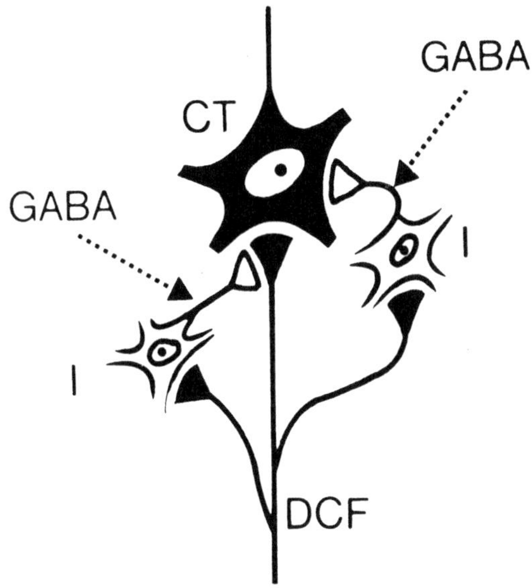

Figure 4.8 Schematic diagram of the presynaptic and postsynaptic inhibition of excitatory transmission from primary afferents (dorsal column fibres, DCF) to cuneothalamic relay cells (CT) in the dorsal column nuclei. The GABAergic interneurons involved in the presynaptic and postsynaptic inhibitory pathways are in white; excitatory neurons are in black

Cerebral cortex

Recurrent inhibition plays an important part in the protection of efferent neurons of the cerebral cortex from overstimulation (Figure 4.9). Two groups of workers, Raabe and Gumnit[27] from USA, and Zakusov *et al.*[40] from Russia, reported that benzodiazepines enhanced recurrent inhibition in the cerebral cortex of experimental animals.

Hippocampus

Activity of hippocampal pyramidal cells is also controlled by the recurrent

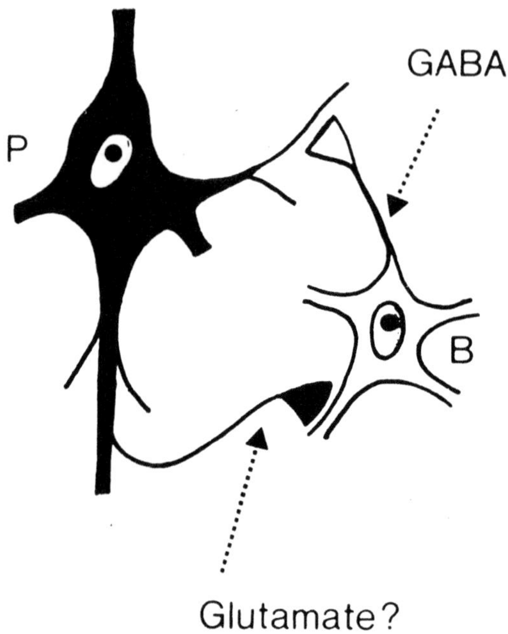

Figure 4.9 Schematic diagram of the recurrent inhibitory pathway in the cerebral cortex. Excitatory pyramidal tract neuron (P) in black, GABAergic basket cell (B) in white

inhibitory feedback mechanisms (see Figure 4.10). This inhibitory circuit seems to be essential for the prevention of paroxysmal activity. Wolf and Haas[39] and Tsuchiya and Fukushima[37] demonstrated that various benzodiazepine derivatives potently enhanced recurrent inhibition in the hippocampus.

Hypothalamus

In the hypothalamus too, principal cells are subject to recurrent inhibition through a GABAergic interneuron; Geller *et al.*[11], working on cultured tuberal cells of the rat, found that diazepam enhanced this recurrent inhibition.

Cerebellar cortex

The cerebellar cortex is a brain structure in which GABAergic neurons prevail (Figure 4.11). Indeed, of the five types of neurons present, four use GABA as transmitter, among them the only efferent neuron, the cerebellar Purkinje cell. Recording the spontaneous activity of cerebellar Purkinje cells in the rat, we found that various benzodiazepines dose-dependently

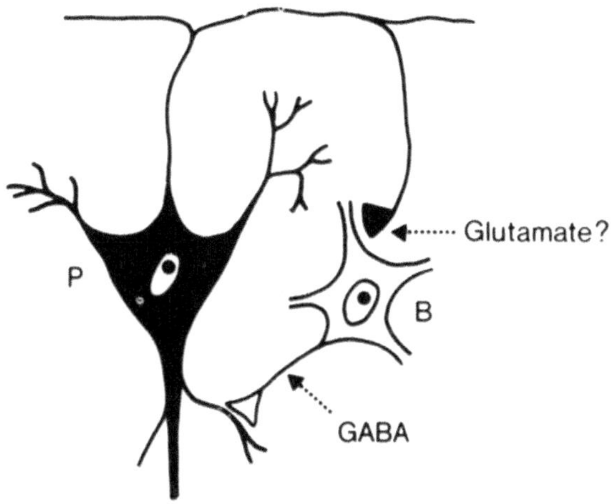

Figure 4.10 Schematic diagram of the recurrent inhibitory pathway in the hippocampus. Hippocampal pyramidal cell (P) in black, the GABAergic basket cell (B) in white

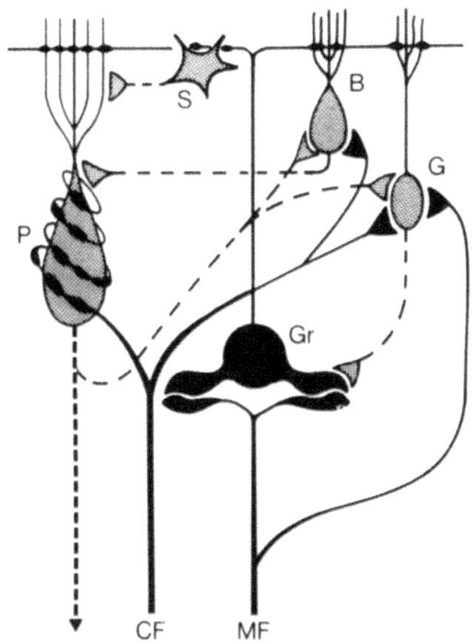

Figure 4.11 Schematic diagram of the main circuits in the cerebellar cortex. The two excitatory inputs to the cerebellar cortex are the climbing fibres (CF) and the mossy fibres (MF). The granule cell (Gr) is the only excitatory neuron in the cerebellar cortex; the Purkinje cell (P) acts as the only (inhibitory) output neuron from the cortex. The Purkinje cell, as well as the 3 interneuron types stellate cell (S), basket cell (B) and Golgi cell (G) are presumably GABAergic. The noradrenergic (inhibitory) input to the cerebellar cortex is omitted in this diagram

reduced the firing rate of these cells[24]. This effect (Figure 4.12) was explained by an enhancement of basket-cell mediated GABAergic inhibition of Purkinje cells. Geller *et al.*[11] directly demonstrated the increased influence of basket cells on single Purkinje cell neurons under the effect of benzodiazepines. The reduced activity of cerebellar cortical neurons is reflected by the dose-dependent decrease of the cerebellar cyclic GMP content after various benzodiazepines (W. P. Burkard, personal communication).

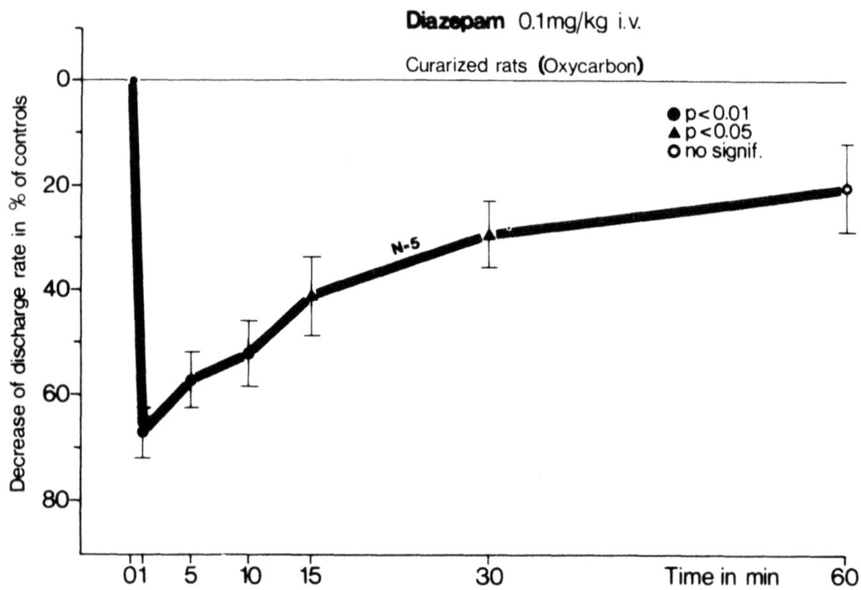

Figure 4.12 Depression by diazepam 0.1 mg/kg i.v. of the spontaneous firing rate of cerebellar Purkinje cells of the rat. The points are the means (plus standard error) of 5 rats (Pieri, unpublished)

Lateral vestibular nucleus of Deiters

One of the sites to which GABAergic Purkinje cells project is the lateral vestibular nucleus of Deiters (Figure 4.13). Applying single shocks to the Purkinje cell axons in the cerebellar white matter of the cat, we recorded a complex evoked potential in Deiters' nucleus, a component of which was abolished by the GABA antagonist, picrotoxin, and, hence, can be regarded as the mass inhibitory synaptic potential. Benzodiazepines restored this potential after its abolition by picrotoxin[17].

Substantia nigra

A GABAergic pathway projects from the caudate nucleus to the substantia nigra, and inhibits the activity of nigral dopaminergic neurons which in

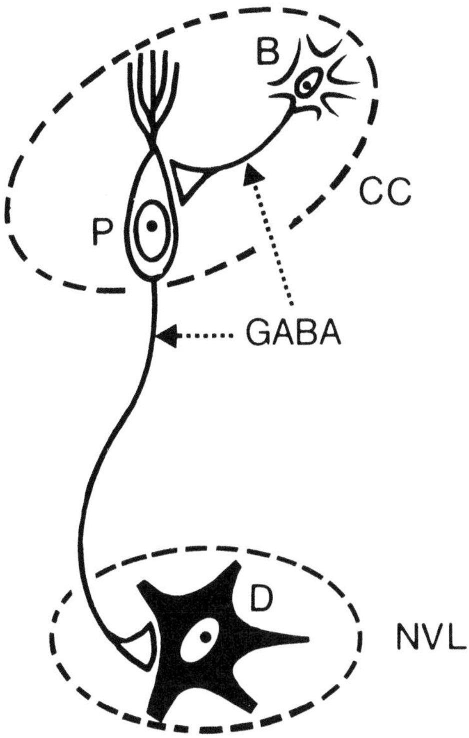

Figure 4.13 Schematic diagram of the connections between cerebellar basket and Purkinje cells and Deiters' neurons (D) in the lateral vesticular nucleus (NVL). CC = cerebellar cortex

turn project to the striatum (Figure 4.14). Single stimuli applied to the caudate nucleus evoked in the substantia nigra a simple potential representing the mass of inhibitory synaptic potentials. We found[16,17] that this evoked potential was depressed and abolished by the GABA antagonists, bicuculline and picrotoxin, but not by the glycine antagonist, strychnine. Benzodiazepines reduced the effect of GABA antagonists, again demonstrating their enhancing action on GABAergic transmission. In accordance with these electropharmacological findings we showed that benzodiazepines potentiated the cataleptic action of neuroleptics and reduced their stimulation of dopamine turnover[18]. This synergistic action of neuroleptics and benzodiazepines is easily explained by the effects of the two groups of drugs on dopaminergic neurons. By blocking dopamine receptors, neuroleptics produce a compensatory increase of the activity of dopamine neurons on the substantia nigra. This increased activity in part overcomes the block of dopamine receptors. Benzodiazepines, by enhancing the inhibitory

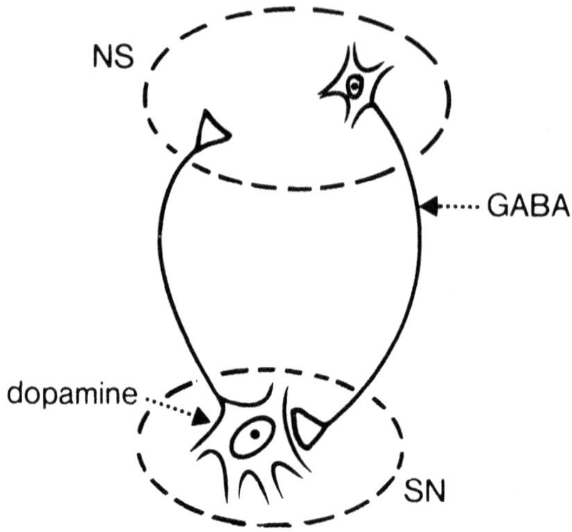

Figure 4.14 Schematic, very simplified, diagram of two pathways interconnecting the neostriatum (NS) and the substantia nigra (SN), the nigrastriatal dopaminergic pathway and the GABAergic striatonigral pathway

effect of the striatonigral pathway on dopamine neurons, partially blocks this compensatory increase of activity. This reduces the increase of dopamine turnover by the neuroleptics and, thereby, makes the block of dopamine receptors more apparent.

Other brain structures
Evidence that benzodiazepines also enhance a GABAergic inhibiting influence on other neurons, has been obtained in our own laboratories and by other workers. This concerns e.g. the serotoninergic neurons in brainstem raphe nuclei and noradrenergic neurons in the locus coeruleus[14].

The benzodiazepine receptors

The view, which emerged from two decades of research, that benzodiazepines had a very specific profile of activity differing from other groups of agents, such as barbiturates and meprobamate, in spite of some common actions, was confirmed beautifully by the recent studies on benzodiazepine receptors.

Braestrup and Squires[4] in Denmark and Möhler and Okada[20] in our laboratories initiated these studies two years ago. The method is relatively simple. A preparation of nerve cell membranes from the brain is incubated with a highly radioactive benzodiazepine, either [^{3}H]diazepam or [^{3}H]flunitrazepam (Figure 4.15). The preparation is then washed on a filter and the

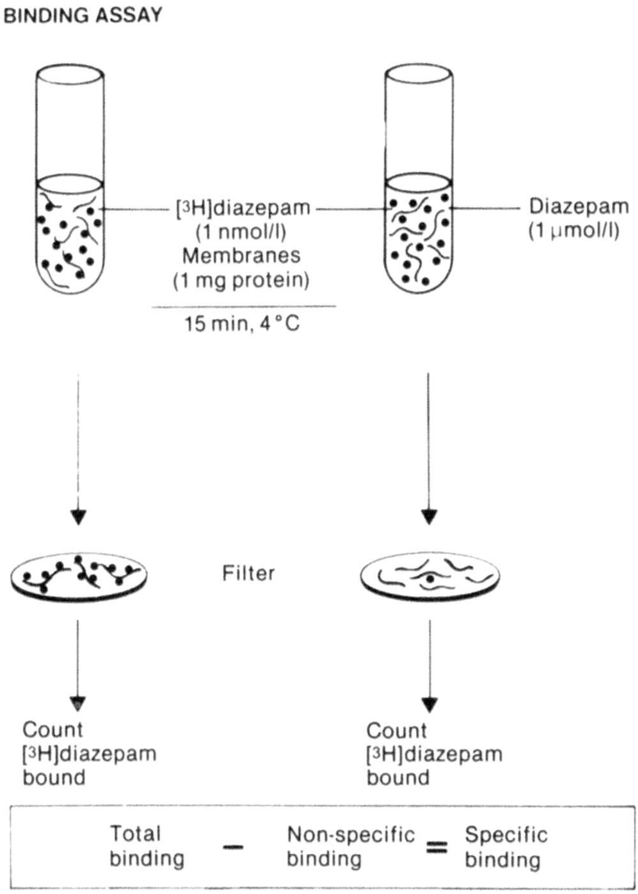

Figure 4.15 Schematic diagram of the *in vitro* binding assay for benzodiazepine receptors

radioactivity which remains bound to the membranes is counted. The radioligand remaining in the membranes may be bound to those specific sites, through which the benzodiazepines initiate their effects, but also to non-specific sites, where no activity is initiated, e.g. lipid structures. To differentiate between these two binding sites, part of the incubation experiments are done in the presence of high concentrations of a non-radioactive benzodiazepine. This non-radioactive molecule should inhibit the binding of the radioligand to the true receptors, but not to the non-specific binding sites. That part of the total binding of the radioligand to the membranes, which remains even in the presence of high concentrations of the cold benzodiazepine, represents the non-specific binding and by subtracting this from the total binding, the so-called 'specific binding' to receptors is obtained (Figure 4.16). As one would expect, the specific binding reaches saturation with increasing concentrations of the radioligand, demonstrating that there is a limited number of binding sites in the membranes. The non-specific binding, however, increases linearly over a wider range of ligand concentrations (Figure 4.16). A mathematical analysis of such binding experiments permits the affinity of the ligand to the receptor as well as the maximal number of receptors present in a given brain tissue

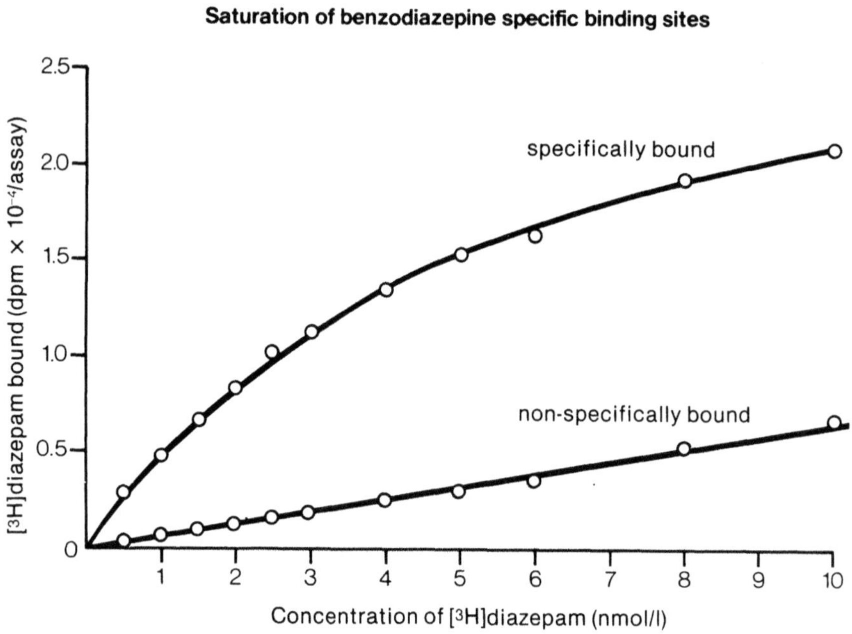

Figure 4.16 Curves for specifically and non-specifically bound [^{3}H]diazepam to rat brain synaptosomes (from Möhler and Okada[21], used by kind permission of *British Journal of Psychiatry*)

to be calculated. The density of benzodiazepine receptors in body tissues was calculated in this way for various species. Benzodiazepine receptors were, most importantly, not found outside the central nervous system. Within the central nervous system,[21] the density of these receptors varies in different regions, being highest in the central cortex, the hippocampus and the cerebellum (Table 4.2).

Binding experiments are simple procedures to determine the affinity of a great number of drugs to the benzodiazepine receptor by determining the concentration required to displace the radioligand from the specific

Table 4.2 [^{3}H]Diazepam binding in various regions of the human brain. Shown are the maximal binding and the apparent affinity (K_D) (from Möhler and Okada[21])

Brain region	*Max. spec. binding (fmol/mg protein)*	K_D *(nmol/l)*
Cerebral cortex	1200	7.0
Cerebellum	730	6.9
Limbic system	720–410	6.7–8.7
Basal ganglia	380–290	8.5–6.2
Brainstem	160–150	14.2–20.9
Corpus callosum	50	6.4

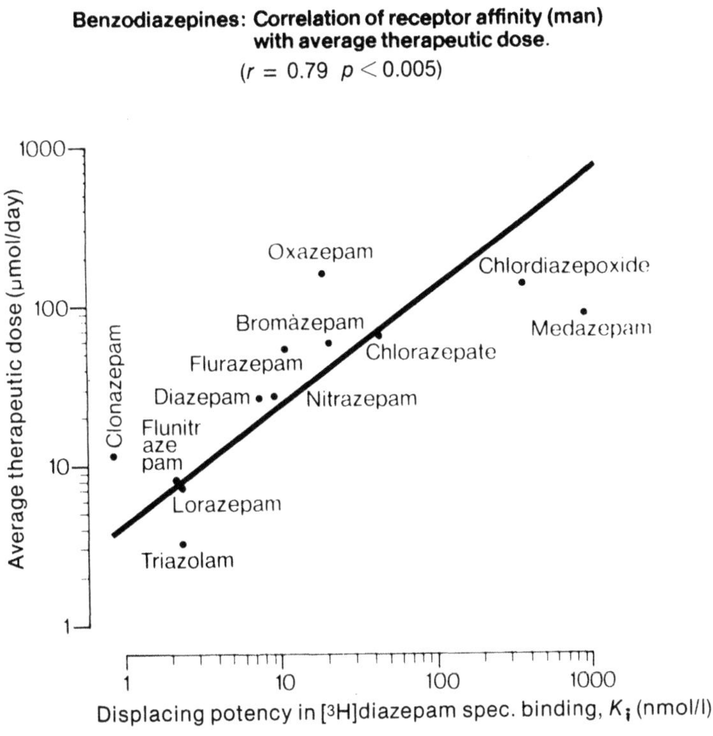

Figure 4.17 Correlation between the *in vitro* affinity of some benzodiazepines to the specific [^{3}H]diazepam binding sites and their average therapeutic dose (from Möhler and Okada[21], used by kind permission of *British Journal of Psychiatry*)

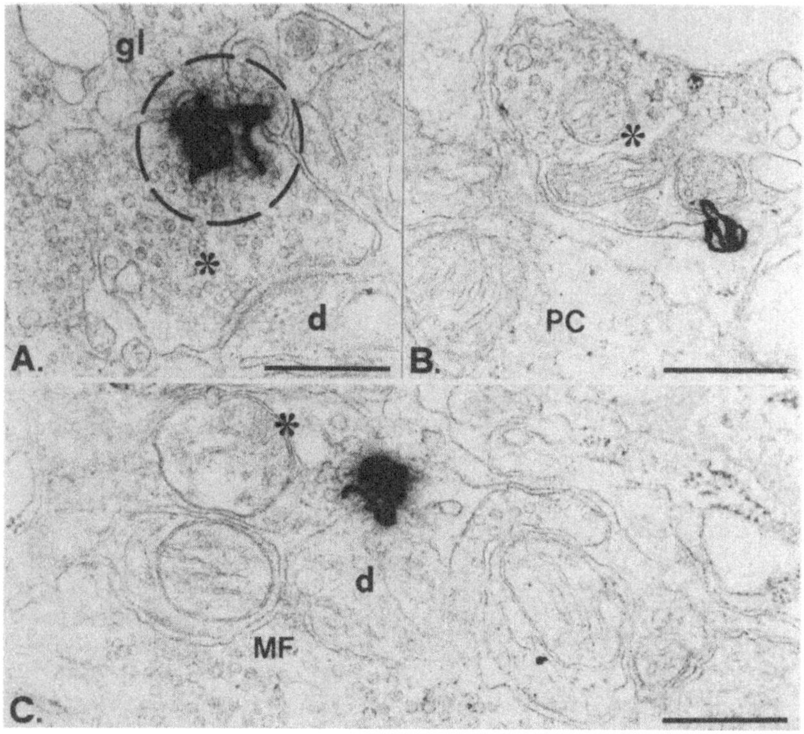

Figure 4.18 Electron microscopic localization of specific benzodiazepine binding sites (receptors) after photoaffinity labelling with [^{3}H]flunitrazepam. Rats were injected i.v. with [^{3}H]flunitrazepam 100μCi and decapitated 2min later. Slices (1.5mm thick) from the cerebral and cerebellar cortex were irradiated for 5 min with u.v. light at 0°C. Unreacted [^{3}H]flunitrazepam was removed by extensive washing. After fixation with glutaraldehyde and postfixation with osmium tetroxide, ultrathin (60nm) sections were coated with Ilford L_4 Nuclear Research emulsion. After exposure at 4°C for 8 weeks, sections were developed, fixed and dried before staining with lead citrate. A: Cerebral cortex. The 66% probability circle around the silver grain suggests that the source of radioactivity is localized on the nerve ending (asterisk) or adjacent glial (gl) structures. B: Cerebellar cortex. A nerve terminal (asterisk) forms a synapse with a Purkinje cell (P) soma. C: Cerebellar cortex. The photaffinity-labelled nerve ending (asterisk) is probably a Golgi cell axon ending, since it is in synpatic contact with the same dendrite (d) as the mossy fibre (MF) ending (from Möhler *et al.*[22])

binding sites. Only benzodiazepines were found so far to have a high affinity for this type of receptor. Barbiturates and meprobamate do not even displace a radioactive benzodiazepine in concentrations that are much higher than those occurring *in vivo*. However, benzodiazepine derivatives displace the radioligand binding in concentrations that are nicely correlated with their potency as anxiolytics and anticonvulsants *in vivo* (Figure 4.17).

The technique of receptor binding has opened new lines of research on benzodiazepines, some of which are mentioned below. They are discussed in more detail in Workshop A.

(a) Binding of active benzodiazepines to their receptors in the animal brain can be measured not only *in vitro*, but also *in vivo*[5,32,38]. A non-radioactive benzodiazepine is administered to an animal; at desired times afterwards a very small dose of a radioactive ligand is then injected intravenously. The brain is then removed and the radioactivity present in different brain areas measured. The amount of radioactivity found is compared with that determined in the absence of a non-radioactive drug, and the difference indicates the amount of benzodiazepine receptors that were occupied at the moment of the removal of the brain. This *in vivo* determination of receptor occupancy permits for the first time the correlation to be made between pharmacological effect and number of receptors occupied by the drug. Comparing drug concentrations at the active receptor sites with total concentration of the drug in the brain and other body tissues will provide us with the badly needed insight into the relationship between drug concentrations in the plasma and at the receptor sites.

(b) Labelling the receptor with a strongly bound radioactive benzodiazepine will enable the localization of benzodiazepine receptors in the electron microscope (Figure 4.18) and the isolation and identification of the receptor protein. Attempts in this direction have been successful very recently in our laboratories[2,22].

(c) A question which arises immediately in connection with the demonstration of specific benzodiazepine receptors in the central nervous system is whether endogenous substances exist that occupy these receptors in physiological or pathological conditions[1,23]. Is there an endogenous 'anti-anxiety substance' in the brain which may prevent abnormal fear developing or is there an 'anxiogenic compound' which may block these receptors and, thereby, induce anxiety?

(d) The question of how the benzodiazepine receptors are involved in the facilitation of GABAergic synaptic transmission by these drugs is actually being studied with great efforts in many laboratories of the world. Two principal possibilities exist[15]: the drugs may act on a presynaptic site of the GABAergic synapse, e.g. by increasing the amount of GABA released by an action potential or by increasing the sensitivity of GABAergic interneurons to excitatory influences. Alternatively, they may act postsynaptically to increase the efficacy of GABA at the subsynaptic membrane[12]. Evidence for both sites of action is presently available and we shall know in the near future which one is solely or predominantly responsible for the facilitation of GABAergic transmission.

Synaptic and molecular pharmacology of benzodiazepines and their actions in man

The goals of experimental pharmacology are not only to detect new active molecules, but also to provide knowledge for a deeper understanding of how neuropsychotropic drugs, by affecting certain neuronal activities, produce useful therapeutic effects in the somatic and psychic domain and possibly also undesired and harmful effects.

The actual knowledge of the mechanism of action of benzodiazepines helps us to understand quite a number of events that occur with these drugs. The fact that benzodiazepines seem to interact in a highly specific manner with a distinct neurotransmitter system, the GABAergic one, shows that these drugs affect in principle most areas of the central nervous system, since the GABAergic synapses are rather ubiquitous. The therapeutic effects are, therefore, likely to result from a concerted action on many central structures. This does not exclude the likelihood that some structures will be more affected by the drugs than others. By enhancing a physiological inhibitory mechanism operating at most neurons, the drugs will affect abnormally overactive parts of the brain more than parts with a low level of activity.

The improved inhibitory protection of neurons can easily be recognized as the mechanism by which benzodiazepines depress paroxysmal epileptiform neuronal activity. Anxiety and other emotional responses are also likely to be due to neuronal hyperactivity, particularly in the limbic system, and may be reduced by an enhanced efficiency of synaptic inhibitory mechanisms. GABAergic pathways have been recently detected in the central control systems for endocrine and autonomic nervous activity, providing an explanation for the central effect of benzodiazepines on autonomic and some endocrine functions. The facilitating effect of benzodiazepines on GABAergic transmission is of moderate intensity at a single synapse and does not increase without limit with increasing doses. This may account for the fact that benzodiazepines produce their desired therapeutic effects already in low doses and that depression of the central nervous function does not increase steeply with incremental doses, as is the case with compounds that also block excitatory transmission, e.g. the barbiturates.

The class of benzodiazepines, recognized over twenty years ago (in the absence of any knowledge of their mechanisms of action) as highly active yet very untoxic drugs, now turn out to be acting by enhancing a physiological and protective mechanism which is indispensable for the normal functioning of the central nervous system. If we had to devise a useful type of neuropsychotropic drug today, based on the present knowledge of synaptic functions and dysfunctions, we would search for drugs like the benzodiazepines if they did not happen to exist already.

Acknowledgement

I gratefully acknowledge the excellent co-operation of my colleagues Drs W. P. Burkard, M. Da Prada, H. H. Keller, H. Möhler, L. Pieri, P. Polc, J. G. Richards and R. Schaffner in our past and present efforts to evaluate the mechanism of action of benzodiazepines.

References

1. Asano, T. and Spector, S. (1979). Identification of inosine and hypoxanthine as endogenous ligands for the brain benzodiazepine-binding sites. *Proc. Natl. Acad. Sci.*, **76,** 977
2. Battersby, M. K., Richards, J. G. and Möhler, H. (1979). Benzodiazepine receptor: photoaffinity labeling and localization. *Eur. J. Pharmacol.*, **57,** 277
3. Boissier, J. R. and Simon, P. (1969). Evaluation of experimental techniques in the psychopharmacology of emotion. *Ann. NY Acad., Sci.*, **159,** 898
4. Braestrup, C. and Squires, R. F. (1977). Brain specific benzodiazepine receptors in rats characterized by high affinity ^{3}H-diazepam binding. *Proc. Natl. Acad. Sci.*, **74,** 3805
5. Chang, R. S. L. and Snyder, S. H. (1978). Benzodiazepine receptors: labeling in intact animals with ^{3}H-flunitrazepam. *Eur. J. Pharmacol.*, **48,** 213
6. Cook, L. and Davidson, A. B. (1973). Effects of behaviorally active drugs in a conflict-punishment procedure in rats. In Garattini, S., Mussini, E. and Randall, L. O. (eds.), *The Benzodiazepines*, pp. 327–345. (New York: Raven Press)
7. Da Prada, M., Pieri, L. and Picotti, G. B. (1979). Effect of midazolam (a water-soluble benzodiazepine) on stress-induced increase of plasma catecholamines. *Proc. 2nd Symposium on Catecholamines and Stress.* September 1979, Smolenice, Czechoslovakia. (In press)
8. Dews, P. B. (1979). Behavioural pharmacology of anxiolytics. In *Handbook of Experimental Pharmacology*. (Berlin: Springer) (In press)
9. Fielding, S. and Lal, H. (eds.) (1979). *Anxiolytics.* (Mount Kisko: Futura Publishing Company)
10. Garattini, S., Mussini, E. and Randall, L. D. (eds.) (1973). *The Benzodiazepines.* (New York: Raven Press)
11. Geller, H. M., Taylor, D. A. and Hoffer, B. J. (1978). Benzodiazepines and central inhibitory mechanisms. *Naunyn-Schmiedeberg's Arch. Pharmacol.*, **304,** 81

12. Guidotti, A., Toffano, G., Baraldi, M., Schwartz, J. P. and Costa, E. (1979). A molecular mechanism for the facilitation of GABA receptor function by benzodiazepines. In Krogsgaard-Larsen, P., Scheel-Krüger, J. and Kofod, H. (eds.), *GABA-Neurotransmitters*, pp. 406–415. (Copenhagen: Munksgaard)
13. Haefely, W. E. (1978). Behavioral and neuropharmacological aspects of drugs used in anxiety and related states. In Lipton, M. A., DiMascio, A. and Killam, K. F. (eds.), *Psychopharmacology: A Generation of Progress*, pp. 1359–1374. (New York: Raven Press)
14. Haefely, W. E., Pieri, L., Polc, P. and Schaffner, R. (1979). General pharmacology and neuropharmacology of benzodiazepines. In *Handbook of Experimental Pharmacology*. (Berlin: Springer) (In press)
15. Haefely, W., Polc, P., Keller, H. H., Pieri, L. and Möhler, H. (1979). Facilitation of GABA-ergic transmission by drugs. In Krogsgaard-Larsen, P., Scheel-Krüger, J. and Kofod, H. (eds.), *GABA-Neurotransmitters*, pp. 357–375. (Copenhagen: Munksgaard)
16. Haefely, W., Kulcsár, A., Möhler, H., Pieri, L., Polc, P. and Schaffner, R. (1975). Possible involvement of GABA in the central actions of benzodiazepines. *Adv. Biochem. Psychopharmacol.*, **14,** 131
17. Haefely, W., Keller, H. H., Pieri, L., Polc, P., Schaffner, R. and Zihlmann, R. (1978). Interaction of minor tranquillizers with synaptic processes mediated by GABA. In Deniker, P., Radouco-Thomas, C. and Villeneuve, A. (eds.), *Neuropsychopharmacology*, pp. 907–916. (Oxford: Pergamon Press)
18. Keller, H. H., Schaffner, R. and Haefely, W. (1976). Interaction of benzodiazepines with neuroleptics at central dopamine neurons. *Naunyn-Schmiedeberg's Arch. Pharmacol.*, **294,** 1
19. Krogsgaard-Larsen, P., Scheel-Krüger, J. and Kofod, H. (eds.) (1978). *GABA-Neurotransmitters*. (Copenhagen: Munksgaard)
20. Möhler, H. and Okada, T. (1977). Benzodiazepines receptor: demonstration in the central nervous system. *Science*, **198,** 849
21. Möhler, H. and Okada, T. (1978). The benzodiazepine receptor in normal and pathological human brain. *Br. J. Psychiatry*, **133,** 261
22. Möhler, H., Battersby, M. K. and Richards, J. G. (1979). Benzodiazepine receptor protein identified and visualized in brain tissue by a novel type of photoaffinity label. *Proc. Natl. Acad. Sci.* (In press)
23. Möhler, H., Polc, P., Cumin, R., Pieri, L. and Kettler, R. (1979). Nicotinamide is a brain constituent with benzodiazepine-like actions. *Nature*, **278,** 563
24. Pieri, L. and Haefely, W. (1976). The effect of diphenylhydantoin, diazepam and clonazepam on the activity of Purkinje cells in the rat cerebellum. *Naunyn-Schmiedeberg's Arch. Pharmacol.*, **296,** 1
25. Polc, P. and Haefely, W. (1976). Effects of two benzodiazepines, phenobarbitone and baclofen on synaptic transmission in the cat cuneate nucleus. *Naunyn-Schmiedeberg's Arch. Pharmacol.*, **294,** 121
26. Polc, P., Möhler, H. and Haefely, W. (1974). The effect of diazepam on spinal cord activities: possible sites and mechanisms of action. *Naunyn-Schmiedeberg's Arch. Pharmacol.*, **284,** 319
27. Raabe, W. and Gumnit, R. J. (1977). Anticonvulsant action of diazepam: increase of cortical postsynaptic inhibition. *Epilepsia*, **18,** 117
28. Roberts, E., Chase, T. N. and Tower, D. B. (eds.) (1976). *GABA in Nervous System Function*. (New York: Raven Press)
29. Scherschlicht, R., Schneeberger, J., Steiner, M. and Haefely, W. (1979).

Delta sleep inducing peptide (DSIP) antagonizes morphine insomnia in cats. *Abstr. 3rd Int. Cong. of Sleep Research*, Tokyo, 1979

30. Schmidt, R. F., Vogel, M. E. and Zimmermann, M. (1967). Die Wirkung von Diazepam auf die präsynaptische Hemmung und andere Rückenmarksreflexe. *Naunyn-Schmiedeberg's Arch. Pharmakol. Exp. Pathol.*, **258,** 69
31. Sepinwall, J. and Cook, L. (1978). Behavioral pharmacology of antianxiety drugs. In Iversen, L. L., Iversen, S. D. and Snyder, S. H. (eds.), *Handbook of Psychopharmacology*, Vol. 13, pp. 345–393. (New York: Plenum Publishing Company)
32. Skolnick, P., Marangos, P. J., Syapin, P., Goodwin, F. K. and Paul, S. M. (1979). CNS benzodiazepine receptors: physiological studies and putative endogenous ligands. *Pharmacol. Biochem. Behav.*, **10,** 815
33. Soubrié, P., Simon, P. and Boissier, J.-R. (1976). An amnesic effect of benzodiazepines in rats. *Experientia*, **32,** 359
34. Soubrié, P., Kulkarmi, S., Simon, P. and Boissier, J.-R. (1975). Effets des anxiolytiques sur la prise de nourriture de rats et de souris placés en situation nouvelle ou familière. *Psychopharmacology*, **45,** 203
35. Soubrié, P., Thiébot, M.-H., Simon, P. and Boissier, J.-R. (1977). Effet des benzodiazépines sur les phénomènes d'inhibition qui contrôlent les comportements exploratoires et le recueil de l'information chez le rat. *J. Pharmacol. (Paris)*, **8,** 393
36. Soubrié, P., Thiébot, M.-H., Simon, P. and Boissier, J.-R. (1978). Benzodiazepines and behavioral effects of reward (water) omission in the rat. *Psychopharmacology*, **59,** 95
37. Tsuchiya, T. and Fukushima, H. (1978). Effects of benzodiazepines and pentobarbitone on the GABAergic recurrent inhibition of hippocampal neurons. *Eur. J. Pharmacol.*, **48,** 421
38. Williamson, M. J., Paul, S. M. and Skolnick, P. (1978). Labelling of benzodiazepine receptors in vivo. *Nature*, **275,** 551
39. Wolf, P. and Haas, H. L. (1977). Effects of diazepines and barbiturates on hippocampal recurrent inhibition. *Naunyn-Schmiedeberg's Arch. Pharmacol.*, **299,** 211
40. Zakusov, V. V., Ostrovskaya, R. U., Kozhechkin, S. N., Markovich, V. V., Molodavkin, G. M. and Voronina, T. A. (1977). Further evidence for GABA-ergic mechanisms in the action of benzodiazepines. *Arch. Int. Pharmacodyn.*, **229,** 313

5

Pharmacokinetics of the Benzodiazepines

S. A. Kaplan

Pharmacokinetics is the study of the rate processes associated with the absorption, distribution, metabolism, and elimination of a drug, i.e. quantitating drug and/or metabolite(s) concentrations in body fluids, tissues and excreta at any time from the moment of administration until elimination from the body is complete.

The primary standard of a pharmacokinetic study is based on the data obtained following intravenous administration. Since the entire dose administered is placed directly into the bloodstream following intravenous administration, the pharmacokinetic parameters obtained are unaffected by all the potential rate limiting and metabolic factors associated with drug absorption. Subsequent to obtaining the primary pharmacokinetic parameters, the drug absorption parameters following other routes of administration may be evaluated and defined in relation to the intravenous standard.

Bioavailability is defined as a measure of the rate and extent of absorption of an administered dose into the systemic circulation. This can be reported in absolute terms based on an intravenous standard or in relative terms by comparison with a standard which may or may not have a known absolute bioavailability. A relative or comparative bioavailability study is also referred to as a bioequivalence study.

In pharmacokinetics one attempts to describe biological events in mathematical terms, usually by developing mathematical models. In the evaluation of intravenous blood, serum, or plasma concentration data the first assumption to be made and tested is that the drug is eliminated exponentially, i.e. via first-order kinetics. This assumption, which is valid in most instances, is easily verified. Benzodiazepines have all been shown to exhibit apparent first-order pharmacokinetic profiles.

First-order kinetics can be demonstrated by plotting the blood, serum or plasma concentrations against time using semi-logarithmic paper and observing visually or by curve-fitting computer techniques that the curve is linear. The pharmacokinetic profile is determined as a function of the number of exponential phases observed in the drug concentration curve. In most instances, the data will be found to be mono-, bi-, or tri-exponential.

The pharmacokinetic parameters obtained following single dose administrations may be used to predict the steady-state blood levels following chronic administration. Such calculations may be used to determine dosing regimens which will maintain a desired blood concentration range, and permit the determination of dosing regimens which may be safely used in a disease state in which the disposition profiles of a drug may be altered.

Clinical pharmacokinetic studies on the 1,4-benzodiazepines require highly sensitive and specific assays for their quantitation since therapeutic doses are usually low[5]. Although electron capture–gas liquid chromatography (EC-GLC) and gas chromatography–chemical ionization–mass spectroscopy (GC-CI-MS) analysis are by far the most sophisticated means of highly sensitive and specific analysis, the utility of other specific GLC detectors, such as the nitrogen specific flame ionization (N/P-FID) detector, high performance liquid chromatography (HPLC) analysis using u.v. fluorescence, polarographic, and mass spectrometric (LC-MS) detection, has not yet been fully realized.

The majority of the assays reported for the determination of specific benzodiazepines in biological fluids use EC-GLC detection due to the presence of an electronegative group in the 7-position of the molecule (usually a halogen or nitro group). A halogen in the 2′-position of the 5-phenyl ring, and a carbonyl group in position 2 of the 1,4-benzodiazepine ring, also contribute to electron capture detector response[6,7].

Radioimmunoassays have recently been developed which are both very sensitive and specific for the parent drug in the presence of its major metabolites and/or other drugs administered concomitantly.

The 1,4-benzodiazepines as a drug class are extensively metabolized. Although some differences occur, the overall metabolic pathways of the benzodiazepines are similar in that:

(1) Substituents are removed from the B ring of the 1,4-benzodiazepine nucleus.

(2) Position 3 is hydroxylated.

(3) The hydroxylated metabolite undergoes conjugation and subsequent elimination in the urine.

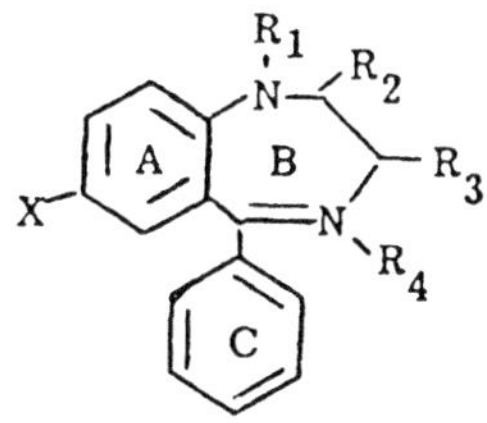

Chlordiazepoxide, diazepam, clorazepate, and prazepam all form nordiazepam by different pathways. Chlordiazepoxide is dealkylated in the liver in two steps with subsequent loss of the oxide to form nordiazepam with all substances contributing to the circulating benzodiazepine pool[8].

Diazepam produces nordiazepam as its major metabolite with both substances contributing to the circulating benzodiazepine pool[15]. The kinetics of formation and elimination of nordiazepam from diazepam reflect the elimination rate of diazepam. The kinetics of the formation of nordiazepam from clorazepate reflect the acidity of the gastric fluids of the patient. Abruzzo *et al.*[1] observed prolongation of blood concentration peak times and a decrease in blood concentration peak heights and areas under the blood concentration curves of nordiazepam in subjects receiving clorazepate with gastric pHs elevated with sodium bicarbonate. Shader *et al.*[24] observed similar effects when patients were administered clorazepate concomitantly with Maalox (Figure 5.1).

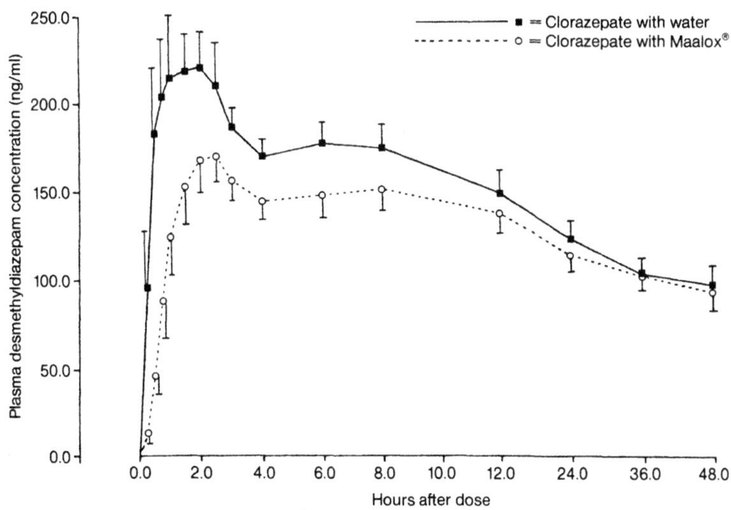

Figure 5.1 Plasma desmethyldiazepam (nordiazepam) concentrations in patients receiving 15 mg oral doses of clorazepate with water and with Maalox[24]

Prazepam differs in that it undergoes virtually complete presystemic dealkylation of the cyclopropylmethyl side chain in the liver to form nordiazepam at a very slow rate. Greenblatt and Shader[13] found no intact prazepam concentrations following single doses of prazepam to fasting volunteers. Following the oral administration of prazepam, plasma concentrations of nordiazepam peaked between 6 to 24 hours post-administration, indicating either slow gastro-intestinal absorption, slow metabolism, or possible binding of prazepam at some site prior to the formation and passage of nordiazepam into systemic circulation. The influence of metabolism on the formation and hence pharmacokinetic profile of nordiazepam exemplifies the many physiological variables associated with drug disposition.

Nordiazepam is hydroxylated by hepatic enzymes in the 3-position to form oxazepam which is subsequently conjugated and excreted in the urine[23]. Temazepam can form its own conjugate or be demethylated in the liver to form oxazepam[23]. Lorazepam, the 2′-chloro derivative of oxazepam, is also metabolized by conjugation[10].

Flurazepam is *N*-desalkylated in two steps[18]. Initially, the secondary amino group is removed to produce the hydroxyethyl metabolite which is subsequently metabolized to *N*-desalkyl flurazepam. The *N*-desalkyl metabolite can be hydroxylated in the 3-position. The 7-nitro groups of clonazepam and of flunitrazepam are reduced to their amino derivatives which are acetylated[17]. All three drug-related components are hydroxylated in the 3-position.

Bromazepam exhibits two major metabolic pathways: hydroxylation at the 3-position with subsequent conjugation of the 3-OH metabolite; and a ring opening to form the benzoylpyridine derivative which is hydroxylated in the 3-position and conjugated[16].

The benzodiazepines as a class of compounds are generally rapidly and completely absorbed following oral administration. A typical absorption evaluation is exemplified by the blood concentration curves of diazepam and nordiazepam following a 10 mg single intravenous and oral dose[15] (Figure 5.2). The comparable areas under the diazepam intravenous and oral blood concentration curves indicate complete absorption, whereas the early and sharp blood concentration peak following oral administration is indicative of rapid absorption. The metabolite, nordiazepam, exhibited blood concentration curves following intravenous and oral administrations of diazepam that are virtually the same, further reflecting the completeness of absorption of diazepam. In most instances, wherever intravenous blood concentration profiles have been obtained as a standard for oral absorption evaluation of the various benzodiazepines, the conclusion is rapid and complete absorption. Departure from such profiles would reflect presystemic biodegradation rather than intrinsic dissolution or permeability rate limited absorption factors.

Autoradiograms with benzodiazepines obtained in several animal species

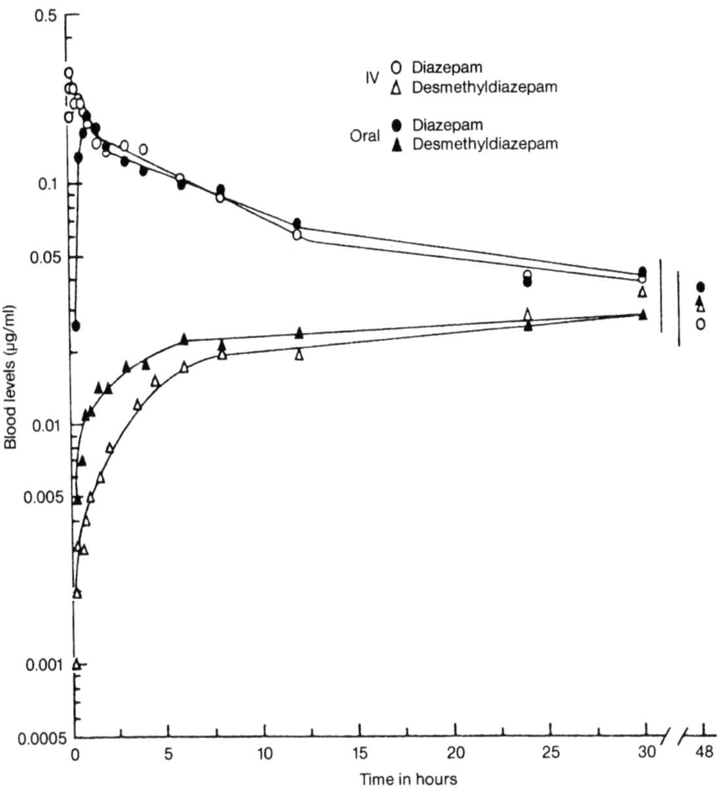

Figure 5.2 Diazepam and desmethyldiazepam (nordiazepam) blood concentration curves in a volunteer receiving single 10 mg i.v. and oral doses[15]

indicated that the labelled compound accumulates very rapidly in the brain. It localizes first in the grey matter, whereas shortly thereafter the radioactivity is primarily concentrated in the white matter[21]. This is exemplified in the autoradiograms obtained from the brain of the cat killed 1 minute after intravenous injection of [^{14}C]diazepam[21]. Initially, when the radioactivity was confined to the grey matter, the highest uptake was found in such sites as thalamus, colliculi, geniculate bodies, midbrain nuclei, cerebral and cerebellar cortex. At this time, the radioactivity in the white matter was low. As time progressed, the concentration of the labelled material tended to become more uniform throughout the whole brain, and the autoradiograms obtained 30 minutes after drug administration did not show marked differences between grey and white matter. One and four hours after the intravenous injection of [^{14}C]diazepam, the radioactivity was much higher in the white than in the grey matter.

It is of interest to contrast these distribution and redistribution findings in the cat with the pharmacokinetics of diazepam in man. Immediately upon intravenous administration of diazepam to man, one observes sedation and amnesia during the first hour which is not observed following comparable oral doses[9]. Such observations reflect the rapid distribution of intravenously administered diazepam into the central nervous system and subsequent redistribution. During this interval following intravenous administration blood concentrations decline to approximately one-half their maximum values; whereas following oral administration blood concentrations are increasing due to absorption. In addition, since metabolite concentrations are very low or non-existent during this interval, the clinical observations must be attributed to the high concentrations of diazepam *per se*.

The benzodiazepine compounds are generally all highly protein bound. Differences are noted in the volumes of distribution of the various benzodiazepines. The more lipophilic the compound, the greater the volume of distribution. Structurally, the $-NHCH_3$ and $N \rightarrow O$ substituents of chlordiazepoxide and the $-OH$ substituents of oxazepam on the benzodiazepine nucleus diminish lipophilicity; whereas diazepam and nordiazepam lack such substituents.

The benzodiazepines are all eliminated from the body by biotransformation via one or several steps. The 'apparent' halflife of elimination of the several benzodiazepines can vary from less than 10 hours to over 100 hours. This variability reflects a composite of physicochemical properties, rates of presystemic metabolism, and the intricacies of the metabolic pathways.

Compounds such as oxazepam[2], lorazepam[20], temazepam[11], chlordiazepoxide[4], and bromazepam[16] are eliminated fairly rapidly with 'apparent' halflives for each ranging from about twenty to under ten hours. It is interesting to note that all of these benzodiazepines have polar functional groups such as a 3-OH, a N_4-oxide, or a pyridine (bromazepam) in place of the 5-phenyl ring. Clonazepam and flunitrazepam with nitro groups in the 7-position exhibit halflives in the 20- to 30-hour range[17]. Diazepam and nordiazepam exhibit much longer halflives probably because they do not possess corresponding polar functional groups. The differences in the apparent elimination rate of nordiazepam when observed after clorazepate, prazepam, or diazepam administration reflect the influence of the formation rate constant on the 'apparent' elimination rate constant of the drug. Flurazepam is rapidly eliminated with a mean halflife of 2.3 hours[12].

The elimination profiles of all the benzodiazepines can be characterized as 'apparent' first-order processes, inferring that the elimination rate is not dose dependent. Confirmation of the apparent first-order elimination kinetics of the benzodiazepines is based on the ability of each of the compounds to achieve predictable multiple dose steady-state drug concentration profiles. Overall, the experimental steady-state concentrations of the

1,4-benzodiazepines can be predicted from the single dose pharmacokinetic parameters. The ability to achieve such profiles confirms the constancy and hence reproducibility of absorption, distribution, metabolism, and elimination from administration to administration.

Interpretation of the pharmacokinetic profiles of the benzodiazepines following multiple dose administration in man must consider their extensive metabolism and accumulation of the parent compounds and metabolites. The administered benzodiazepines are absorbed, accumulate to steady-state concentrations, and are metabolized at different rates while their respective metabolites are subsequently formed, metabolized, and excreted at rates differing from those of the parent compound. For some benzodiazepines, the metabolites are pharmacologically and pharmacokinetically unimportant following single dose administrations, but become significant following chronic dosing schedules.

Several investigators have studied the disposition profiles of diazepam and its major metabolite, nordiazepam, following chronic administration of diazepam to man. Pharmacokinetic constants obtained after single dose intravenous studies allowed for the prediction of the typical oral steady-state blood concentration profile of diazepam, presented in Figure 5.3, obtained on a 10 mg once daily oral dosing regimen over 15 days. Steady-state diazepam blood concentrations were achieved within seven days and the steady-state maximum and minimum blood concentrations are approximately twice the corresponding blood concentrations observed following single dose studies. The calculated elimination rate constant,

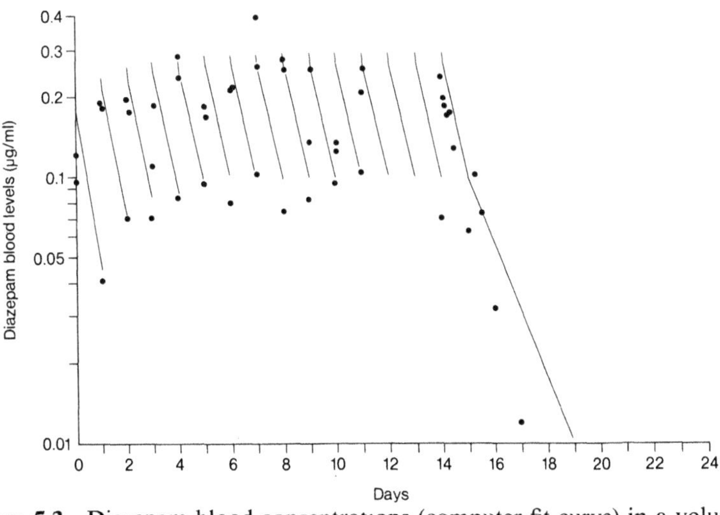

Figure 5.3 Diazepam blood concentrations (computer fit curve) in a volunteer receiving 10mg oral doses once daily for 15 days[15]

observed following the last dose during chronic administration, approximated the corresponding rate constant observed following single dose administration. The corresponding nordiazepam profile is presented in Figure 5.4. The steady-state concentrations of nordiazepam following the administration of diazepam are essentially equivalent to the mean steady-state blood levels of diazepam. The small range of maximum to minimum blood concentrations of nordiazepam is a reflection of the drug's slow formation and elimination following the administration and metabolism of diazepam.

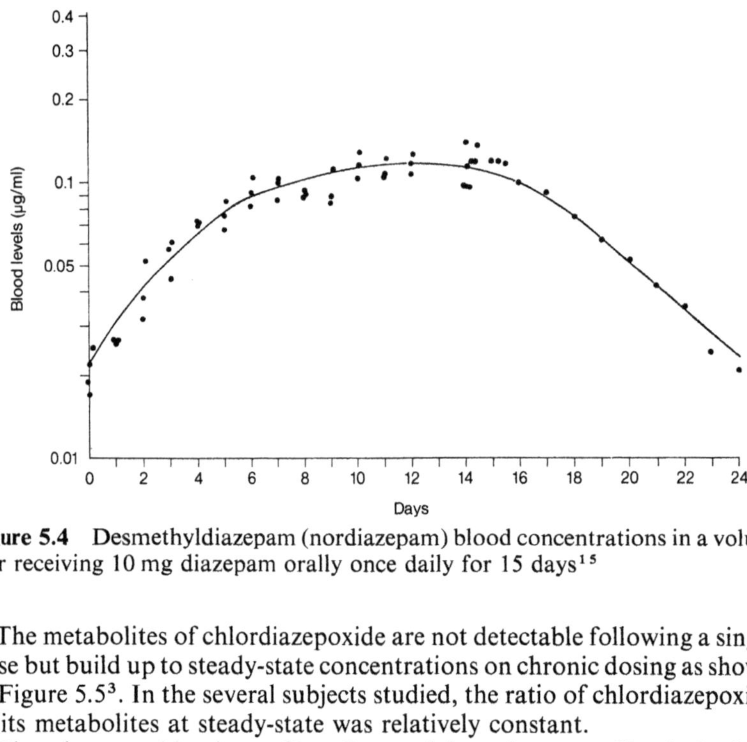

Figure 5.4 Desmethyldiazepam (nordiazepam) blood concentrations in a volunteer receiving 10 mg diazepam orally once daily for 15 days[15]

The metabolites of chlordiazepoxide are not detectable following a single dose but build up to steady-state concentrations on chronic dosing as shown in Figure 5.5[3]. In the several subjects studied, the ratio of chlordiazepoxide to its metabolites at steady-state was relatively constant.

The pharmacokinetic profiles discussed have been profiles in healthy volunteers. However, in a clinical setting, patients of various age groups may possess a variety of pathological, genetic, and environmental characteristics. Age, disease state, and drug interactions may also affect the physiological disposition profile of a drug. Such changes may be reflected in specific pharmacokinetic parameters which, in turn, may influence the clinical profile of the drug. For example, metabolic reactions such as oxidations, reductions, hydrolyses, and conjugations, which readily occur within the liver of children and adults, are negligible in newborns[25].

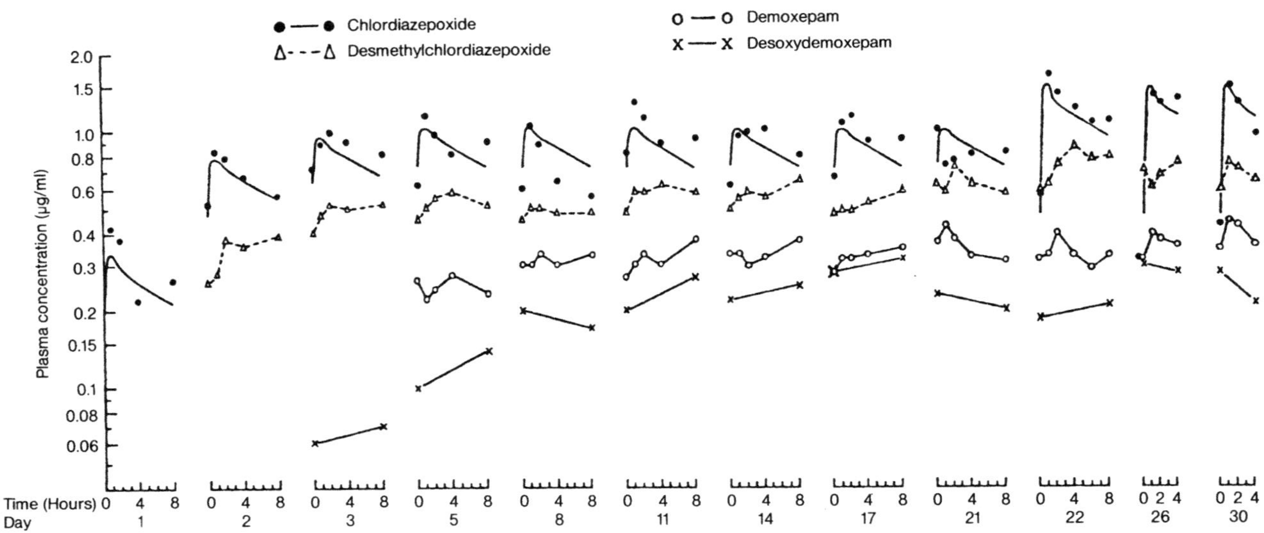

Figure 5.5 Plasma concentrations of chlordiazepoxide and metabolites in a volunteer receiving 30 mg chlordiazepoxide daily for 36 days (10 mg every 8 hours on days 1–21; 30 mg once daily on days 22–36)[3] (Used by kind permission of Plenum Publishing Corporation)

Hydroxylation and glucuronidation capabilities, which are major metabolic pathways for the benzodiazepines, appear to be related to the degree of maturation. Such alterations in metabolism are reflected in the pharmacokinetic parameters of these drugs.

The urinary excretion profiles of diazepam metabolites in prematures of 8 to 81 days old, full term infants of 4 to 162 days old, and children, 3.5 to 8 years old, are presented in Figure 5.6[25]. The three groups all have the ability to demethylate diazepam to form nordiazepam. However, the ability to hydroxylate and conjugate is limited in the premature and full term infant but not in older children.

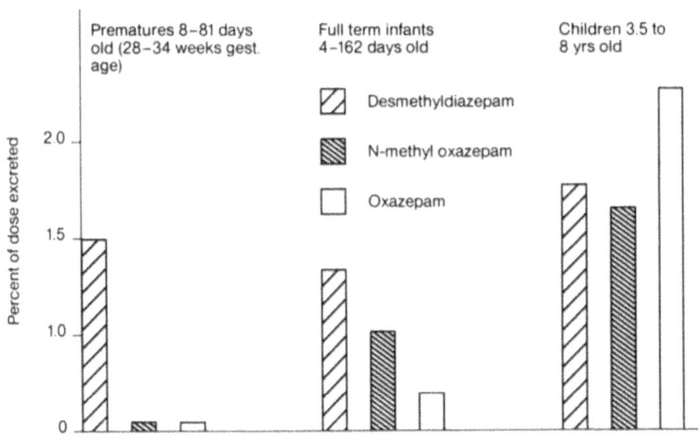

Figure 5.6 Urinary excretion of diazepam metabolites in children of different age group[25]

The pharmacokinetic parameters of diazepam in prematures, children and adults are presented in Table 5.1[22]. The long halflife of elimination of diazepam in prematures reflects hepatic immaturity. The volume of distribution (V_d) is less for newborns than for adults. Differences in V_d may reflect the lesser amount of plasma proteins and protein binding capacity in newborns and/or their differences in body composition, e.g. greater body water, low fat content.

Table 5.1 Pharmacokinetic parameters of diazepam

Subjects	$t_{1/2}(h)$	$V_d(l/kg)$
Prematures (8–81 days)	40–100	1.10
Children (3–7 years)	20–45	1.99
Adult (25–43 years)	21–46	1.86

The pharmacokinetic parameters of halflife and volume of distribution that differ in the infant also differ in geriatric patients when both groups are compared to young adults. The correlation between the halflife of elimination of diazepam and age is shown in Figure 5.7[19]. There is a marked

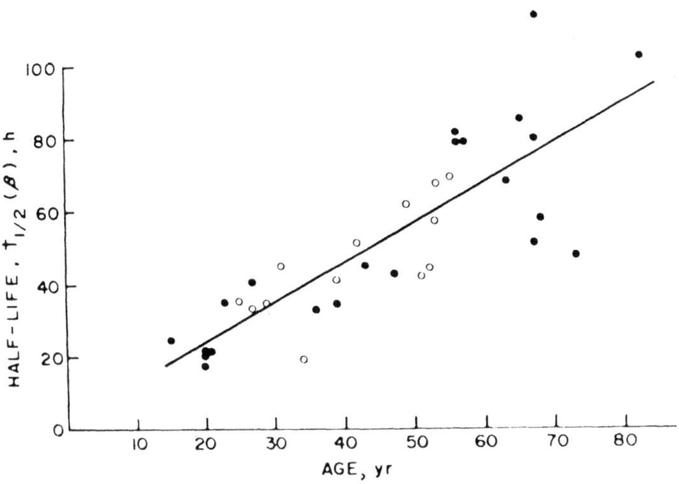

Figure 5.7 Diazepam halflife of elimination as a function of age[13] (Used by kind permission of *Journal of Clinical Investigation*)

increase in diazepam halflife with age. Figure 5.8 demonstrates that there is also an increase in volume of distribution of diazepam with age. Although these are the same diazepam pharmacokinetic parameters that were altered in newborns, these parameters are probably changing in the geriatric subject for different reasons. The prolonged halflives of the benzodiazepines in ageing normal subjects reflect alterations in distribution characteristics, V_d, rather than hepatic dysfunction or alterations in protein binding. Such pharmacokinetic observations may be reflecting normal physiological changes on ageing, such as diminishing lean body mass.

The pharmacokinetics of drugs may be altered in the presence of hepatic disease requiring adjustments in dosing schedules. The pharmacokinetic parameters affected by liver disease include protein binding, extraction ratio, hepatic clearance, and halflife of the administered drug. Renal dysfunction also results in a reduction of plasma proteins. Once the influence of disease state on the pharmacokinetic parameters is established, a new dosing regimen may be calculated to yield desired plasma concentrations. Therefore, in spite of changes in the pharmacokinetic parameters of the benzodiazepines due to age, hepatic or renal dysfunction or other pathological states, new dosing regimens may be readily calculated to assure plasma concentrations associated with clinical efficacy and safety of the drugs.

A clinical manifestation of a long halflife of elimination of the benzodiazepine compound and/or their active metabolites is an intrinsic 'tapering-off' of drug concentration which may minimize or negate the withdrawal syndromes[13] and rebound insomnia[14] generally observed with rapidly eliminated anxiolytic and hypnotic drugs.

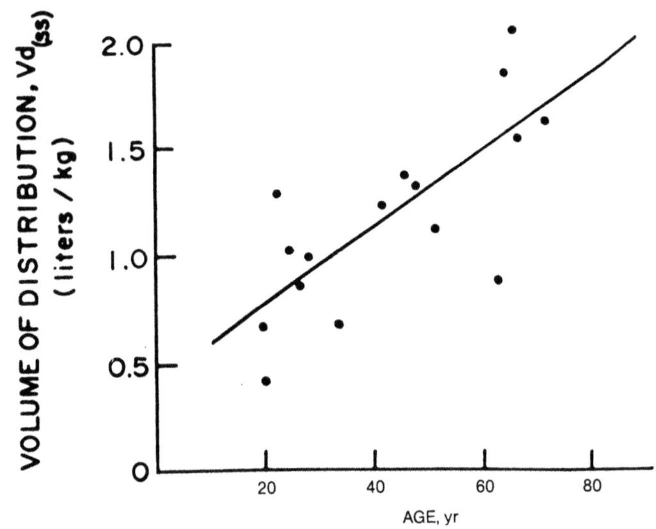

Figure 5.8 Diazepam volume of distribution as a function of age[19] (Used by kind permission of *Journal of Clinical Investigation*)

In conclusion, the application of pharmacokinetics and comparison of these profiles for the several benzodiazepines, in use today and under development, provide quantitative precision for our understanding of their clinical performance characteristics. One can anticipate that the application of pharmacokinetic insights to the synthesis and evaluation of new benzodiazepines will be a major factor in the successful development of the next generation of benzodiazepine compounds.

References

1. Abruzzo, C.W., Macasieb, T., Weinfeld, R.W., Rider, J.A. and Kaplan, S.A. (1977). Changes in the oral absorption characteristics in man of dipotassium clorazepate at normal and elevated gastric pH. *J. Pharmacokin. Biopharm.*, **5**, 377

2. Alvan, G., Sievers, B. and Vessman, J. (1977). Pharmacokinetics of oxazepam in healthy volunteers. *Acta Pharmacol. Toxicol.*, **40 Suppl. 1,** 40
3. Boxenbaum, H. G., Geitner, K. A., Jack, M. L., Dixon, W. R. and Kaplan, S. A. (1977). Pharmacokinetic and biopharmaceutic profile of chlordiazepoxide HCl in healthy subjects: multiple-dose administration. *J. Pharmacokin. Biopharm.*, **5,** 25
4. Boxenbaum, H. G., Geitner, K. A., Jack, M. L., Dixon, W. R., Spiegel, H. E., Symington, J., Christian, R., Moore, J.D., Weissmann, L. and Kaplan, S. A. (1977). Pharmacokinetic and biopharmaceutic profile of chlordiazepoxide HCl in healthy subjects: single dose studies by the intravenous, intramuscular and oral routes. *J. Pharmacokin. Biopharm.*, **5,** 3
5. de Silva, J. A. F. (1976). In Kellaway, P. and Petersen, I. (eds.) *Quantitative Analytic Studies in Epilepsy*, pp. 11–38. (New York: Raven Press)
6. de Silva, J. A. F. (1978). Electron capture–GLC in the quantitation of 1,4-benzodiazepines. In Pippenger, C. E., Penry, J. K. and Kutt, H. (eds.) *Antiepileptic Drugs: Quantitative Analysis and Interpretation*, pp. 111–138. (New York: Raven Press)
7. de Silva, J. A. F., Bekersky, I., Puglisi, C. V., Brooks, M. A. and Weinfeld, R. E. (1976). Determination of 1,4-benzodiazepines and -diazepin-2-ones in blood by electron-capture gas-liquid chromatography, *Anal. Chem.*, **48,** 10
8. Dixon, R., Brooks, M. A., Postma, E., Hackman, M. R., Spector, S., Moore, J. D. and Schwartz, M. A. (1976). *N*-desmethyl diazepam; a new metabolite of chlordiazepoxide in man. *Clin. Pharmacol. Ther.*, **20,** 450
9. Driscoll, E., Smelack, Z., Lightbody, P. and Fiorucci, R. (1972). Sedative with intravenous diazepam, *J. Oral Surg.*, **30,** 332
10. Elliott, H. (1976). Metabolism of lorazepam. *Br. J. Anaesth.*, **48,** 1017
11. Fuccella, L. M., Tosolini, G., Moro, E. and Tamassia, V. (1972). Study of physiological availability of temazepam in man. *Int. J. Clin. Pharmacol. Ther. Toxicol.*, **6,** 303
12. Glover, W., Early, J., Dellaney, M. and Dixon, W. (1980). Flurazepam: RIA and plasma levels in man. *J. Pharm. Sci.*, **69,** 601
13. Greenblatt, D. J. and Shader, R. T. (1978). Pharmacokinetics understanding of antianxiety drug therapy. *South. Med. J.*, **7. (Suppl. 2)**
14. Kales, A., Scharf, M. S. and Kales, J. D. (1978). Rebound insomnia: a new clinical syndrome. *Science*, **201,** 1039
15. Kaplan, S. A., Jack, M. L., Alexander, K. and Weinfeld, R. W. (1973). Pharmacokinetic profile of diazepam in man following single intravenous and oral and chronic oral administration. *J. Pharm. Sci.*, **62,** 1789
16. Kaplan, S. A., Jack, M. L., Weinfeld, R. W., Glover, W., Weissman, L. and Cotler, S. (1976). Biopharmaceutical and clinical pharmacokinetic profile of bromazepam. *J. Pharmacokin. Biopharm.*, **4,** 1
17. Kaplan, S. A., Alexander, K., Jack, M. L., Puglisi, C. V., de Silva, J. A. F., Lee, T. and Weinfeld, R. (1974). Pharmacokinetic profiles of clonazepam. *J. Pharm. Sci.*, **63,** 527
18. Kaplan, S. A., de Silva, J. A. F., Jack, M. L., Alexander, K., Strojny, N., Weinfeld, R., Puglisi, C. and Weissman, L. (1973). Blood level profile in man following chronic oral administration of flurazepam hydrochloride. *J. Pharm. Sci.*, **62,** 1932
19. Klotz, U., Avant, G. R., Hoyumpa, A., Schenker, S. and Wilkinson, G. R.

(1975). The effect of age and liver disease on the disposition and elimination of diazepam in adult man. *J. Clin. Invest.*, **55,** 347

20. Kyriakopoulos, A. A., Greenblatt, D. J. and Shader, R. I. (1978). Clinical pharmacokinetics of lorazepam: a review. *J. Clin. Psychiatry*, **39,** 16
21. Morselli, P., Cassano, G., Placidi, G., Muscettola, G. and Rizzo, M. (1973). Kinetics of the distribution of ^{14}C-diazepam and its metabolites in various areas of cat brain. In Garattini, S., Mussini, E. and Randall, L. O. (eds.) *The Benzodiazepines*, pp. 129–145. (New York: Raven Press)
22. Morselli, P. L., Principi, N., Tognoni, G., Reali, E., Belvedere, G., Standen, S. M. and Sereni, F. (1973). Diazepam elimination in premature and full term infants, and children. *J. Perinat. Med.*, **1,** 133
23. Schwartz, M. (1973). Pathways of metabolism of the benzodiazepines. In Garattini, S., Mussini, F. and Randall, L. O. (eds.) *The Benzodiazepines*, pp. 53–74. (New York: Raven Press)
24. Shader, R. I., Georgotas, A., Greenblatt, D. J., Harmatz, J. S. and Allen, M. D. (1978). Impaired absorption of desmethyldiazepam from clorazepate by magnesium aluminium hydroxide. *Clin. Pharmacol. Ther.*, **24,** 308
25. Vest, M. F. and Rossier, R. (1963). Detoxification in the newborn: The ability of the newborn infant to form conjugates with glucuronic acid, glycine, acetate, and glutathione. *Ann. NY Acad. Sci.*, **111,** 183

6

Importance of Pharmacokinetic Data for Clinical Practice

R. Amrein and B. Leishman

Introduction

By the early 1960s, when Librium and Valium were first introduced onto the market, pharmacokineticists had already begun to be interested in the benzodiazepines. They were especially drawn to two properties of benzodiazepines which they had not yet discovered in their investigations with other drugs, namely their extraordinarily broad margin of safety, and the ease with which clinical efficacy can be ascertained even after single doses.

It would appear fitting at this point to give some consideration to the ways in which the practising physician has benefited from these 20 years of pharmacokinetic studies. In doing so, we are confronted with the impressive fact that several hundred papers have been written, all dealing with some aspect of the pharmacokinetics of benzodiazepines.

Definition

Pharmacokinetics aims to describe in quantitative terms the behaviour of a substance in the human body and, for this purpose, accurate determinations must be made. This is made extremely difficult by the necessity of determining plasma concentrations in nanograms, since benzodiazepines are effective even in small doses (0.25–10 mg as a single dose) and are widely distributed in the human body.

The lengths of the halflives of benzodiazepines are well-known to clinicians. Many benzodiazepines differ only slightly in the length of their halflives: chlordiazepoxide[27], diazepam[33], nitrazepam[48, 49] and bromazepam[45] have a halflife of 20 to 40 hours. Oxazepam[20] and pinazepam[13] are usually credited with a halflife of 5 to 15 hours. Flurazepam, triazolam and midazolam have a short halflife. For reasons which will be discussed later, flurazepam is regarded today more as a long-acting benzodiazepine.

These figures ought to concern us, since there are two benzodiazepines with a longer halflife, nitrazepam and flunitrazepam, which are used almost exclusively as hypnotic agents.

Experience in thousands of cases to date has shown that, in suitable dosage, nitrazepam (Mogadon), flunitrazepam (Rohypnol) or diazepam (Valium) can be administered as hypnotic agents for many consecutive nights at a constant dosage without resulting in a prolonged action or 'hangover' effect.

Supposing that the behaviour of the benzodiazepines could be completely explained in terms of their halflife period, and also supposing that there is a connection between plasma concentrations and effect, then patients

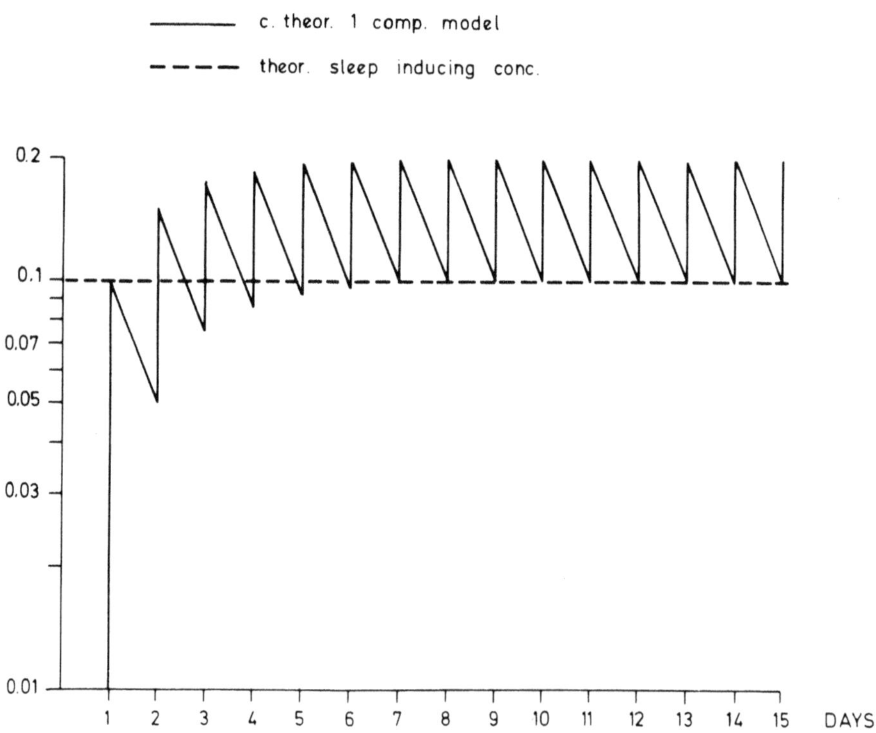

Figure 6.1 Theoretical plasma concentration–time curve following multiple doses of a benzodiazepine

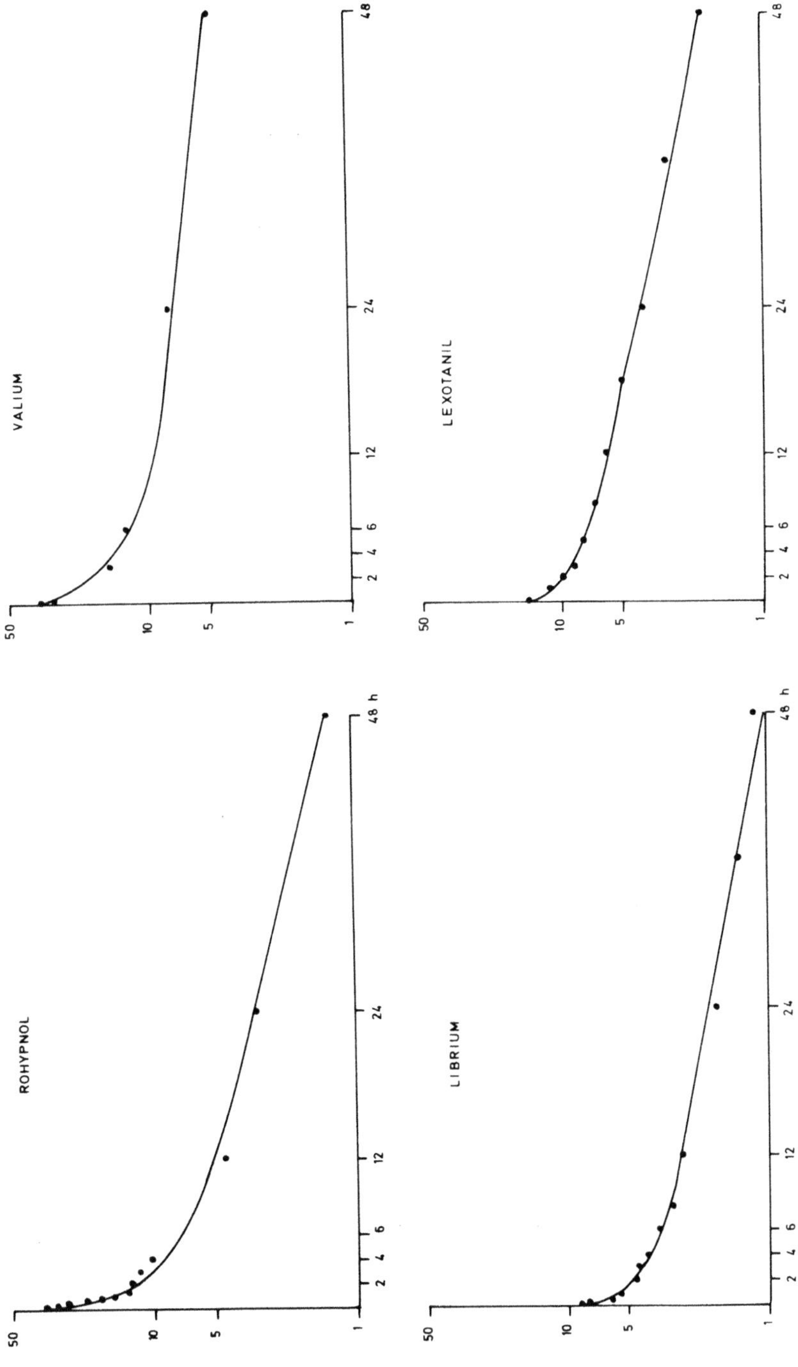

Figure 6.2 Plasma concentration–time curves following intravenous injection of a benzodiazepine

taking benzodiazepines as hypnotics would all fall into a permanent sleep within a few days (Figure 6.1).

While halflives are important in the description of certain pharmacokinetic aspects[40, 44, 50], to use them as the sole standard by which to gauge pharmacokinetic behaviour must necessarily give a misleading picture. A more complex approach would correspond more faithfully to the real situation.

To illustrate this approach, let us examine what occurs after intravenous

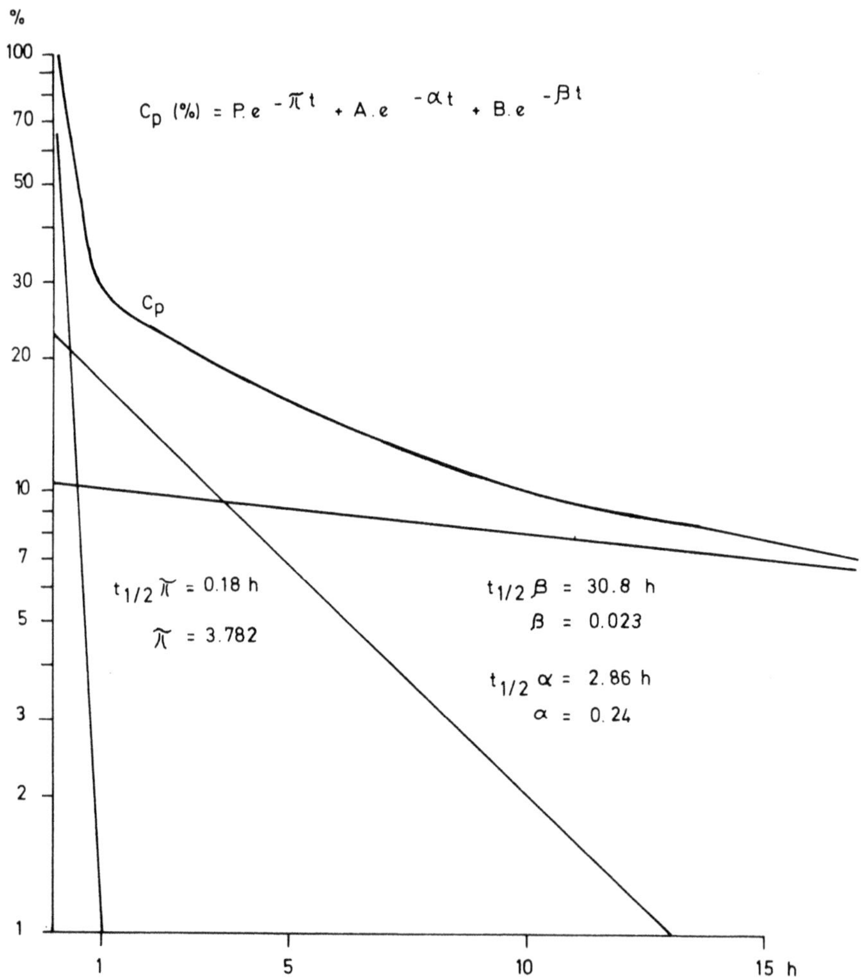

Figure 6.3 The three-compartment model is represented by a tri-exponential equation to describe the post-intravenous injection data

injection of flunitrazepam. We note the plasma concentrations at short intervals and present the results semilogarithmically (Figure 6.2). It is immediately apparent that this preparation cannot be adequately described in terms of its halflife alone. Many other benzodiazepines, such as diazepam (Valium)[32, 33], chlordiazepoxide (Librium)[23–27] and bromazepam (Lexotanil)[45, 46] behave in a similar way: presented semilogarithmically, the plasma concentration curve is clearly non-linear (Figure 6.2). The final section in the semilogarithmic presentation, described by means of the β-halflife, starts in the case of flunitrazepam (Rohypnol) at around the 20th hour[11], that is, at a time when the therapeutically useful sleep-inducing and sedative action has long since disappeared. While the fall in plasma concentration in the terminal phase is due entirely to elimination – which in the case of the benzodiazepines described here involves both metabolic breakdown and excretion – in the initial phase, the distribution phenomena are essentially, or even chiefly, responsible for the changes in plasma concentration.

The concentration curve can be presented as the sum of several processes (Figure 6.3). The mathematical formula is expressed as a bi- or tri-exponential term in which the halflife is also found. The pharmacokineticist associates such a bi- or tri-exponential expression with the concept of a 2- or 3-compartment model, in which, grossly simplified, the body is represented as a system of 2 or 3 loosely connected vessels (Figure 6.4). By definition, the plasma is a part of the first compartment. It is usually assumed that elimination takes place from this central compartment.

Shortly after administration of the substance, there is a considerable concentration gradient between the compartments. In this initial phase, the disappearance of the benzodiazepine from the central compartment is

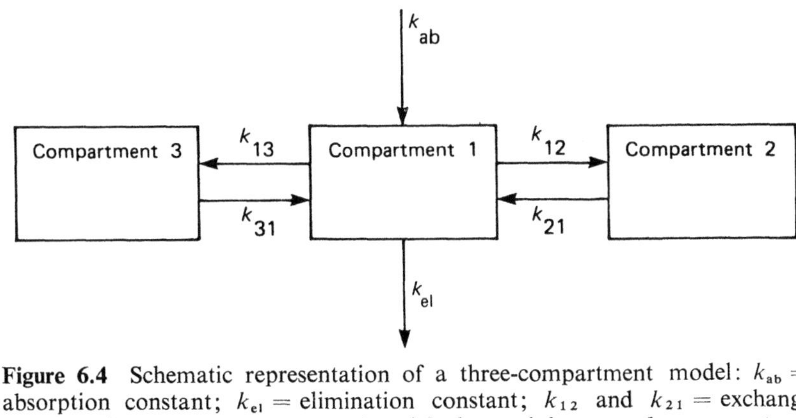

Figure 6.4 Schematic representation of a three-compartment model: k_{ab} = absorption constant; k_{el} = elimination constant; k_{12} and k_{21} = exchange constants between compartments 1 and 2; k_{13} and k_{31} = exchange constants between compartments 1 and 3

not primarily attributable to metabolism but to redistribution into the deeper compartments (Figure 6.5). One hour after injection of Rohypnol, around 7% of the dose administered has been metabolized, but the drug concentration has already dropped to 33% of the original level.

Without exception, all the benzodiazepines are easily fat-soluble and therefore have no difficulty in passing the blood–brain barrier. It is therefore assumed that the receptors for the benzodiazepines form part of the central compartment. Distribution processes are also of great importance as they give the body a means of rapidly reducing the concentration of a drug at the site of action.

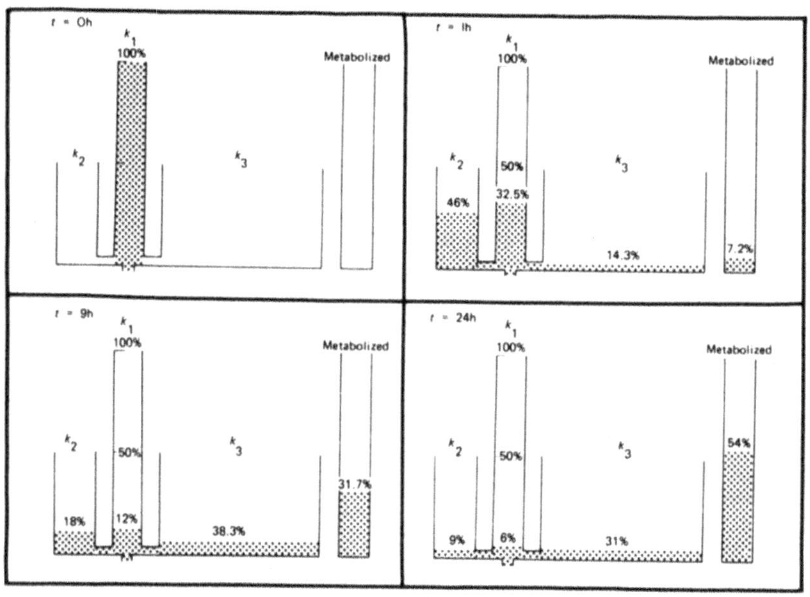

Figure 6.5 Schematic representation of the relative amounts of flunitrazepam present in the three compartments (k_1, k_2, k_3) at various times. The plasma is included in the central compartment k_1 (reprinted from Priest, R.G., Pletscher, A. and Ward, J. (eds), *Sleep Research* (Lancaster: MTP Press))

Earlier, mention was made of the course of plasma concentration of Rohypnol, Valium, Librium and Lexotanil. In pharmacological experiments, these four have all been shown to possess sedative, anxiolytic, muscle relaxant and anticonvulsant properties[1]. Rohypnol, administered orally, is however used only as an hypnotic agent. Valium is also often used for the same purpose. The anxiolytic, muscle relaxant and anticonvulsant properties of diazepam are also used therapeutically very frequently. Librium is used chiefly, and Lexotanil exclusively, for anxiolytic therapy. Let us have another brief look at the plasma curve for the four benzodiazepines: Figure 6.6. These four benzodiazepines all have β-halflives of almost equal length ($\simeq$20h) but differ in the distribution phase. In the case of Rohypnol, the rapid drop in plasma concentration in the first couple of hours after drug intake is caused almost exclusively by distribution processes. With Valium, these distribution processes are also chiefly responsible for the drop in plasma concentration in the period immediately following drug intake. They are of less significance for Librium and Lexotanil. Thus it appears to be less the differences in pharmacological behaviour and rather more the variations in distribution behaviour in the human body which are responsible for the variety of clinical applications of benzodiazepines with a longer β-halflife: benzodiazepines with a strongly pronounced distribution phase are used chiefly as hypnotic agents, while benzodiazepines with a less pronounced distribution phase are employed mainly as anxiolytics.

Metabolism

We have already said that benzodiazepines are removed from the body chiefly by metabolism in the liver. Direct elimination in urine and elimination in bile[42] or gastric juices is of practically no significance[17,54]. The metabolism of benzodiazepines varies greatly. A certain proportion of the drug is always glucuronidated and the pharmacologically inactive glucuronide is subsequently excreted in the urine. Oxazepam[18,20,38] for example is eliminated almost exclusively in the form of the glucuronide. Other benzodiazepines such as diazepam and chlordiazepoxide form desmethyl- and hydroxy-compounds. Amino compounds can also be formed but are mostly pharmacologically inactive.

These primary metabolites are in turn further metabolized, either to inactive secondary metabolites or to pharmacologically active secondary decomposition products such as oxazepam, which is formed by the metabolism of both Valium and Librium. Metabolites are, it is true, usually less active than the unaltered drug, but they still serve to prolong the active life of the benzodiazepines.

Clorazepate (Tranxene) is so unstable that, even in the stomach, it hydrolyses almost completely to desmethyldiazepam. After Tranxene administration, although it is not possible to measure plasma concentrations of clorazepate, the metabolite desmethyldiazepam certainly can be detected. In this case, the duration of action depends entirely on the activity of the metabolites[6,12]. With flurazepam (Dalmane), the unaltered active ingredient has a halflife of about one hour. Through a series of metabolites, some active, *N*-desalkylflurazepam is formed and later eliminated with a halflife of around 50 hours.

From these few examples, it should be clear that it is not sufficient to

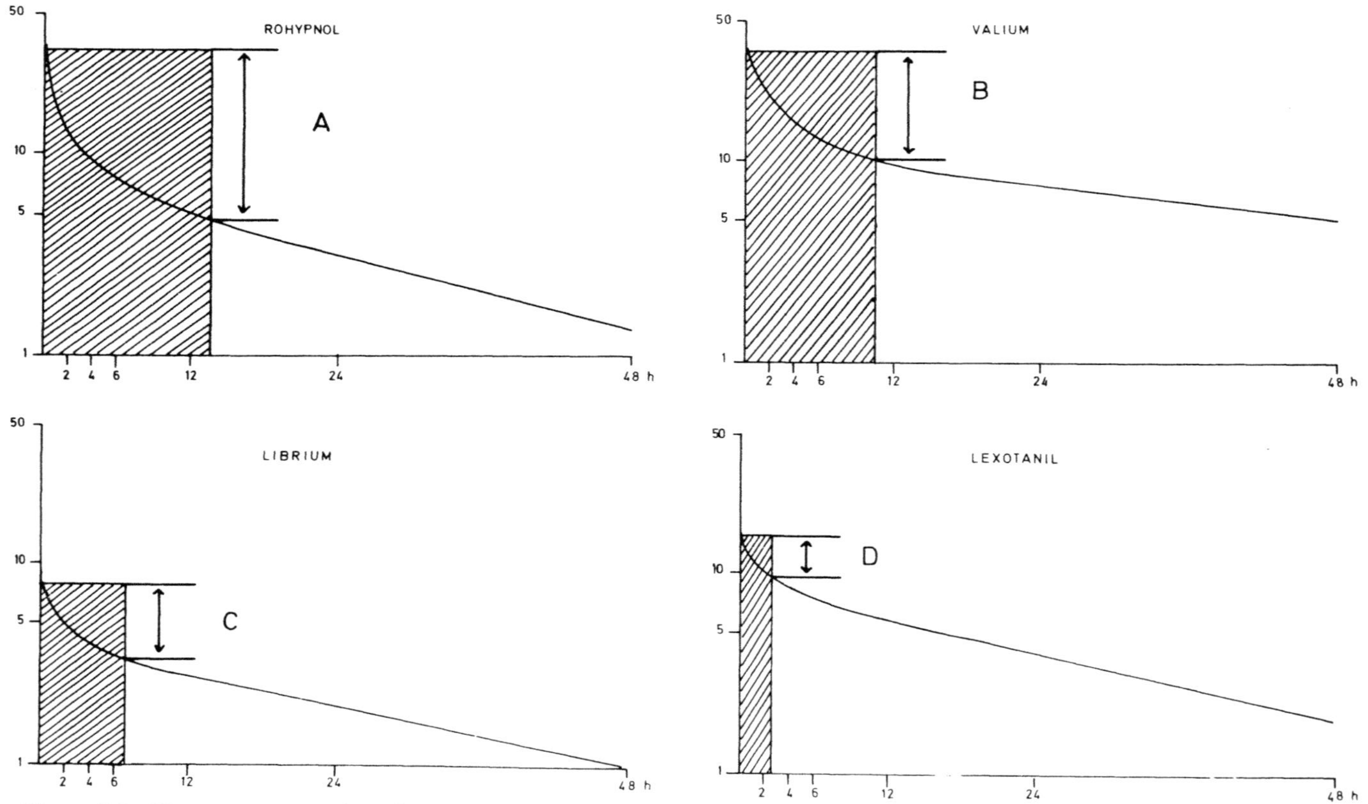

Figure 6.6 Plasma concentration–time curves following an intravenous injection. The hatching represents the duration of the distribution phase

describe the duration of action of a preparation in terms of the pharmacokinetics of the unaltered substance. It would, however, be equally wrong to regard the halflife of a slowly eliminated metabolite such as desalkylflurazepam as being typical of and responsible for the activity as a whole. Unfortunately, we still lack a recognized procedure to present in a rational manner the sum total of the effects. In most cases, the efficacy of the metabolites has not been compared with that of the original substance in man and, in this respect, animal experiments have given contradictory results which offer little reliable guidance.

In very general terms, the duration of action of benzodiazepines is prolonged and the activity profile somewhat flattened by the active metabolites: metabolites are formed in direct proportion to the disappearance of the unaltered substance. Therapeutically, this process can be put to very good use, especially if a suitable special pharmaceutical form is available.

Relation of pharmacokinetic parameters to age, sex, smoking habits, liver function, protein binding: interactions

The pharmacokinetic behaviour of benzodiazepines is not only complicated but demonstrates great individual variations[2, 9]. In the last few years it has been possible to discover some of the reasons for this variability[39, 51]. As an example of this, it has been said that the halflife of diazepam increases with age[14, 22, 37, 41, 50], this increase being about one hour per year of life. Diazepam clearance is, however, not age-related, since lengthening of the halflife occurs as a result of an increased distribution volume.

In patients with cirrhosis of the liver, the halflife is markedly longer and clearance reduced[5, 10, 22, 28, 29, 34–37, 43]. Sex-specific variation in pharmacokinetic behaviour[22, 27] and the influence of smoking on benzodiazepines have also been investigated, although these differences are less significant than the others mentioned above. The literature available on this subject also provides somewhat contradictory reports. Benzodiazepines are highly protein-bound. Thus, in the plasma, diazepam is 95–97.5% bound to plasma protein.

In severe hypalbuminaemia (liver cirrhosis, terminal renal insufficiency), binding of the benzodiazepines to plasma protein decreases somewhat, although these alterations appear to have limited therapeutic significance[1, 21, 47].

In longterm administration of barbiturates, the liver enzyme system is induced[52] and, in consequence, the breakdown of the barbiturates accelerated. When benzodiazepines are administered simultaneously, the benzodiazepine metabolism is also accelerated because of this pre-existing enzyme induction[29, 30]. This is above all significant in the treatment of epilepsy, since combination therapy of this disease is today more the rule than the exception. According to statistics, patients receiving Rivotril as monotherapy have a much better therapeutic result than those who receive Rivotril as part of a combination therapy. In the case of the latter, the poorer result may partly be due to enzyme stimulation by barbiturates or hydantoin derivatives.

Consequences for therapy

An increasing number of more precise relationships between benzodiazepine plasma concentration and clinical parameters has been discovered in recent years: quantitative EEG changes, degree of sedation, performance of tasks and muscle relaxation have been successfully related to the prevailing plasma concentration[3,4,7–9,15,16,19,31,53]. Very often, the relationships have been established in healthy subjects: usually, relationships between plasma concentration and clinical effect have been able to be determined only for the first 3–12 hours after drug intake.

Most authors describe very wide individual variations of the effective plasma concentration. The wide margin of safety of benzodiazepines, the variability of the effective dose from patient to patient, the often rapidly changing therapeutic situation and the rapid onset of a clearly marked clinical effect are factors which make it advisable to adjust the dosage of benzodiazepines to individual patient response. In patients with sleep disorders, an initial dose of around 15 mg Dalmane is prescribed but, should this prove inadequate, the dosage can be raised without hesitation. In epilepsy, an attempt is made to interrupt attacks with 10 mg Valium i.v.; when success is only short-lasting, it is reasonable to give an additional dose. Where a patient who has previously suffered daily from frequent petit-mal attacks can successfully control his condition with a certain daily dose of Rivotril, it would be of purely academic interest to investigate at what plasma concentration this particular individual therapeutic goal is attained. Apart from in the treatment of epilepsy, there are only a few therapeutic situations in which benzodiazepines are administered long-term at a constant dose and at constant dosage intervals.

Where the therapeutic effect of the initial recommended dose is inappropriate, it can be changed to a level which will bring about the desired effect in the individual patient.

Since the benzodiazepine dosage is checked for its successful action and adjusted to the situation, pharmacokinetic measurements or considerations play only a very limited role in the therapy of individual cases. Here a pragmatic approach is usually much more efficient and cost-saving than complicated roundabout methods involving measurement of concentrations. However, in extreme therapeutic situations, such measurements can sometimes be helpful: for example, when, completely contrary to expectations, there is no clear therapeutic response, plasma concentration can be measured in order to determine whether the patient is making some serious mistake in medication or whether a grossly abnormal metabolic condition has been overlooked.

Pharmacokinetics can also make a useful contribution when it comes to discovering a new indication or method of administration for a benzodiazepine, or designing a new pharmaceutical form. In this context, bioavailability has become a fashionable term in recent years. Bioavailability is concerned with the extent and rate at which the administered drug reaches the systemic circulation and can, within certain limits, be influenced and deliberately controlled. In recent years, description of the bioavailability of the benzodiazepines has mainly stressed the available amount. It is probably generally accepted that, in practical terms, it is of little importance to know whether the bioavailability of a certain benzodiazepine is 85% or 95%. Naturally, it is possible to aim for complete bioavailability.

If a benzodiazepine is very rapidly absorbed on oral administration, then the distribution phase is pronounced and, in the first hours after administration, massive changes in plasma concentration occur. In parallel to this, there will be rapid qualitative and quantitative changes in the clinical effects, so that, shortly after administration, it is possible for a strong sedative, muscle relaxant effect to occur and then diminish in the next few hours, to be replaced by a mainly anxiolytic effect. However, should the same benzodiazepine be absorbed very slowly, then the distribution phase is almost imperceptible; much smaller peak concentrations would be reached and the fluctuations in concentration would be much more limited. In this way, the preparation's profile of action could be basically changed, meaning that, for example, with unchanged or even prolonged anxiolytic effect, there would be very much less sedation and muscle relaxation. Roche has recently developed a special form of Valium (Valium CR) which allows full absorption of the active ingredient, but at a controlled rate, slower than that of the usual marketed forms. After Valium CR administration, the distribution phase is only slightly in evidence, resulting in a definite change in the profile of action: the anxiolytic effect remains constant while muscle relaxation and sedation are greatly reduced. In this way, the necessary prerequisites are provided for one single administration of the entire daily dose.

Thus, in this case, pharmacokinetic knowledge and pharmaceutical know-how have helped to provide Valium with significant new therapeutic attributes nearly 20 years after its introduction. In many situations in the future, Valium CR will serve to simplify and improve the design of therapeutic regimens and will, as a result, improve patient compliance.

In conclusion

The pharmacokinetics of benzodiazepines is very complicated and can be influenced by many factors. One cannot describe the benzodiazepines in terms of their elimination or β-halflife alone; furthermore, in spite of known connections between plasma concentrations and clinical effect, benzodiazepines should continue to be prescribed according to the established patterns which are efficient when they are based on the individual situation and response to treatment. The usefulness of pharmacokinetics lies, above all, in the ability to characterize benzodiazepines or special pharmaceutical forms, to help design rational schemes of therapy and to aid the assessment of new indications and product formulations.

References

1. Abel, J. G., Sellers, E. M., Naranjo, C. A., Shaw, J., Kadar, D. and Romach, M.K. (1979). Inter- and intrasubject variation in diazepam free fraction. *Clin. Pharmacol. Ther.*, **26**, 247
2. Alvan, G. (1978). Individual differences in the disposition of drugs metabolised in the body. *Clin. Pharmacokin.*, **3**, 155
3. Amrein, R., Cano, J. P. and Hügin, W. (1976). Pharmakokinetische und pharmakodynamische Befunde nach einmaliger intravenöser, intramuskulärer und oraler Applikation von 'Rohypnol'. In Hügin, W., Hossli, G. and Gemperle, M. (eds.). *Bisherige Erfahrungen mit 'Rohypnol' (Flunitrazepam) in der Anästhesiologie und Intensivtherapie*, pp. 39–56. (Basel: Editiones Roche)
4. Amrein, R., Cano, J. P., Hartmann, D., Ziegler, W. H. and Dubuis, R. (1979). Clinical and psychometric effects of flunitrazepam observed during the day in relation to pharmacokinetic data. In Priest, R. G., Pletscher, A. and Ward, J. (eds.). *Sleep Research*, pp. 83–98. (Lancaster: MTP Press Limited)
5. Andreasen, P. B., Hendel, J., Greisen, G. and Hvidberg, E. F. (1976). Pharmacokinetics of diazepam in disordered liver function. *Eur. J. Clin. Pharmacol.*, **10**, 115
6. Aymard, N. and Soulairac, A. (1978). Chronobiologic changes in pharmacokinetics of dipotassic clorazepate, a benzodiazepine. *Chronobiologica*, **5**, 187
7. Baird, E. S. and Hailey, D. M. (1972). Delayed recovery from a sedative; correlation of the plasma levels of diazepam with clinical effects after oral and intravenous administration. *Br. J. Anaesth.*, **44**, 803
8. Bliding, A. (1974). Effects of different rates of absorption of two benzodiazepines on subjective and objective parameters. Significance for clinical use and risk of abuse. *Eur. J. Clin. Pharmacol.*, **7**, 201
9. Booker, H. E. and Celesia, G. G. (1973). Serum concentrations of diazepam in subjects with epilepsy. *Arch. Neurol.*, **29**, 191
10. Branch, R. A., Morgan, H. and James, J. (1976). Diazepam administration in chronic liver disease. *Gastroenterology*, **70**, 979
11. Cano, J. P., Soliva, M., Hartmann, D., Ziegler, W. H. and Amrein, R. (1977). Bioavailability from various galenic formulations of flunitrazepam. *Arzneim. Forsch.*, **27**, 2383
12. Carrigan, P. J., Chao, G. C., Barker, W. M., Hoffmann, D. J. and Chun, A. H. C. (1977). Steady-state bioavailability of two clorazepate dipotassium dosage forms. *J. Clin. Pharmacol.* **17**, 18

13. Corni, L., Palmarin, R., Gervasi, G. B., Comi, V. and Fossati, A. (1976). Cinetica ematica e prove di accumulo nell'uomo di una nuova benzodiazepina (pinazepam) dopo somministrazione orale. *Clin. Ter.*, **78,** 111
14. Crooks, J., O'Malley, K. and Stevenson, I. H. (1976). Pharmacokinetics in the elderly. *Clin. Pharmacokin.*, **1,** 280
15. Dasberg, H. (1974). The clinical change due to oral diazepam (Valium) and N-desmethyl diazepam in relation to their plasma levels in anxious patients and normals. *J. Pharmacol.* (*Paris*), **5,** Suppl. 2, 23
16. Dasberg, H. (1975). Effects and plasma levels of N-desmethyl-diazepam after oral administration in normal volunteers. *Psychopharmacologia* (*Berlin*), **43,** 191
17. Gibaldi, M. (1977). Drug distribution in renal failure. *Am. J. Med.*, **62,** 471
18. Glenne, P. O., Pilbrant, A., Sundwall, A. and Vessmann, J. (1972). Relationship between bioavailability and dissolution rate of oxazepam. *Acta Pharmacol. Toxicol.*, **31,** Suppl. 1, 90
19. Gottschalk, L. A. and Cohn, J. B. (1978). The relationship of diazepam and ketazolam. Blood levels to anxiety and hostility in chronic alcoholics. *Psychopharmacol. Bull.*, **14,** 39
20. Greenblatt, D. J., Shader, R. I. and Koch-Weser, J. (1975). Pharmacokinetics in clinical medicine: oxazepam versus other benzodiazepines. *Clin. Pharmacol. Unit, Dis. Nerv. Syst.*, **36,** 6
21. Greenblatt, D. J., Harmatz, J. S. and Shader, R. I. (1978). Sex differences in diazepam protein binding in patients with renal insufficiency. *Pharmacology* (*Basel*), **16,** 26
22. Greenblatt, D. J., Harmatz, J. S. and Shader, R. I. (1978). Factors influencing diazepam pharmacokinetics. Age, sex and liver-disease. *Int. J. Clin. Pharmacol. Biopharm.*, **16,** 177
23. Greenblatt, D. J., Shader, R. I., Koch-Weser, J. and Franke, K. (1975). Clinical pharmacokinetics of chlordiazepoxide. *Psychopharmacol. Bull.*, **11,** 34
24. Greenblatt, D. J., Shader, R. I., Harmatz, J. S. and Franke, K. (1976). Influence of magnesium and albumin hydroxide mixture on chlordiazepoxide absorption. *Clin. Pharmacol. Ther.*, **19,** 234
25. Greenblatt, D. J., Shader, R. I., MacLeod, S. M. and Sellers, E. M. (1978). Clinical pharmacokinetics of chlordiazepoxide. *Clin. Pharmacokin.*, **3,** 381
26. Greenblatt, D. J., Shader, R. J., Harmatz, J. S., Franke, K. and Koch-Weser, J. (1977). Absorption rate, blood concentrations and early response to oral chlordiazepoxide. *Am. J. Psychiatry*, **134,** 559
27. Greenblatt, D. J., Shader, R. I., Franke, K., MacLaughlin, D. S., Ransil, B. J. and Koch-Weser, J. (1977). Kinetics of intravenous chlordiazepoxide, sex differences in drug distribution. *Clin. Pharmacol. Ther.*, **22,** 893
28. Hendel, J., Elsass, P., Andreasen, P. B., Gymoese, E. and Hvidberg, E. F. (1976). Neuropsychologic effects of diazepam related to single dose. Kinetics and liver function. *Psychopharmacology*, **48,** 11
29. Hepner, G. W., Vesell, E. S., Lipton, A., Harvey, H. A., Wilkinson, G. and Schenker, S. (1977). Disposition of aminopyrine antipyrine diazepam and indocyanine green in patients with liver disease or on anti-convulsant drug therapy; diazepam breath test and correlation in drug elimination. *J. Lab. Clin. Med.*, **90,** 440

30. Hvidberg, E. F. (1976). Plasma levels, anti-epileptics and anti-depressants. *Arzneim. Forsch.*, **26,** 1259
31. Itil, T. M. (1976). Bioequivalency and pharmacodynamics of psychotropic drugs based on computer-analysed ECG. *Psychopharmacol. Bull.*, **12,** 60
32. Kanto, J. (1975). Plasma concentrations of diazepam and its metabolites after peroral, intramuscular and rectal administration. *Int. J. Clin. Pharmacol. Biopharm.*, **12,** 427
33. Kaplan, S. A., Jack, M. L., Alexander, K. and Weinfeld, R. E. (1973). Pharmacokinetic profile of diazepam in man following single intravenous and oral and chronic oral administrations. *J. Pharm. Sci.*, **62,** 1789
34. Klotz, U. (1976). Pathophysiological and disease induced changes in drug distribution volume; pharmacokinetic implications. *Clin. Pharmacokin.*, **1,** 204
35. Klotz, U., Antonin, K. H., Bruegel, H. and Bieck, P. R. (1977). Disposition of diazepam in patients with liver disease. *Clin. Pharmacol. Ther.*, **21,** 430
36. Klotz, U., Avant, G. R., Wilkinson, G. R., Hoyumpa, A. and Schenker, S. (1973). Altered disposition and elimination of diazepam in patients with liver disease. *Gastroenterology*, **65,** A-28/552
37. Klotz, U., Avant, G. R., Hoyumpa, A., Schenker, S. and Wilkinson, G. R. (1975). The effects of age and liver disease on the disposition and elimination of diazepam in adult man. *J. Clin. Invest.*, **55,** 347
38. Knowles, J. A. and Ruelius, H. W. (1972). Absorption and excretion of 7-chloro-1,3-dihydro-3-hydroxy-5-phenyl-*2H*-1,4-benzodiazepin-2-one (oxazepam) in humans. Determination of the drug by gas-liquid chromatography with electron capture detection. *Arzneim. Forsch.*, **22,** 687
39. Korttila, K., Mattila, J. J. and Linnoila, M. (1976). Prolonged recovery after diazepam sedation: the influence of food, charcoal ingestion and injection rate on the effects of intravenous diazepam. *Br. J. Anaesth.*, **48,** 333
40. Kurz, H. (1977). Kumulation und Dosisfindung. *Arzneim. Forsch.*, **27,** 250
41. MacLeod, S. M., Giles, H. G., Bengert, B., Liu, F. F. and Sellers, E. M. (1979). Age-related and gender-related differences in diazepam pharmacokinetics. *J. Clin. Pharmacol.*, **19,** 15
42. Mahon, W. A., Inaba, T., Umeda, T., Tsutsumi, E. and Stone, R. (1975). Studies on the biliary elimination of ^{14}C-diazepam in man. Data on file. (Basel: F. Hoffmann-La Roche & Co. Ltd.)
43. Mendenhall, C. L., Robinson, J. D. and Morgan, D. D. (1975). Chlordiazepoxide, Librium (L). Therapy in hepatic insufficiency. *Gastroenterology*, **69,** A-45/845
44. Mutschler, E. (1976). Die Bedeutung der Pharmakokinetik für die medikamentöse Therapie. *Therapiewoche*, **26,** 8019, 8023, 8026
45. Raaflaub, J. (1977). On the pharmacokinetics of bromazepam in man. In Antonelli, F. (ed.). *Psychopharmacology of Somatization, Biological and Psychological Assessments. 3. Congr. Mondiale del International College of Psychosomatic Med.*, pp. 57–60. (Rome: Pozzi)
46. Raaflaub, J. and Speiser-Courvoisier, J. (1974). Zur Pharmakokinetik von Bromazepam beim Menschen. *Arzneim. Forsch.*, **24,** 1841
47. Reidenberg, M. M. (1977). The binding of drugs to plasma proteins and the interpretation of measurements of plasma concentration of drugs in patients with poor renal function. *Am. J. Med.*, **62,** 466

48. Rieder, J. (1973). Plasma levels and derived pharmacokinetic characteristics of unchanged nitrazepam in man. *Arzneim. Forsch.*, **23,** 212
49. Rieder, J. and Wendt, G. (1973). Pharmacokinetics and metabolism of the hypnotic nitrazepam. In Garattini, S., Mussini, E. and Randall, L. D. (eds.). *The Benzodiazepines*, pp. 99–127. (New York: Raven Press)
50. Shader, R. I. and Greenblatt, D. J. (1977). Clinical implications of benzodiazepine pharmacokinetics. *Am. J. Psychiatry*, **134,** 652
51. Shader, R. I. and Greenblatt, D. J. (1977). Absorption and disposition of chlordiazepoxide in young and elderly male volunteers. *J. Clin. Pharmacol.*, **17,** 709
52. Stjernholm, M. R. and Katz, F. H. (1975). Effects of diphenylhydantoin phenobarbital diazepam on the metabolism of methyl prednisolone and its sodium succinate. *J. Clin. Endocrinol. Metab.*, **41,** 887
53. Tansella, M., Zimmermann-Tansella, C., Ferrario, L., Preziati, L., Tognoni, G. and Lader, M. (1978). Plasma concentrations of diazepam, nordiazepam and amylobarbitone after short-term treatment of anxious patients. *Pharmakopsychiat. Neuro-Psychopharmakol.*, **11,** 68
54. Verbeeck, R., Tjandramaga, T. B., Verberckmoes, R. and De Schepper, P. (1976). Biotransformation and excretion of lorazepam in patients with chronic renal failure. *Br. J. Clin. Pharmacol.*, **3,** 1033

7

The Benzodiazepines: A Clinical Review

R. G. Priest

Clinical use of benzodiazepines

The introduction of benzodiazepines has been one of the major advances in medicine. Time will tell whether it will eventually be regarded as more important than the discovery of penicillin. I mention penicillin firstly because I work at St Mary's Hospital in London, which has recently celebrated the memory of Fleming's discovery there fifty years ago. I mention it secondly because the introduction of penicillin altered the attitude of men towards pharmacotherapy and has widely been regarded as ushering in the new era of powerful drugs that dramatically alter the outcome of illness.

The benzodiazepines are famous for their actions on anxiety and insomnia. These two symptoms are widespread. It is not always appreciated how common and troublesome they are. Even among psychiatrists there is confusion about their prevalence. This is such an important topic that I should like at this stage to explain some new understanding of psychiatric diagnosis.

Mental illnesses can be broadly divided into neuroses and psychoses. It is accepted that in psychoses severe distortions of reality occur, such as delusions and hallucinations[14]. In the neuroses the illnesses are closer to the reactions that we all have from day to day and they include obsessive–compulsive disorders, hysteria, anxiety states and depressive illnesses[15].

For many years, then, there has been an implicit assumption in the textbooks that if you have bizarre delusions you have a psychosis (e.g. schizophrenia), but if you have for example a combination of apprehension, tremor, excessive perspiration and tension pains then the mental illness is an anxiety state – a neurosis. Collections of symptoms appropriate to each diagnosis were handed on from one text to another.

There came a time when a group of clinical psychologists led by Graham Foulds decided to investigate whether patients conformed to these descriptions. They collected a list of eighty questions called the Symptom–Sign Inventory, covering the commoner neuroses and psychoses, and they asked a series of newly admitted psychiatric inpatients if they had each symptom.

What they found was that in some ways the textbooks were not so far from the truth. The neurotic subjects on the whole had the symptoms that they were supposed to have to justify the diagnosis. The surprise came with the psychoses. The psychotic subjects did have the symptoms that corresponded to their case-note diagnosis. However, in addition, psychotic patients had neurotic symptoms in significant numbers. In fact, they had as many neurotic symptoms as did the patients with neurosis alone. So, if you were a schizophrenic, you had not only bizarre delusions, but also maybe a combination of tremor, palpitations, apprehension and insomnia. The diagnosis of psychosis could be made positively on the basis of the appropriate hallucinations and delusions. The diagnosis of neurosis in the light of these findings has now to be made, in part, positively, for instance demonstration of the appropriate obsessional symptoms. It also has to be justified negatively, by demonstrating that the patient did *not* have delusions, hallucinations or other psychotic phenomena.

It is interesting to speculate why it had not been more widely realized in the past that psychotics suffer from neurotic symptoms. One explanation may be that put forward by Foulds[5]. He quotes Shakespeare's play *King Lear*:

> 'Where the greater malady is fixed
> the lesser is scarce felt.'

Relevance to benzodiazepines

Why is this question of diagnosis so crucial to the understanding of the importance of benzodiazepines? One reason is this. It was found in the work of Foulds, which has been confirmed by further studies[1,2,5–7], that virtually *all* acute mental illnesses carry with them a vulnerability to anxiety and insomnia. Anxiety and insomnia are two of the commonest features of emotional reactions requiring treatment.

The pathological emotional reactions themselves are seen in every branch of medicine. They are found not just in the psychiatric clinic. It is now well recognized that they form a high proportion of the disorders treated by general practitioners. They form maybe a third of the population of outpatients seen by general hospital physicians.

Many of these disorders are self-limiting and clear up spontaneously in the course of time. The underlying cause is often obscure, or specific psychodynamic treatment is neither practicable nor available. What the patient needs is relief from the distress until his illness remits. Benzodiazepines can be used to relieve his anxiety by day and his insomnia by night.

When the diagnosis is a more serious one, such as a psychosis, the patient will usually be given neuroleptic medication, lithium, electroconvulsive therapy (E.C.T.) or some other physical treatment to relieve the mental illness itself. However, even in these cases, the patient will often receive benzodiazepines as well. I believe that it is not appreciated how widely benzodiazepines are required in these other disorders. Dr Thomas Pastor has analysed the patients receiving inpatient treatment in the psychiatric wards of St Mary's Hospital and he was astonished to find that two-thirds of all the patients are receiving benzodiazepines, whatever the underlying diagnosis. I can assure you that very few of these inpatients are suffering from simple anxiety states.

What are the alternatives?

There are a number of drugs used to relieve anxiety and insomnia that are not of the benzodiazepine group[11, 13]. They include the traditional sedatives and hypnotics like barbiturates, paraldehyde, chloral, glutethimide, methyprylon and ethchlorvynol. The neuroleptic drugs, or major tranquillizers, including the phenothiazines and the butyrophenones, are also sometimes used for this purpose. There is a fundamental distinction between traditional sedatives like barbiturates and the neuroleptic drugs (e.g. chlorpromazine). In very low doses the actions are similar – a reduction in anxiety and the possibility (though not the certainty) of some drowsiness. It is in the large doses that the effects are dissimilar. Barbiturates produce a progressive reduction in consciousness, until eventually coma or even death results. If the patient does not fall asleep after a large dose, then he suffers from ataxia, dysarthria, diplopia and nystagmus. After prolonged administration physical dependence may occur, with the characteristic withdrawal syndromes of grand mal type convulsions or delirium tremens[4].

These features do not characteristically occur with neuroleptics. Other drugs have been shown to produce the same effects as the barbiturates, including not only those mentioned in the traditional sedative group above, but also meprobamate (in earlier years regarded as a tranquillizer) and the more recently introduced methaqualone[13]. Another drug that can produce ataxia, coma and even death in acute intoxication, and in the longer term physical dependence complicated by fits and delirium tremens on withdrawal, is of course alcohol. The type of addiction induced is now sometimes referred to as the barbiturate–alcohol type of dependence.

Compared with these two major classes of drug, where do the

benzodiazepines come? In high doses they are very much safer than the barbiturate group. The benzodiazepines are commonly used in suicide attempts. Although they may form part of a lethal mixture swallowed by the patient when combined with more toxic drugs, they are rarely fatal when taken alone (some would say never). This safety factor is of immense benefit, since suicidal feelings so often accompany anxiety and insomnia[12]. By contrast overdoses of barbiturates are a common cause of death.

Ataxia and slurred speech can occur with very high doses of benzodiazepines, but again the therapeutic ratio seems to be much more favourable than that of traditional sedatives.

What about addiction? Here the neuroleptics come out best, since dependence is not in practice a problem with them. However, many have unwanted extrapyramidal and autonomic side-effects, and their action on anxiety and insomnia is relatively weak – it is their effect on the psychoses that largely accounts for their present place in the psychiatrist's armamentarium. We have seen how seriously addicting the traditional sedatives are, so much so that there are powerful campaigns to restrict very tightly the prescription of barbiturates. There is no doubt that the benzodiazepines produce *psychological* dependence in some patients. *Physical* dependence seems to be much more rare. Fits can occur after withdrawal from very high doses in experimental situations[8, 9]. I have yet to see a convincing case of delirium tremens in the literature on benzodiazepine withdrawal. In one report by Malatinsky *et al.*[10], high doses of diazepam were used in the treatment of tetanus and two patients developed a delirious syndrome after withdrawal, but here one must consider the possible predisposing noxious effect of tetanus itself on the central nervous system.

It looks as if under certain circumstances physical dependence on the benzodiazepines can occur, but when one bears in mind the extent to which the drugs are used, reports of addiction in ordinary clinical practice are relatively scarce. Again the benzodiazepines are clearly much safer than the barbiturates.

Other uses

We can now say that there is ample justification for using benzodiazepines for the treatment of anxiety[15] and for insomnia[13, 16]. What of other uses? The third property that is characteristic of benzodiazepines is their muscle relaxant activity, which is a separate effect that does not merely result from lowered anxiety levels. This is a useful action in the relief of muscular spasm. The fourth main property is that of anticonvulsant activity. It seems that, with doses of compounds that are equipotent for the relief of anxiety there are wide variations in effectiveness between drugs in these last two actions[3]. Thus diazepam and clonazepam are particularly useful in the treatment of spasticity, and the same drugs (together with several others) are especially effective as anticonvulsants.

Side-effects

What is a therapeutic effect for one patient is a side-effect for another. The patient who is prescribed benzodiazepines for excessive anxiety may resent any drowsiness he experiences by day, or the unsteady sensation in his legs produced by muscular relaxation. It may be that future advances will enable us to develop benzodiazepines that are more specific for each of the four main actions.

There is a fifth action that is well known as a side-effect but which can scarcely be regarded as a therapeutic effect *per se*. That is loss of inhibition. Some patients taking benzodiazepines show the same lack of control over their emotional impulses as does the intoxicated alcoholic or the patient in early stages of general anaesthesia. It may be this unwanted effect that accounts for the occasional reports of patients who show a paradoxical outburst of violence. It could also be the reason for some road traffic accidents. I should say, however, that it has yet to be demonstrated that the increased frequency of road accidents among patients who have been prescribed tranquillizers[17] is due to the tranquillizer rather than due to the psychologically vulnerable population taking the drugs, or that there is any causal relationship whatsoever.

Nevertheless I am sure that in the ideal world clinicians would like to have available a minor tranquillizer that is free from the potential disadvantage of behavioural disinhibition.

Summary

The benzodiazepines have gained an unprecedented reputation in clinical psychopharmacology for safety and efficacy. They have proved to be useful in the treatment of muscle spasm and epilepsy. They have become the standard treatment for those emotional and psychiatric disorders in which anxiety is the dominant symptom. They are widely regarded as the drugs of choice in various sleep disorders, of which insomnia is the most prevalent.

The benzodiazepines are selective in action. As with other tranquillizers (but in contrast to barbiturates) there is no strict dose-dependent relationship to the level of consciousness resulting from their action. Unlike many other psychotropic drugs extrapyramidal and anticholinergic side-effects are not a problem in their clinical use.

They have superseded a previous generation of sedative drugs. Serious physical dependence on the benzodiazepines is a rarity. The characteristic physical withdrawal syndrome found with addiction to the barbiturate–alcohol group of sedatives is delirium tremens (DTs). Evidence of addiction, followed by DTs, is now known to be a problem not only with the barbiturates and alcohol themselves, but also with chloral, paraldehyde, glutethimide, ethchlorvynol, meprobamate and methaqualone. A similar withdrawal syndrome to benzodiazepines is rarely, if ever, observed in ordinary clinical practice.

As well as being relatively free from chronic abuse potential the benzodiazepines are remarkably safe in acute misuse. The toxicity of barbiturates in overdosage is notorious, and still accounts for many suicidal deaths each year. Benzodiazepines are much safer, and it is usually only when they are combined with other drugs that they prove fatal.

Their great value in relieving anxiety and in sleep induction means that, as well as being prized as a single item of treatment, the benzodiazepines are very much in demand as an adjunct to treatment given simultaneously with other psychotropic drugs.

Conclusions

The benzodiazepines are very widely used in clinical practice, in the ways that I have mentioned and in other ways that there is no space to cover. I regret to say that despite current advances in our knowledge about them there is still a great deal of misunderstanding among physicians about their properties. There is also a great deal of prejudice, prejudice which one may feel would make it difficult for some doctors to contemplate comparing the benefits of benzodiazepines with the benefits of penicillin.

These drugs are certainly not always used wisely. I hope that in the future doctors will become more discriminating in their use. That is not to say that less will necessarily be prescribed in total quantity. It remains to be seen whether the reduction in the amount that is at present handed out in some quarters in poorly justified and excessive use will be outweighed by the effects of recognizing that much distress and pointless agony that at present remains undiagnosed and untreated could be promptly and effectively relieved by benzodiazepines.

To address the title of this book, it may be that in various ways tomorrow will be greater for the benzodiazepines than today.

References

1. Bagshaw, V.E. (1977). A replication study of Foulds' and Bedford's hierarchical model of depression. *Br. J. Psychiatry*, **131**, 53
2. Bedford, A. and Foulds, G. (1978). *Manual of the Delusions–Symptoms–States Inventory*. (Windsor: NFER Publishing Co.)
3. *Drugs & Therapeutics Bulletin* (1978). Therapeutic differences between benzodiazepines, **16** (12), 46
4. Ewart, R.B.L. and Priest, R.G. (1967). Methaqualone addiction and delirium tremens. *Br. Med. J.*, **3**, 92
5. Foulds, G.A. (1965). *Personality and Personal Illness*. (London: Tavistock Publications)

6. Foulds, G. A. and Bedford, A. (1975). Hierarchy of classes of personal illness. *Psychol. Med.*, **5,** 181
7. Foulds, G. A., Bedford, A. and Csapo, K. G. (1975). Class change in the personal illness hierarchy. *Br. J. Psychiatry*, **127,** 316
8. Hollister, L. E., Motzenbecker, F. P. and Degan, R. O. (1961). Withdrawal reactions from chlordiazepoxide ('Librium'). *Psychopharmacologia (Berlin)*, **2,** 63
9. Isbell, H. and Chrusciel, T. L. (1970) Dependence liability of 'non-narcotic' drugs. *Suppl. Bull. WHO*, **43**
10. Malatinsky, J., Prochazka, M. and Kadlic, T. (1975). Transient psychological syndrome following diazepam therapy for tetanus. *Postgrad. Med. J.*, **51,** 860
11. Priest, R. G. (1973). A new approach to sleep disorders. *Gazzetta Sanitaria*, **22,** 3
12. Priest, R. G. (1977). Recognition of the suicidal patient. *J. Int. Med. Res.*, **5,** Suppl. 1, 157
13. Priest, R. G. (1978). Sleep and its disorders. In Gaind, R. G. and Hudson, B. (eds.), *Current Themes in Psychiatry*. (London: Macmillan Press)
14. Priest, R. G. and Steinert, J. (1977). *Insanity: A Study of Major Psychiatric Disorders*. (Plymouth: Macdonald & Evans)
15. Priest, R. G. and Woolfson, G. (1978). *Minski's Handbook of Psychiatry*, 7th Edn. (London: Heinemann)
16. Priest, R. G., Pletscher, A. and Ward, J. (eds.) (1979). *Sleep Research*. (Lancaster: MTP Press)
17. Skegg, D. C. G., Richards, S. M. and Doll, R. (1979). Minor tranquillizers and road accidents. *Br. Med. J.*, **1,** 917

8

The Psychophysiological Effects of Benzodiazepines

V. Gentil Filho

Introduction

The characteristic psychophysiological effects of benzodiazepines are few but important. At therapeutic doses, most of their actions are centrally mediated. Before I review the most important psychophysiological changes observed in anxious patients and the effects of benzodiazepines on these parameters, I would like to spend a few moments on some of the basics of psychophysiology.

Anxiety

Anxiety is a subjective experience which is difficult to quantify objectively, in which emotional and physical discomfort are associated with increases in central and autonomic nervous activity. Consequently, some somatic expressions of anxiety are manifested as pallor, sweating, palpitation, respiratory distress, gastro-intestinal disorders, tremor, dizziness, dry mouth, muscle tension, weakness, insomnia etc. These responses are attributable, in part, to an excessive discharge of the sympathetic autonomic nervous system. The ensuing release of catecholamines results in tremor, vasoconstriction, a positive inotropic and chronotropic effect, dilatation of pupils etc. The release of acetylcholine into post-ganglionic fibres, on the other hand, results for example in excessive sweating.

Psychophysiological methods

The goal of psychophysiology is to quantify physiological changes associated with emotions by measuring physiological parameters whose changes could be correlated to psychological or behavioural events in man[5]. The most frequently used psychophysiological parameters can be classified as central and peripheral.

Examples of central parameters are: the electroencephalogram (EEG), the critical flicker fusion threshold and the sedation threshold. Examples of peripheral parameters are: skin conductance, the electromyogram (EMG), tremor at rest, arterial blood pressure, respiratory function, pupil diameter, salivation and peripheral blood flow. Psychophysiologists are interested in changes of these parameters triggered by both internal (emotion, ideas) and external stimuli. Subjects must as far as possible be in a condition of physiological neutrality in terms of any stimuli foreign to the research study in progress.

Psychophysiological changes in anxiety

Patients with anxiety manifest a degree of central and autonomic arousal which is not proportional to the objective needs of the moment. Therefore, their ability to adapt is reduced. Even at rest, such patients show an increase in skin conductance indicating an increase in the autonomic activity related to sweat glands. Their electroencephalogram reveals a reduction of the α (7.5–13.5 Hz) activity which is known to be associated with states of quiet and relaxation. In responses triggered by auditory stimuli, they tend to show shorter latency and higher amplitudes in components ranging between 50 and 250 ms, indicating a state of heightened cerebral arousal. Heart rate is higher than that of normal controls. Although the same is true of respiratory rate, the amplitude of respiratory movement is decreased.

Muscle activity increases can be demonstrated by the electromyogram. Contrary to a popular misconception, the tremor these patients show at rest is not substantially different from the normal subject. The change occurs only in amplitude and not in frequency distribution[8]. Pupil diameter under soft lighting is similar to that of controls, although anxious patients show less of a constrictor response to bright light, a fact which has been attributed to an excess of sympathetic tonus with reduced ability to adapt[2]. Indirect signs of excessive arousal are: greater vasodilatation and bradycardia observed in anxious patients during sleep. Further, they need higher doses of intravenous barbiturates to induce sleep due to a higher sedation threshold. This increased basal physiological activity in anxious patients, which results in a higher threshold of response to some psychophysiological tests, explains their relatively low response to stimuli which would elicit adequate responses in control subjects.

Experimental anxiety

In experimental anxiety, changes in several psychophysiological parameters can be elicited in normal subjects with a significant anxiety component submitted to stressing procedures. The resulting subjective feeling of anxiety can be quantified by means of self-evaluation scales. This presents us with a very useful model to test anxiolytic drugs. The use of placebo as a comparative substance is ethically acceptable as it is necessary to exclude placebo effect which can represent up to 50% of the positive results.

Correlations between psychophysiological measures and anxiety

Tyrer and Lader[10] submitted 36 healthy volunteer subjects to a battery of stress-inducing stimuli to determine whether psychophysiological parameters correlated with subjective evaluation of anxiety. They reported that, centrally, the rate of α-waves, and, peripherally, skin conductance and heart rate, correlated the most closely with the state of anxiety. However, the coefficient of correlation remained less than 0.51, suggesting therefore that none of the parameters measured could be considered specific for anxiety. On the other hand, there is a significant relationship between psychophysiological change and the clinical response of anxious patients treated with benzodiazepines[3]. Although these correlations are no higher than 0.52, they are better than that found between the serum levels of benzodiazepines and therapeutic response[7].

The effect of benzodiazepines

What then are the effects of benzodiazepines on these psychophysiological parameters?

In normal therapeutic doses, benzodiazepines reduce central arousal[6, 9]. At high doses, peripheral effects such as anticholinergic effects may also exceptionally be observed. The psychophysiological effects of benzodiazepines are summarized in Table 1. Some of these parameters, however, deserve special attention. For example, the rise in β-activity in the EEG is a sensitive indicator of the effect of benzodiazepines and is one of the few objective parameters which correlates with serum nitrazepam levels[1]. The mechanism responsible for the increase of β-activity induced by benzodiazepines (and barbiturates) is still unknown. These drugs would, however, be expected to slow down rather than activate cerebral activity. A significant contribution has also been made by benzodiazepines to the understanding of the physiology of sleep. It appears that benzodiazepines not only reduce the proportion of REM sleep but also practically suppress stage 4 of sleep. The effect on the REM sleep diminishes while suppression of stage 4 persists. Since stage 4 is first to be reinstated after sleep deprivation and its duration is inversely related to the individual's age, we may ascribe an important role to stage 4 in the restorative function of sleep.

Table 8.1 The psychophysiological effects of benzodiazepines

1. EEG	*Spectrum Analysis* Decrease in low frequency activity Increase in high frequency activity *Evoked Response (Auditory)* Decrease in amplitude *Contingent Negative Variation* Decrease in amplitude *EEG in Sleep* Increase in total sleep time Increase in phase 2 Sharp decrease in phase 4 Moderate decrease in REM sleep
2. SKIN CONDUCTANCE	Modest decrease of mean conductance Decrease in the number of fluctuations
3. EMG	Decrease in muscle tone
4. CRITICAL FLICKER FUSION	Decrease in fusion threshold
5. TREMOR	Decrease due to lower central arousal
6. ARTERIAL BLOOD PRESSURE	Decrease due to arousal reduction
7. HEART RATE	Decrease due to arousal reduction
8. SKIN VASCULAR DIAMETER	Delation due to arousal reduction
9. BREATHING	Decrease in RR and increase in amplitude due to arousal reduction
10. SALIVATION	Increase due to arousal reduction

On this basis one would therefore expect sleep induced by benzodiazepines to be less restful than normal sleep. This is, however, not the case. An explanation for this apparent paradox has been suggested by Feinberg and colleagues[4]. The increase in total sleep time and the significant extension of stage 2 allow the total number of δ-waves to remain unaltered although their amplitude is lower than during stage 4.

In conclusion, psychophysiological parameters can be used to quantify the pharmacological effect of drugs. It is to be hoped that either new parameters or more sensitive techniques of measurement will be discovered in the near future so that understanding of the psychophysiological basis of mental activity will be improved.

References

1. Bond, A.J. and Lader, M.H. (1973). The residual effects of flurazepam. *Psychopharmacologia (Berlin)*, **32,** 223
2. Bond, A.J., James, D.C. and Lader, M.H. (1974). Physiological and psychological measures in anxious patients. *Psychol. Med.*, **4,** 364

3. Bond, A. J., James, D. C. and Lader, M. H. (1974). Sedative effects on physiological and psychological measures in anxious patients. *Psychol. Med.*, **4,** 374
4. Feinberg, I., Fein, G., Walker, J. M., Price, L. J., Floyd, T. C. and March, J. D. (1977). Flurazepam effects on slow-wave sleep: stage 4 suppressed but number of delta waves constant. *Science*, **198,** 847
5. Lader, M. (1975). *The Psychophysiology of Mental Illness*, p. 270. (London: Routledge & Kegan Paul)
6. Nakano, S., Gillespie, H. K. and Hollister, L. E. (1978). Propranolol in experimentally induced stress. *Psychopharmacology*, **59,** 279
7. Tansella, M., Zimmermann-Tansella, C., Ferrario, L., Preziati, L., Tognoni, G. and Lader, M. (1978). Plasma concentrations of diazepam, nordiazepam and amylobarbitone after short-term treatment of anxious patients. *Pharmakopsychiat. Neuro-Psychopharmakol.*, **11,** 68
8. Tyrer, P. J. and Lader, M. H. (1974). Tremor in acute and chronic anxiety. *Arch. Gen. Psychiatry*, **31,** 506
9. Tyrer, P. J. and Lader, M. H. (1974). Clinical response to propranolol and diazepam in somatic and psychic anxiety. *Br. Med. J.*, **2,** 14
10. Tyrer, P. J. and Lader, M. H. (1976). Central and peripheral correlates of anxiety: A comparative study. *J. Nerv. Ment. Dis.*, **162,** 99

Bibliography

Circulation

Ashton, H., Millman, J. E., Telford, R. and Thompson, J. W. (1978). A comparison of some physiological and psychological effects of motival (fluphenazine and nortriptyline) and diazepam in normal subjects. *Br. J. Clin. Pharmacol.*, **5,** 141

Cote, P., Gueret, P. and Bourassa, M. G. (1974). Systemic and coronary hemodynamic effects of diazepam in patients with normal and diseased coronary arteries. *Circulation*, **50,** 1210

Dalen, J. E., Evans, G. L., Banas, J. S., Brooks, H. L., Paraskos, J. A. and Dexter, L. (1969). The hemodynamic and respiratory effects of diazepam (Valium). *Anesthesiology*, **30,** 259

D'Amelio, G., Dalla Volta, S. and Celon, E. (1974). Influenza del diazepam sul contegno della pressione arteriosa e sulla eliminazione urinaria di adrenalina e di noradrenalina in situazione di stress nella ipertensione essenziale stabilizzata. *Minerva Med.*, **65,** 2459

De Alvarez, R. R. and Zighelboim, I. (1969). Diazepam during labour. *Penn. Med.*, **72,** 93

Haldemann, G., Wüest, H. P., Hossli, G. and Schaer, H. (1976). Die Wirkung von Flunitrazepam (Rohypnol) als Praemedikation und Anaesthetikum auf die Haemodynamik bei kreislaufgesunden Patienten. In Hügin, W., Hossli, G. and Gemperle, M. (eds.). *Bisherige Erfahrungen mit 'Rohypnol' (Flunitrazepam) in der Anaesthesiologie und Intensivtherapie*, pp. 74–83. (Basel: Editiones 'Roche').

Healy, T. E. J. (1969). Intravenous diazepam for cardiac catheterisation. *Anaesthesia*, **24,** 537

Hempelmann, G., Seitz, W. and Piepenbrock, S. (1978). Diazepam (Valium). Ein Beitrag zu Haemodynamik, myokardialem Sauerstoffverbrauch und Gefässeffekt. *Anaesthesist*, **27,** 357

Hvidberg, E. F., Harder, F., Elsass, P., Hendel, J. and Hjoerting Hansen, E. (1975). Single dose diazepam kinetics and continuous reaction times in man. In *6th International Congress of Pharmacology, 20–25 July 1975*. Helsinki, Abstr. No. 121, p. 58. (Helsinki: Finnish Pharmacol. Soc.)

Jenkinson, J. L., MacRae, W. R., Scott, D. B. and Gould, J. F. (1974). Haemodynamic effects of diazepam used as a sedative for oral surgery. *Br. J. Anaesth.*, **46**, 294

Kaneko, Y. *et al.* (1973). Cardiorespiratory effects of intravenous minor tranquilizer and non-narcotic analgesic combinations as an adjuvant agent in local anesthesia. *Jpn. J. Anaesthesiol.*, **22**, 33

Knapp, R. B. and Dubow, H. S. (1970). Diazepam as induction agent for patients with cardiopulmonary disease. *South. Med. J.*, **63**, 1451

Kroenig, B., Dufey, K., Moergel, K., Michaelis, J. and Jahnecke, J. (1974). Telemetrische Untersuchungen zur Wertigkeit eines Basalblutdruckes bei Hochdruckkranken. *Klin. Wochenschr.*, **52**, 809

Morales, E. S., Krumperman, L. W. and Cohen, J. G. (1973). Bronchoscopy under diazepam anesthesia. *Anesth. Analg. Curr. Res.*, **52**, 414

Nakano, S., Ogawa, H., Kawazu, Y., Osato, E. and Miyamoto, M. (1973). Human pharmacological study. Bromazepam, diazepam, placebo. *Jpn. Psychosom. Soc.*, **13**, 111

Ogawa, N., Asano, C., Yamaguchi, T., Osato, E., Sakata, T., Fuchimoto, H. Tanaka, H., Toyama, Y., Nakano, S., Tanaka, M., Goto, M. and Uesaka, H. (1974). The effect of antianxiety agent (medazepam) for essential hypertensions. *Jpn. J. Clinl Pharmacol.*, **5**, 294

Pekkarinen, A. (1973). The effect of diazepam (D) on the heart rate (HR) during oral examination of pharmacology (EP). *Acta Physiol. Scand.*, **89**, Suppl. 396, 135

Pozenel, H., Bückert, A. and Amrein, R. (1975). The antihypertensive effect of bromazepam (Lexotan). – A new benzodiazepine derivative. Presented at *3. International Kongress für psychosomatische Medizin*, September 16–20, Rome.

Pozenel, H., Bückert, A. and Amrein, R. (1977). The antihypertensive effect of bromazepam (Lexotan). – A new benzodiazepine derivative. Further haemodynamic investigations. In Antonelli, F. (ed.). *Psychopharmacology of Somatization, Biological and Psychological Assessments. 3. Congr. Mondiale del-l'International College of Psychosomatic Med.*, pp. 48–56. (Rome: Pozzi).

Raiski, V., Rozonov, Y. and Chichkanov, G. (1972). Diazepam and the cardiovascular system. *Soviet Sci. Rev.*, **3**, 215

Raiski, V., Rosonow, J. and Tschitschkanow, G. (1972). Diazepam und das Herz- und Gefässystem. *Ideen Exakt. Wiss.*, **1972**, 13

Raiski, V. A., Rozonov, Y. B. and Chichkanow, G. G. (1973). Nature and mechanism of seduxen effect on some indices of the blood circulation. *Ter. Arkh.*, **45**, 35

Ruy de Oliveira, G. and Teixetra Lopes, A. (1974). Ro 5–4200. – Seus efeitos sôbre a dinamica circulatoria e condução cardiaca. *Rev. Bras. Anest.*, **24**, 44

Ryder, W. (1970). Cardiovascular changes during dental anaesthesia and sedation. *Dent. Pract. Dent. Rec.*, **21**, 89

Schaller, K. (1973). Der Einfluss des Tranquilizers Faustan auf das Mechanokardiogramm im akuten Versuch. *Dtsch. Gesundh.-Wes.*, **28**, 1886

Ueno, K., Kitanaka, T., Mizushima, N., Miyabo, S., Hisada, T., Kishida, S.,

Ogawa, N. *et al.* (1977). The alleviating effects of medazepam on psychologically induced rise in the blood pressure of essential hypertensives. *Jpn. J. Clin. Pharmacol.*, **8,** 17

Wheatley, D. (1977). Circulatory manifestations of soma and psyche. In Antonelli, F. (ed.). *Therapy in Psychosomatic Medicine. Proc. 3rd Congr. Intern. College of Psychosomatic Med. Rome/It., September 1975*, Vol. 2, Symposia, pp. 163–7. (Rome: Pozzi)

Wheatley, D. (1977). Antianxiety drug trials in hypertension. *Psychopharmacol. Bull.*, **13,** 27

Wheatley, D. and Hordern, A. (1977). Antianxiety drugs in the treatment of hypertension. In Wheatley, D. (ed.). *Stress and the Heart, Interactions of the Cardiovascular System, Behavioral State and Psychotropic Drugs*, pp. 175–92. (New York: Raven Press)

Whitehead, W. E., Blackwell, B. and Robinson, A. (1977). Why physicians prescribe benzodiazepines in essential hypertension. – A phase IV study. *Biol. Psychiatry*, **12,** 597

Yamane, A., Itoh, S., Iwasaki, T., Tanimoto, M., Yasutomi, S., Makihata, S. and Ohyagi, M. (1977). Clinical application of stabilitin, one of benzodiazepines, to circulatory anxiety symptom. *Bas. Pharmacol. Ther.*, **5,** 1857

Critical flicker frequency

Grove-White, I. G. and Kelman, G. R. (1971). Critical flicker frequency after small doses of methohexitone, diazepam and sodium 4-hydroxybutyrate. *Br. J. Anaesth.*, **43,** 110

Holmberg, G. and Livstedt, B. (1971). Fortsatta flicker-fusion-førsøk med sedativa inkl. fenemal. *Nord. Psykiat. T.*, **25,** 391

Korttila, K. and Linnoila, M. (1974). Skills related to driving after intravenous diazepam, flunitrazepam or droperidol. *Br. J. Anaesth.*, **46,** 961

Korttila, K. and Linnoila, M. (1975). Skills related to driving after intramuscular diazepam and pethidine. Presented at the *Vth Intern. Conf. for the Int. Assoc. for Accident and Traffic Med. and the 3rd Int. Conf. on Drug Abuse of the Intern. Council on Alcohol and Addictions*, September 1–5, London.

Ogle, C. W., Turner, P. and Markomihelakis, H. (1976). The effects of high doses of oxprenolol and of propranolol on pursuit rotor performance, reaction time and critical flicker frequency. *Psychopharmacologia (Berlin)*, **46,** 295

Smith, J. M. and Misiak, H. (1976). Critical flicker frequency (CFF) and psychotropic drugs in normal human subjects. – A review. *Psychopharmacology*, **47,** 175

Turner, P. (1973). Section A. Clinical pharmacological studies on lorazepam. *Curr. Med. Res. Opin.*, **1,** 262

Electrodermal activity

Beer, B. and Migler, B. (1975). Effects of diazepam on galvanic skin response and conflict in monkeys and humans. In Sudilovsky, A. Gershon, S. and Beer, B. (eds.). *Predicability in Psychopharmacology, Preclinical and Clinical Correlations*, pp. 143–57. (New York: Raven Press)

Björkstrand, P. A. and Dureman, I. (1971). Relaxation transfer in electrodermal activity as affected by a new minor tranquillizer (4306CB). *Psychopharmacologia (Berlin)*, **20**, 288

Bond, A. J. and Lader, M. H. (1975). Residual effects of flunitrazepam. *Br. J. Clin. Pharmacol.*, **2**, 143

Cullen, J. and Fischer, I. (1974). The psychopharmacological study of Ro 5–3350 using normal volunteers. Presented at the *10th European Conference on Psychosomatic Research*, September 15–20, Edinburgh.

Danielsen, A., Haffner, J. F., Morland, J., Setekleiv, J., Frivik, P. T. and Strømsaether, C. E. (1975). Effects of diazepam and ethanol on heart rate and galvanic skin responses. *Arch. Pharmacol. Toxicol.*, **36**, 113

Monti, J. M., Altier, H., Prandro, M. and Gil, J. L. (1975). The actions of flunitrazepam (Rohypnol) on heart and respiratory rates and skin potential fluctuations during the sleep cycle in normal volunteers and neurotic patients with insomnia. *Psychopharmacologia (Berlin)*, **43**, 187

Perkins, R. and Baker, M. (1976). Changes in skin potential level during sleep in psychiatric patients. *Postgrad. Med. J.*, **52**, 37

Salkind, M. R. and Silverstone, J. T. (1972). The clinical and psychophysiological effects of a beta-adrenergic blocking agent (Sotalol) in anxiety. *Psychopharmacologia (Berlin)*, **26**, Suppl. 72

Electroencephalography

Baust, W., Joerg, J., Wortmann, R. and Zimmermann, A. (1977). Untersuchungen zur Beeinflussung kortikaler somatosensorischer Reizantwortpotentiale durch Pharmaka. *Arzneim. Forsch.*, **27**, 440

Dumermuth, G. (1976). Possibilities of electronic EEG processing in epileptology. In *Epileptology, Proceedings 7th Intern. Symp. on Epilepsy, Berlin, June 1975*, pp. 364–72. (Stuttgart: Georg Thieme)

Dumont-Girard, P. (1978). La TRH. Revue des données actuelles et étude polygraphique après injection intra-veineuse. Diss., Facultés A et B de Médecine, Nancy 1978.

Enderlein, J. and Mitschke, H. (1977). EEG-Veränderungen durch Diazepam. – Ein diagnostisches Hilfsmittel. *Dtsch. Gesundh.-Wes.*, **32**, 1279

Escande, M., Goldberger, E. and Fabre, J. M. (1975). Benzodiazépines et électroencéphalogramme. *Actualités Psychiatriques*, **6**, 77

Faingold, C. L. (1978). Brainstem reticular formation mechanisms subserving generalized seizures. – Effects of convulsants and anticonvulsants on sensory-evoked responses. *Progr. Neuro-Psychopharmacol.*, **2**, 401

Fincham, R. W., Yamada, T., Schottelius, D. D., Hayreh, S. M. and DaMascio, A. (1975). Electroencephalographic absence status with minimal behavior change. *Arch. Neurol. (Chic.)*., **36**, 176

Fink, M. (1969). Drugs, EEG, and behavior. In Black, P. (ed.). *Drugs and the Brain*, pp. 149–60. (Baltimore: Johns Hopkins University Press)

Fink, M. (1975). Prediction of clinical activity of psychoactive drugs. Application of cerebral electrometry in phase-I studies. In Sudilovsky, H., Gershon, S. and Beer, B. (eds.). *Predicability in Psychopharmacology, Preclinical and Clinical Correlations*, pp. 65–87. (New York: Raven Press)

Fink, M. (1978). Psychoactive drugs and waking EEG, 1966–76. In Lipton, M. A.,

DiMascio, A. and Killam, K. F. (eds.). *Psychopharmacology, a Generation of Progress*, pp. 691–8. (New York: Raven Press)

Fink, M. (1978). EEG and psychopharmacology. In Cobb, W. A. *et al.* (eds.). *Contemporary Clinical Neurophysiology, Clin. Neurophysiol.*, **Suppl. 34,** 41

Fisher, C., Kahn, E., Edwards, A. and Davis, D. M. (1973). A psychophysiological study of nightmares and night terrors. *J. Nerv. Ment. Dis.*, **157,** 75

Hartmann, E. (1974). Effect of psychotropic drugs on desynchronized sleep. *Mod. Probl. Pharmacopsych.* Vol. 8, pp. 216–27. (Basel: Karger)

Itil, T. M. (1968). Electroencephalography and pharmacopsychiatry. *Mod. Probl. Pharmacopsych.* Vol. 1, pp. 163–94. (Basel: Karger)

Itil, T. M. (1969). Invited discussion of Dr. M. Fink's paper. – Human psychopharmacology and functional electroencephalography. In Efron, D. H. (ed.). *Psychopharmacology, a review of Progress 1957–67, Proc. 6th Ann. Meet. Am. Coll. of Neuropsychopharmacol., San Juan/Puerto Rico, Dec. 12–15, 1967*, pp. 509–22. (Washington: US Govt. Printing Off.)

Itil, T. M. (1974). Quantitative pharmaco-electroencephalography (Use of computerized cerebral biopotentials in psychotropic drug research). *Mod. Probl. Pharmacopsych.* Vol. 8, pp. 43–75. (Basel: Karger)

Itil, T. M. (1975). Electroencephalography in psychiatry. In Denber, H. C. (ed.). *Psychopharmacological Treatment, Symp. Univ. Florida, Gainesville/Fla. Feb. 1973*, pp. 241–62. (New York: Dekker)

Itil, T. M. (1975). Computer EEG profiles of antidepressants. – Quantitative pharmaco-EEG in the development of new antidepressive drugs. In Fielding, S. (series ed.). Fielding, S. and Lal, H.(eds.). *Antidepressants. Industrial Pharmacology*, Vol. 2, pp. 319–51. (Mount Kisco: Futura)

Itil, T. M. (1976). Discrimination between some hypnotic and anxiolytic drugs by computer-analyzed sleep. In Williams, R. L. and Karacan, I. (eds.). *Pharmacology of Sleep*, pp. 225–38. (New York: Wiley)

Itil, T. M. and Herrmann, W. M. (1978). Effects of hormones on computer-analyzed human electroencephalogram. In Lipton, M. A., DiMascio, A. and Killam, K. F. (eds.). *Psychopharmacology, a Generation of Progress*, pp. 729–43. (New York: Raven Press)

Itil, T. M., Saletu, B. and Akpinar, S. (1974). Classification of psychotropic drugs based on digital computer sleep prints. *Mod. Probl. Pharmacopsych.* Vol. 8, pp. 193–215. (Basel: Karger)

Johnson, L. C., Hanson, K. and Bickford, R. G. (1976). Effect of flurazepam on sleep spindles and K-complexes. *Electroencephalogr. Clin. Neurophysiol.*, **40,** 67

Jovanovic, U. J. (1978). Vigilanzverlauf und Schlafqualitäten unter Einwirkung von Flunitrazepam. In Ahnefeld, F. W., Bergmann, H., Burri, C. *et al.* (eds.). *Rohypnol (Flunitrazepam): pharmakologische Grundlagen, klinische Anwendung*, pp. 25–53. (Berlin: Springer)

Kaim, S. C. (1974). Prevention of delirium tremens. Use of phenothiazines versus drugs cross-dependent with alcohol. In Forrest, I. S., Carr, C. J. and Usdin, E. (eds.). *Phenothiazines and Struct. Related Drugs. Adv. Biochem. Psychopharm.* Vol. 8, pp. 585–90. (New York: Raven Press; Amsterdam: North-Holland Publ.)

Karacan, I., Anch, A. M. and Williams, R. L. (1976). Recent advances in the psychophysiology of sleep and their psychiatric significance. In Grenell, R. G. and Gabay, S. (eds.). *Biological Foundations of Psychiatry.* Vol. 1, pp. 449–98. (New York: Raven Press)

Karbowksi, K. (1975). Absenzen und absenzartige Krisen. *Schweiz. Med. Wochenschr.*, **105,** 1006

Killam, E. K., Killam, K. and Longo, V. G. (eds.) (1977). Section IV. EEG effects of antipsychotics, tranquilizers and antidepressants. In Remond, A. (series ed.). *Handbook of Electroencephalography and Clinical Neurophysiology*, Vol. 7, Part c, pp. 40–56. (Amsterdam: Elsevier)

Killam, E. K. and Longo, V. G. (eds.) (1977). Section VII. EEG effects of convulsants and anticonvulsants in man. In Remond, A. (series ed.). *Handbook of Electroencephalography and Clinical Neurophysiology*, Vol. 7, Part c, pp. 78–87. (Amsterdam: Elsevier)

Kugler, J., Doenicke, A., Suttmann, H., Laub, M., Spaeth, M. and Woeller, L. (1978). Einfluss von Flunitrazepam auf Verhalten und Psyche. In Ahnefeld, F. W., Bergmann, H., Burri, C. *et al.* (eds.). *Rohypnol (Flunitrazepam): pharmakologische Grundlagen, klinische Anwendung*, pp. 54–61. (Berlin: Springer).

Lader, M. (1977). Human pharmacology of antidepressives. *Br. J. Clin. Pharmacol.*, **4,** Suppl. 2, 135S

Laguna, J. F. and Korein, J. (1972). Diagnostic value of diazepam in electroencephalography. *Arch. Neurol.*, **26,** 265

Levratti, M. G. and Pastena, L. (1977). Studio comparativo dell'azione di alcune benzodiazepine (clonazepam, diazepam, nitrazepam). *Riv. Neurol.*, **47,** 282

Masland, R. L. (1976). The diagnosis and treatment of little seizures. *Hosp. Med.*, **12,** 85, 87, 92, 93, 100, 103, 106, 107, 111

McDowall, D. G. (1976). Monitoring the brain. *Anesthesiology*, **45,** 117

McFarland, H. R. (1975). The effect of drugs on the electroencephalogram. – A review with commentary. *Clin. Electroencephalogr.*, **6,** 178

Meldrum, B. S. (1976). Experimental epilepsy. – Its relation to clinical problems. In Bradford, H. F. and Marsden, C. D. (eds.). *Biochem. and Neurol. Proc. of a Conf. Organized by the Neurochem. Group of the Biochem. Soc. and Held at Nottingham Univ. April 1975*, pp. 143–61. (New York: Academic Press)

Oswald, I. and Brezinova, V. (1976). Some physiological effects of psychotropic drugs. *Br. J. Clin. Pharmacol.* **1976,** Suppl. 45

Saletu, B. (1974). Classification of psychotropic drugs based on human evoked potentials *Mod. Probl. Pharmacopsych.* Vol. 8, pp. 258–85. (Basel: Karger)

Shagass, C. (1969). Pharmacology of evoked potentials in man. In Efron, D. H. (ed.). *Psychopharmacol., a Review of Progr. 1957–67. Proc. 6th Ann. Meet. Am. Coll. of Neuropsychopharmacol., San Juan/Puerto Rico, Dec 12–15, 1967*, pp. 483–92. (Washington: US Govt. Printing Off.)

Shagass, C. (1974). Effects of psychotropic drugs on human evoked potentials. *Mod. Probl. Pharmacopsych.* Vol. 8, pp. 238–57. (Basel: Karger)

Tamai, M. (1973). Activation in electroencephalography with drugs. *Gendai Iryo*, **5,** 1141

Electromyography

Budzynski, T. H., Stoyva, J. M., Adler, C. S. and Mullaney, D. J. (1973). EMG biofeedback and tension headache. – A controlled outcome study. *Psychosom. Med.*, **35,** 484

Cirignotta, F., Rasi, F., Sacquegna, T., Forte, A. and Lugaresi, E. (1974). Studio poligrafico sugli effetti ipnotici del farmaco Ro 5–6901 (flurazepam). In

Lubaresi, E. and Coccagna, G. (eds.). *Le insonnie, clinica e terapia. Symp. Intern. Bologna, May 1974*, pp. 127–33. (Bologna: University)
De White, C. B. (1974). Comparison of thymoxamine and diazepam in patients with spasticity. *Br. J. Clin. Pharmacol.*, **1**, 347P
Lapierre, Y. D., Elie, R. and Tetreault, L. (1973). Diazepam and benzoctamine, effects on certain objective parameters of muscular spasticity. *Curr. Ther. Res.*, **15**, 521
Ludin, H. P. and Dubach, K. (1971). Action of diazepam on muscular contraction in man. *Z. Neurol.*, **199**, 30
Ludin, H. P. and Robert, F. (1974). The action of diazepam on human skeletal muscle. *Eur. Neurol.*, **11**, 345
Runion, H. I. and Fowler, F. N. (1978). A double blind study of chlordiazepoxide and hydroxyzine HCl therapy in acute alcohol withdrawal utilizing chronic electromyography for tremor assessment. *Proc. West. Pharmacol. Soc.*, **21**, 303

Respiration

Aukburg, S. J., Miller, J. and Smith, T. C. (1976). Interaction between meperidine and diazepam on the ventilatory response to carbon dioxide. *Clin. Res.*, **24**, 506A
Benke, A., Balogh, A. and Reich-Hilscher, B. (1975). Der Einfluss von Flunitrazepam (Rohypnol) auf die Atmung. *Wien. Klin. Wochenschr.*, **87**, 656
Cegla, U. H. (1973). The use of CO_2 response curves to determine the respiration-depressant action of drugs with diazepam as an example. *Pneumonologie*, **149**, 219
Cohen, R., Finn, H. and Steen, S. N. (1969). Effect of diazepam and meperidine, alone and in combination on respiratory response to carbon dioxide. *Anesth. Analg. Curr. Res.*, **48**, 353
De Biasi, S., Dalfino, L., Brienza, A., Fiore, T. and Carreras, B. (1973). Effetto del diazepam endovenoso sulla ventilazione polmonare e sulla risposta ventilatoria al CO_2. *Minerva Anest.*, **39**, 481
De Biasi, S., Dalfino, L., Brienza, A., Fiore, T. and Carreras, B. (1973). Effetto del nitrazepam endovenoso sulla ventilazione polmonare e sulla risposta ventilatoria al CO_2. *Minerva Anest.*, **39**, 498
Denaut, M., Yernault, J. C. and De Coster, A. (1975). Double-blind comparison of the respiratory effects of parenteral lorazepam and diazepam in patients with chronic obstructive lung disease. *Curr. Med. Res. Opin.*, **2**, 611
Dieckmann, W., Frank, W. and Schlotter, C. (1976). Der Einfluss von 'Rohypnol' auf die Atmung. In Hügin, W., Hossli, G. and Gemperle, M. (eds.). *Bisherige Erfahrungen mit 'Rohypnol' (Flunitrazepam) in der Anaesthesiologie und Intensivtherapie*, pp. 64–73. (Basel: Editiones Roche)
Dodson, M. E., Yousseff, Y., Maddison, S. and Pleuvry, B. (1976). Respiratory effects of lorazepam. *Br. J. Anaesth.*, **48**, 611
Doenicke, A., Suttmann, H. and Sohler, W. (1978). Der Einfluss von Flunitrazepam und Lormetazepam auf die Blutgase. In Ahnefeld, F. W., Bergmann, H. Burri, C. *et al.* (eds.). *Rohypnol (Flunitrazepam): pharmakologische Grundlagen, klinische Anwendung*, pp. 93–8. (Berlin: Springer)
Fernandez-Guardiola, A., Salgado, B. A., Landazuri, M. and Ayala, F. (1975). Estudio poligráfico del efecto de fármacos tranquilizantes (clobazam vs.

diazepam) en humanos, durante una tarea de monitoreo. *Invest. Med. Int.*, **2**, 240

Gasser, J.C. and Bellville, J.W. (1976). The respiratory effects of hydroxyzine, diazepam and pentazocine in man. *Anaesthesia*, **31**, 718

Geddes, D.M., Rudolf, M. and Saunders, K.B. (1976). Effect of nitrazepam and flurazepam on the ventilatory response to carbon dioxide. *Thorax*, **31**, 548

Hudson, L.D., Lakshminarayan, S., Sahn, S.A. and Weil, J.V. (1974). Diminished hypoxic ventilatory drive following diazepam. *Am. Rev. Resp. Dis.*, **109**, 694

Knapp, R. and Remen, D. (1977). An evaluation of the cardiopulmonary safety and efficacy of triazolam, flurazepam, and placebo as oral hypnotic agents. *Clin. Pharmacol. Ther.*, **21**, 107

Kronenberg, R.S., Cosio, M.G., Stevenson, J.E. and Drage, C.W. (1975). The use of oral diazepam in patients with obstructive lung disease and hypercapnia. *Ann. Intern. Med.*, **83**, 83

Mahlich, J., Keller, R. and Herzog, H. (1972). Die Wirkung von Diazepam auf die Atmung des gesunden Menschen. *Pneumologie*, **148**, 39

Olt, I. (1975). Der Einfluss von Flunitrazepam (Rohypnol) auf die Atmung. Presented at *Zentraleuropaeischer Anaesthesie-Kongress*, September, Bremen.

Pateisky, K. and Wessely, P. (1973). Polygraphic examination during fast and slow intravenous injection of the same dose of diazepam. *Elektroenceph. Clin. Neurophysiol.*, **34**, 738

Patrick, J.M. and Sempik, A.K. (1978). The effect of diazepam on the threshold of the ventilatory response to CO_2. *Br. J. Clin. Pharmacol.*, **6**, 462

Schmitz, J.E., Lotz, P., Bock, K.H., Fisseler, A. and Ahnefeld, F.W. (1978). Auswirkungen des Flunitrazepam auf die Atmung. In Ahnefeld, F.W., Bergmann, H., Burri, C. *et al.* (eds.). *Rohypnol (Flunitrazepam): pharmakologische Grundlagen, klinische Anwendung*, pp. 67–81. (Berlin: Springer)

Tandon, M.K. (1974). Effect of diazepam, chloropromazine and haloperidol on respiration in cases with chronic airways obstruction. *Aust. NZ J. Med.*, **4**, 311

Zsigmond, E.K., Flynn, K. and Martinez, D.A. (1974). Diazepam and meperidine on arterial blood gases in healthy volunteers. *J. Clin. Pharmacol.*, **14**, 377

Salivation

Fourestier, J., Gacon, J., Esvan, J., Le Stir, A. and Morcelet, J.L. (1973). Scintigraphie salivaire: intérêt dans le traitement des bouches sèches provoquées par les médicaments psychotropes. *Nouv. Presse Méd.*, **2**, 839

Steiner, J.E., Cohen, S., Scheinok, F. and Birnbaum, D. (1969). The effect of diazepam on volume and ionic composition of unstimulated and stimulated secretion of human saliva. Presented at the *Sci. Meet. Israel Physiol. Pharmacol. Soc.*, June 13, Jerusalem

Steiner, J.E., Birnbaum, D. Karmeli, F. and Cohen, S. (1970). Effect of diazepam on human salivary secretion. *Digestion*, **3**, 262

Tremor

Cantor, F.K. (1975). Adrenergic mechanisms in benign essential tremor. *Neurology (Minneap.)*, **25**, 376

Critchley, E. (1972). Clinical manifestation of essential tremor. *J. Neurol. Neurosurg. Psychiatry*, **35**, 365

Klapetek, J. (1970). Extrapyramidaler Tremor und Vitamin B6 in hohen Dosen. Eine therapeutische Anmerkung. *Nervenarzt*, **41**, 251

Lader, M.H. (1977). Mechanisms of stress and anxiety. In Kielholz, P. (ed.). *Beta-Blockers and the Central Nervous System, Intern. Ciba-Geigy Symp. St. Moritz, Switz. Jan. 1976*, pp. 47–52. (Bern: Huber)

Loeb, C. and Priand, A. (1977). Preliminary evaluation of the effects of clonazepam on parkinsonian tremor. *Eur. Neurol.*, **15**, 143

Runion, H.I. and Fowler, F.N. (1978). A double blind study of chlordiazepoxide and hydroxyzine HCl therapy in acute alcohol withdrawal utilizing chronic electromyography for tremor assessment. *Proc. West. Pharmacol. Soc.*, **21**, 303

Tyrer, P. and Lader, M.H. (1974). Physiological response to propranolol and diazepam in chronic anxiety. *Br. J. Clin. Pharmacol.*, **1**, 387

Villemos, P. Behandling av følјdtillstand efter excessiv alkoholkonsumtion med nitrazepam Mogadon. *Nord. Psykiat. Tidsskr.*, **23**, 36

9

Clinical Experience with Benzodiazepines in Psychosomatic Disorders

D. Kelly

Psychosomatic disorders

Illness in general, of whatever type, is a reaction by the person to a variety of changing events both in the internal and external environments. In this broad sense all illness is psychosomatic, physical and psychological changes being part of the total response of the patient. The effect of an external stimulus will, to a large extent, depend upon the genetic make-up of the individual, a relatively weak environmental stress producing marked changes in a predisposed individual, whilst in others the same stimulus would produce no effect. Illness is usually multifactorially determined; for instance in bronchial asthma an attack will often only result when a number of allergic, emotional and infective factors combine to trigger the attack.

The psychosomatic disorders are a heterogeneous group of illnesses in which psychosocial events can be shown to have a direct relationship to the production of the symptoms and signs of an otherwise apparently physical disorder. The capacity to react to changing circumstances determines whether the person remains healthy, falls ill, recovers or dies. The genetic vulnerability of a particular organ system determines where psychosocial stress will alter normal functioning, which we then recognize as illness. In the cardiovascular system this may manifest itself as hypertension or coronary thrombosis. The gastro-intestinal tract may react to stress by peptic ulceration, ulcerative colitis or the irritable bowel syndrome. The skin may break down into areas of eczema, psoriasis or urticaria.

To understand the proper clinical use of benzodiazepines in the treatment of psychosomatic disorders, it is necessary to appreciate *how* stress affects target organs in normal health and the way in which this can be ameliorated by benzodiazepines.

The benzodiazepines are the most widely prescribed drugs in medical practice. In the United States in 1977, 8 thousand tons of benzodiazepines were consumed with 54 million prescriptions for diazepam and 13 million prescriptions for chlordiazepoxide. Surveys of outpatient psychotropic drug use suggest that the benzodiazepines and other minor tranquillizers are more often used by individuals with complaints referable to particular organ systems than in those with primary psychiatric diagnoses, and that 16% of the annual use in the United States is for cardiovascular disease of which a major proportion is presumably for hypertension.

The cardiovascular system

The benzodiazepines affect blood pressure mainly through their action on the hypothalamus. Animal experiments have shown that they block the pressor response to hypothalamic stimulation. A recent study asked why physicians prescribed benzodiazepines in essential hypertension, seeking to determine if this was because of concurrent psychological complaints or because of elevations in blood pressure or both. The results suggested that psychological complaints in hypertensive patients reliably lead to the prescription of tranquillizers and that such prescribing is followed by a reduction in psychological complaints. In fact only one third of patients had psychological complaints, the other two thirds had shown a large increase in diastolic blood pressure since the last clinic visit. Prescription of a benzodiazepine was followed by a blood pressure reduction in 62% of cases, the average diastolic fall being 6.7 mmHg, which was clinically significant[5].

Starling's Law of the Heart (1918) stated that the energy of contraction of the heart, other things being equal, depended upon the stretch of the muscle fibres. Increasing the stretch increases the performance to a certain point, but beyond this the fibres are overstretched and performance, manifest as cardiac output, falls. Nixon[4] conceives of psychosocial stress in an analogous way, with increasing arousal enhancing performance in good health. 'The qualities required for success, namely rapid and flexible thought, originality, vigour, expansion and capacity for sustained effort, are abundant.' When the top of the human function curve is reached, however, exhaustion sets in, and the high level of arousal is associated with a number of biochemical changes. These include *increases* in sympatho-adrenal and thyroid activity, serum cholesterol, triglycerides, blood coagulability, heart rate and blood pressure. Fluid retention is common particularly in women. Cardiac arrhythmias, heightened awareness of the heartbeat and neurotic symptoms such as chest pain are common. Impending cardiac breakdown can be diagnosed by the abnormal palpable and audible atrial sound over a distended left ventricle. Diazepam can be used for reducing arousal by day and nitrazepam can prevent sleep deprivation at night. If the warning signs are not heeded or treated, the 'pre-infarction syndrome' can progress to the 'intermediate coronary syndrome' with an acute onset or worsening of angina pectoris or acute coronary insufficiency finally leading to myocardial infarction. The quickest way of reducing arousal is to put the patient into a comfortable sleep with an intravenous infusion of diazepam, which can be life-saving in acute coronary illness. An intravenous drip is put up and boluses of 5 to 10 mg of diazepam injected as often as required to keep the patient free from pain and to allay anxiety which increase the demands upon the heart and hence aggravate coronary insufficiency. Boluses of 50 mg of pethidine may also be needed in the early stages. 'The drowsiness is interrupted for food and toilet purposes, but the regimen is continued until the patient can be wide awake without pain which in extreme cases may take 2 or 3 weeks. When a "preinfarction" or "intermediate coronary syndrome" has been treated by reduction of arousal, the blood pressure, lipid, uric acid and sugar levels usually fall to normal.'

Many studies have demonstrated the value of benzodiazepines in intensive care units (ICUs) where procedures which are potentially life-saving are frequently perceived by the anxious patient as indices of deteriorating clinical condition and impending death. Sensory overstimulation or emotional irritability in the ICU may be produced by sleep deprivation, pain, multiple needle punctures, sounds from respirators and cardiac monitors. Difficulty in communication due to intubation may also increase fear as well as the arrival of new or dying patients, the sudden activity of medical and nursing staff when emergencies arise and the distress of neighbouring patients. Intravenous diazepam has also been found to reduce the frequency of 'psychiatric reactions' following open heart surgery[3]. These usually arise after a lucid interval in the ICU and are manifest as severe anxiety, nervous tension, disorientation, confusion, depression, hostility and even hallucinations.

Intravenous diazepam can also be used for cardioversion, and cardiac catheterization. Psychological studies have demonstrated significant changes in the mood of anxious patients after 10 mg of intravenous diazepam. The patients were significantly less 'Dizzy' ('sick to the stomach, dizzy, jittery and shaky') and less 'Unhappy' ('sad, downhearted, troubled and worried'). The patients were less anxious on self and observer rating scales, and this was accompanied by a significant reduction in physiological arousal, as evidenced by a fall in forearm blood flow, and heart rate, the maximum effect being seen 20–30 minutes after the administration of diazepam. In a group of normal controls who had 5 mg of intravenous diazepam, blood pressure, respiration, and sweat gland activity were not significantly affected, but there was an increase in finger pulse amplitude, indicating cutaneous vasodilatation. Pain at the site of injection radiating down the arm, due to the acidity of the diazepam solution irritating the venous endothelium, can be reduced by first withdrawing an equal volume of blood into the syringe, so that its contents are diluted and well mixed with blood, before diazepam is injected into the vein. Subsequent phlebitis is also less likely to occur, which can be of considerable advantage if a course of injections is given e.g. for treating a phobic condition, or the vein is needed for further investigations or treatment[2].

Lorazepam can also be used in cardiovascular disorders and can also allay stress-induced angina pectoris. It is often used in combination with digoxin, theophylline, anti-arrhythmic agents and coronary dilators.

The benzodiazepines also can play a useful part in the management of the post-myocardial infarction syndrome to protect the heart from the full impact of sudden or unacceptable psychosocial stress.

The cardiovascular system has been considered in detail because it shows the close relationship between mind and body. Cardiovascular abnormalities have been induced experimentally in man and animals by stimulating cortical as well as subcortical areas of the brain. The Western Way of Death is to have a heart attack, and no less than one half of adult male deaths in North America and Britain are due to coronary heart disease. There seems little doubt that the stress of modern urban living is one of the major causes of this alarming state of affairs. Heart attacks are three times commoner in those who live in the cities compared with those who live in the country, and professionals living particularly stressful lives such as airline pilots and doctors are most vulnerable. High blood pressure predisposes to coronary thrombosis and the ability of the benzodiazepines to modify the blood pressure rise produced by stress is very important.

The recent discovery of benzodiazepine receptors in the human brain is of great significance, and this and their wide margin of safety are probably the main reasons for their popularity with the medical profession and the public. It has been shown that certain 'emotional' strains of mice have a decreased number of benzodiazepine receptors compared with 'non-emotional' strains. Similarly, in the rat, 'fearful' strains have fewer receptors compared with 'non-fearful'. It has been suggested that the anti-anxiety action of benzodiazepines is a result of enhancing the effect of the inhibitory neurotransmitter GABA (γ-aminobutyric acid), thus enabling it to 'quiet the brain'. If there are fewer benzodiazepine receptors in the brains of some people compared with others, this might explain why these predisposed individuals are more 'anxiety prone'. Furthermore, since GABA has the capacity to 'quiet' brain cell activity, the benzodiazepines could be expected to enhance this effect, even if there are fewer receptors, and hence to reduce unacceptable and potentially harmful levels of neurophysiological arousal. The locus coeruleus has been postulated as important in the development of anxiety, because stimulation of this part of the brain in animals can produce 'anxiety-like' behaviour, which can be blocked by diazepam. The value of the benzodiazepines in a wide range of psychosomatic disorders would also be explained.

Gastro-intestinal disorders

Stress can produce an increase in gastric hypermotility and acidity, and hence predispose to the development of gastritis and gastric and duodenal ulceration. The benzodiazepines have been used, usually in conjunction with other types of medication, to improve these disorders. The recent discovery of cimetidine, the H_2 receptor antagonist, which has a much more specific effect in reducing gastric acid secretion, has transformed the medical treatment of duodenal ulceration, which was well known for its association with psychosocial stress. Ulcerative colitis, nervous diarrhoea and the irritable bowel syndrome have also been treated with benzodiazepines as adjuncts to therapy because of the long established recognition that many intestinal disorders are made worse by stress. Lorazepam, for example, does not produce any adverse interactions with standard medications used for gastro-enterological disorders.

Respiratory disorders

Anxiety increases the rate of respiration, and can also lead to dyspnoea and bronchospasm. Asthma is, par excellence, a psychosomatic disorder. Lorazepam, diazepam and many other benzodiazepines have been used to reduce the frequency and severity of asthmatic attacks. As discussed previously, infective and allergic factors need to be taken into account and antibiotics, specific bronchodilators, sodium cromoglycate, and if needed steroids, used as well. Reduction in anxiety by a benzodiazepine can, for selected patients, lead to diminished doses of other medication being prescribed for asthma and bronchitis with bronchospasm. Because of the well-known side-effects of steroids, this may be especially advantageous. Some workers have suggested that lorazepam produces less respiratory depression than diazepam and hence may be preferable[1].

Rheumatological disorders

Anxiety can produce an increase in muscular contraction and the perception of pain. In dogs, the effect of electric chocks is attenuated by pretreatment with a benzodiazepine. In rheumatology not only have benzodiazepines been used to reduce pain, but their specific and separate muscle relaxant properties have been employed in rheumatoid arthritis to improve stiffness, spasm and cramps. Diazepam or lorazepam can be used if more sedation is required, otherwise chlordiazepoxide. Mobility and hence daily activity are thereby increased. For ankylosing spondylitis, pain and early morning stiffness can be treated with nocturnal nitrazepam or diazepam with indomethacin.

Low back pain is said to afflict 2.4% of the population. Bed-rest and benzodiazepines can reduce spasm and the acute pain of a prolapsed intervertebral disc lesion, intravenous diazepam being employed in an emergency.

Dermatoses

Anxiety, irritability and sleep disturbances can exacerbate many skin conditions characterized by pruritus, urticaria, hyperhidrosis, eczema and angioneurotic oedema. Benzodiazepines have been used for many skin patients to allay anxiety and improve sleep, and some dermatologists are impressed with the degree of their antipruritic effect.

Sexual disorders

Performance anxiety can induce impotence or premature ejaculation in the most robust of males, and psychological tensions can produce dyspareunia, vaginismus and frigidity in females. The anxiolytic and muscle relaxant properties of benzodiazepines have made them effective drugs for treating sexual disorders. Premenstrual tension, irritability, the menopausal syndrome, dysmenorrhoea and stress-induced amenorrhoea as well as urinary frequency have all responded to benzodiazepines, in carefully selected patients.

Neurological conditions

Benzodiazepines can reduce muscle spasm and have found an established place in the treatment and prevention of tension and migraine headaches.

Summary

Psychosocial factors can be responsible for the precipitation or exacerbation of a wide variety of psychosomatic disorders. The benzodiazepines, which can reduce the effect of stress, have several distinct properties which have led to their great popularity with the medical profession and the general public. The ability to reduce the rise in emotionally induced blood pressure and other cardiovascular effects have led to their use as an adjunct in the treatment of hypertension, coronary artery disease, as well as for specific procedures such as cardiac catheterization, cardioversion, and sedation in cardiac emergencies and widespread use in intensive care units. The use of benzodiazepines for gastro-intestinal disorders, respiratory disease, rheumatology, the dermatoses, sexual dysfunction as well as other conditions are discussed.

References

1. Dodson, M. E., Yousseff, Y., Maddison, S. and Pleuvry, B. (1976). Respiratory effects of lorazepam. *Br. J. Anaesth.*, **48,** 611
2. Kelly, D., Pik, R., Chen, C. N. (1973). A psychological and physiological evaluation of the effects of intravenous diazepam. *Br. J. Psychiatry*, **122,** 419
3. McClish, A., Andrews, D. and Tetreault, L. (1968). Intravenous diazepam for psychiatric reactions following open-heart surgery. *Can. Anaesth. Soc. J.*, **15,** 63
4. Nixon, P. G. (1976). The human function curve. With special reference to cardiovascular disorders–Part I/Part II, *Practitioner*, **217,** 765/935
5. Whitehead, W. E., Blackwell, B. and Robinson, A. (1977). Why physicians prescribe benzodiazepines in essential hypertension. *Biol. Psychiatry*, **12,** 597

Bibliography

Dermatology

Borelli, S. (1976). Medizinische Rehabilitation und Heilverfahren bei Hautkranken und Allergikern aus arbeits- und sozialmedizinischer Sicht. *Arbeitsmed. Sozialmed. Präventivmed.*, **11,** 70

Borelli, S. (1976). Haut und Psyche. *Musik Medizin*, **7,** 12, 16

Borelli, S. and Schellert, P. (1967). Zur Wirksamkeit von Psychopharmaka bei atopischer Neurodermitis. Vergleichende Untersuchung von Diazepam (Valium), Promethazin (Phenergan) und Placebo. *Dermatologica*, **135,** 485

Borelli, S. and Etter, H. (1971). Zur antidepressiven Therapie bei der atopischen konstitutionellen Neurodermitis. *Dermatologica*, **142,** 154

Muston, H., Felix, R. and Shuster, S. (1979). Differential effect of hypnotics and anxiolytics on itch and scratch. Presented at *SID/ESDR Joint Meeting 1979*, June 12, Amsterdam.

Nurse, D. S. (1975). Urticaria: diagnosis and management. *Drugs*, **9,** 292

Nurse, D. S. (1976). Itch: causes and management. *Curr. Ther.*, **17,** 61, 65, 69

Schröpl, F. (1979). Rezidivierende Urtikaria. *Z. Allg. Med.*, **55,** 378

Tokuda, Y. and Tokuda, Y. (1973). Effects of Ro 5-3350 on dermatological psychosomatic symptoms: With special reference to cholinergic hives and alopecia areata. *Clin. Med.*, **15,** 284

Gastrointestinal disorders

Ament, M. E. (1975). Inflammatory disease of the colon. – Ulcerative colitis and Crohn's colitis. *J. Pediatr.*, **86,** 322

Amure, B. O. (1974). Clinical evaluation of Valium and propantheline with propantheline alone on duodenal ulcer patients. Presented at the *World Congress of Gastroenterology*, October, Mexico.
Auden, R. R. and Barrowman, J. A. (1976). Konservative Therapie des Magenkarzinoms. *Leber Magen Darm*, **6**, 108
Baume, P. and Cuthbert, J. (1973). The effect of medazepam in relieving symptoms of functional gastrointestinal distress. *Aust. NZ J. Med.*, **3**, 457
Baume, P., Tracey, M. and Dawson, L. (1975). Efficacy of two minor tranquilizers in relieving symptoms of functional gastrointestinal distress. *Aust. NZ J. Med.*, **5**, 503
Blaha, L. and Wieck, H. H. (1978). Psychopharmaka bei der Behandlung der Ulkuskrankheit. *Mod. Med.*, **6**, 1360
Carvalho, F. A., De Luna, J. A., Machado, M. P. and Lima, M. G. (1975). Ensaio clínico do Ro 5-3350 (Lexotan) em portadores de úlcera gastroduodenal. *Folha Méd.*, **70**, 45
Copelman, H. (1974). Uso de uma associação de medazepam e clidinio (Ro 10-7453) no tratamento de distúrbios funcionais do aparelho digestivo. *Rev. Bras. Clin. Ter.*, **3**, 11
De Pergola, E. (1974). La terapia del dolore addominale e del dolore articolare. *Clin. Ter.*, **70**, Suppl. 129
Doyle, P. J., McKay, A. J. and Browne, M. K. (1979). Failure to thrive in adolescence due to inflammatory bowel disease. *Practitioner*, **22**, 253
Freyberger, H. and Leutner, V. (1974). Die psychosomatische Therapie des Magen- und Zwölffingerdarm-Geschwürs. *Therapiewoche*, **24**, 278
Gardner, R. C. (1977). Pharmacotherapy of inflammatory bowel disease. In Miller, R. R. and Greenblatt, D. J. (eds.), *Drug Therapy Reviews*, Vol. 1, pp. 238–253. (New York: Masson)
Gueller, R. (1976). Die Refluxkrankheit. Konzept der Pathogenese und Therapie des gastroösophagialen Refluxes. *Praxis*, **65**, 945
Gulisano, G., Interlandi, A. and Vandea, I. (1973). Effetti del diazepam sulla motilità biliare extraepatica. (Ricerche con radioisotopi.) *G. Med. Pneumol.*, **22**, 345
Hisano, N., Kasugai, T. and Ito, K. (1973). The effects of medazepam on the psychosomatic syndrome accompanied with gastrointestinal diseases. *J. New Remed. Clin.*, **22**, 739
Issel, W. (1977). Psychopharmaka in der Inneren Medizin. *Fortschr. Med.*, **95**, 21
Kasich, A. M., Richards, D. J. and Vanov, S. K. (1976). Lorazepam in the management of anxiety associated with chronic gastrointestinal disease. – A double-blind study. *Curr. Ther. Res.*, **19**, 292
Kawakami, K. and Sasaki, D. (1974). Therapy of gastritis. – How to use parasympatholytic drugs. *Gendai Iryo*, **6**, 779
Lasagna, L. (1977). The role of benzodiazepines in nonpsychiatric medical practice. *Am. J. Psychiatry*, **134**, 656
Leickert, K. H. (1977). Lexotanil. – Ein neuer Benzodiazepin-Tranquilizer mit stimmungsaufhellenden Eigenschaften. *Med. Welt*, **28**, 1317
Liss, J. L., Alpers, D. and Woodruff, R. A. (1973). The irritable colon syndrome and psychiatric illness. *Dis. Nerv. Syst.*, **34**, 151
Masuda, M., Hosokawa, K., Kondo, M., Kato, T., Yamaguchi, M. and Nishiyama, J. (1972). Clinical effects of Ro 5-4556 (Nobrium) on gastro-intestinal

diseases. – Comparison with diazepam by double-blind method. *Clin. Med.*, **14,** 1299
Meirelles Filho, J.S. and Moraes Filho, J.P. (1978). Clínica e terapêutica das gastrites. *Rev. Bras. Clin. Ter.*, **7,** 265
Nakamura, K., Urayama, S., Matsuura, H., Okazawa, H. and Matsubara, T. (1974). Therapy of nervous gastrointestinal diseases by medazepam (Resmit). *Clin. Med.*, **16,** 1958
Nakayama, T., Yamazoe, A., Konagawa, A., Hisajima, K., Yamaguchi, H. and Nonaka, H. *et al.* (1977). Clinical effect of medazepam (Resmit) on the diseases of gastric tract. *Jpn. J. Clin. Exp. Med.*, **54,** 1631
Niada, R., Omini, C., Prino, G., Folco, G.C., Milani, S. and Berti, F. (1978). Synergistic interaction between diazepam and octatropine-methyl-bromide at the gastrointestinal level. *Pharmacol. Res. Commun.*, **10,** 951
Roberts, D.M. and Oldrey, T.B. (1975). The effect of diazepam on pentagastrin-stimulated and nocturnal (sleeping) gastric secretion in man. *Am. J. Gastroenterol.*, **63,** 396
Ruoff, M. (1973). Clinical management of the irritable colon syndrome. In Lindner, A.E. (ed.), *Emotional Factors in Gastrointestinal Illness. International Congress Series no. 304*, pp. 163–165. (Amsterdam: Excerpta Medica)
Santero, M. and Barba, C. (1977). L'associazione bromazepam e propantelina (Ro 10-9618) nel trattamento dei disturbi gastroenterici di natura psicosomatica. *Policlin. Sez. Med.*, **84,** 489
Schofield, P.F. (1977). Diseases of the colon and rectum. *Update*, **14,** 1315
Schonecke, O.W. and Schueffel, W. (1977). Bromazepam (Lexotanil) in the psychosomatic treatment of patients with functional abdominal disorders. In Antonelli, F. (ed.) *Psychopharmacology of Somatization, Biological and Psychological Assessments. 3. Congr. Mondiale dell'International College of Psychosomatic Med.*, pp. 79–86. (Rome: Pozzi)
Smits, B.J. (1974). The irritable bowel syndrome. *Practitioner*, **213,** 37
Thompson, W.G. (1974). The irritable colon. *Can. Med. Ass. J.*, **111,** 1241
Vetter, D. (1974). Die konservative Therapie des peptischen Ulkus. *Ther. Umsch.*, **31,** 896
Vicari, F., Jeanpierre, R.E. and Laurent, J.X. (1974). Place du Valium 'Roche' en gastro-entérologie. *J. Med. Nord Est*, **11,** 119
Waye, J.D. (1977). Colonoscopy. – Guidelines and techniques for diagnosis and therapy. In Glass, G.B.J. (ed.), *Progress in Gastroenterology*, Vol. 3, pp. 991–1013. (New York: Grune and Stratton)
Weingart, J., Fischer, L.I., Frimberger, E., Seib, H.J. and Ottenjann, R. (1978). Bedeutung der Koloskopie bei Colitis ulcerosa and Morbus Crohn. *Euromedicine*, **18,** 868

Headache

Budzynski, T.H., Stoyva, J.M., Adler, C.S. and Mullaney, D.J. (1973). EMG biofeedback and tension headache. – A controlled outcome study. *Psychosom. Med.*, **35,** 484
Critchley, E.M. (1975). Migraine. *Update*, **10,** 11
Deffeminis, H.A. and Medici, M. (1976). Tratamiento de las cefaleas vasculares con dimetotiazina y clonazepam. Presented at *Congreso de Neurología*, October, Lima-Arequipa, Perú.

Diamond, S. (1975). Severe headaches. – Understanding types and treatments. *Drug Ther.*, **5,** 81
Duvoisin, R. C. (1972). The cluster headache. *J. Am. Med. Assoc.*, **222,** 1403
Dyken, P. R. (1975). Headaches in children. *Am. Fam. Physician*, **11,** 105
Eadie, M. J. (1975). The management of migraine. *Med. J. Aust.*, **1975/I,** 752
Feuerstein, M., Adams, H. E. and Beiman, I. (1976). Cephalic vasomotor and electromyographic feedback in the treatment of combined muscle contraction and migraine headaches in a geriatric case. *Headache*, **16,** 232
Gayral, L. F. (1975). Les 1,4-benzodiazépines en neurologie. *Actual. Psychiatr.*, **6,** 93
Hedri, A. (1975). Rivotril bei Migräne. *Praxis*, **64,** 1062
Kowa, H. (1973). Drug treatment of chronic headache and direction of life. *Med.*, **10,** 1798
Leon-Sotomayor, L. A. (1974). Cardiac migraine-report of twelve cases. *Angiology*, **25,** 161
Morris, R. W. (1974). The nature and treatment of headache. *Pharmindex*, **16,** 6
Mumenthaler, M. (1975). Therapie der Kopf- und Gesichtsschmerzen. *Inform. Arzt*, **3,** 95
Murata, T. (1975). Clinical study of Nobrium (medazepam) with special reference to cardiac neurosis and tension headache. *Clin. Med.*, **17,** 115
One, Y., Takeya, C. and Tanaka, T. (1973). Muscle contraction headache. *J. Ther.*, **55,** 1224
Paci, A. and Vittori, O. (1975). Terapia psicotropa attuale. – Studico clinico di un nuovo preparato benzodiazepinico. *Settim. Osp.*, **17,** 73
Parkes, J. D. (1975). Diseases of the central nervous system. Relief of pain – headache, facial neuralgia, migraine, and phantom limb. *Br. Med. J.*, **2,** 90
Patten, J. P. (1973). Atypical migraine. *Practitioner*, **211,** 304
Paulson, G. W. and Klawans, H. L. (1974). Benign orgasmic cephalalgia. *Headache*, **13,** 181
Ritschl, A. (1976). Folge eines peripheren muskulären Hypertonus. *Med. Trib.*, **9,** 9
Salmon, M. A. (1976). Antikonvulsiva helfen gegen Migräne bei Kindern. *Prax. Kur.*, **14,** 35
Scherzer, E. B. (1975). Ueber den sogenannten posttraumatischen Kopfschmerz. *Fortschr. Neurol.-Psychiatr. Grenzgeb.*, **43,** 271
Seyfeddinipur, N. and Philipp, M. (1976). Das Antiepileptikum Clonazepam (Rivotril) als Schlafmittel. *Fortschr. Med.*, **94,** 1370
Stensrud, P. and Sjaastad, O. (1978). Clonazepam (Rivotril) in migraine prophylaxis. Presented at *Scandinavian migraine meeting.*
Thiroloix, P. (1976). Premiers résultats du traitement de la migraine commune par le clonazépam. *Nouv. Presse Méd.*, **5,** 1838
Troquereau, F. (1976). Utilisation du clonazépam dans le traitement des céphalées en particulier vasculaires. *Diss.*, Bordeaux/Fr., 1976, pp. 161
Vazquez de Negrotto, O., Dalmas, F. and Negrotto, A. (1975). Cefaleas vasculares: tratamiento con clonazepan. Presented at *La Sociedad de Neurología del Uruguay*, December.
Wessely, P. and Quatember, R. (1976). Posttraumatische Kopfschmerzformen. Aetiologie, Pathomechanik und Therapie. *Prakt. Arzt*, **13,** 1464
Wessely, P., Schnaberth, G. and Maly, J. (1975). Der psychogene Kopfschmerz. *Prakt. Arzt*, **12,** 1409

Wilkinson, M. (1976). The treatment of acute migraine attacks. *Headache*, **15**, 291
Woerz, R., Baar, H., Draf, W., Garcia, J., Gerbershagen, U., Gross, D., Magin, F., Rieble, R., Ritter, K., Scheifele, J. and Scholl, W. (1975). Zur Mehrfaktorenbehandlung bei Dauerkopfschmerzen. *Nervenarzt*, **46**, 640

Hypertension

Beale, M. G., Salcedo, J. R. and Chan, J. C. (1974). Management of hypertension in children on chronic hemodialysis and following renal transplantation. *Clin. Proc. Child. Hosp. Nat. Med. Cent.*, **30**, 265
Bear, R. A. and Erenrich, N. (1978). Essential hypertension and pregnancy. *Can. Med. Assoc. J.*, **118**, 936
Chamberlain, G. V., Lewis, R. J., Swiet de, M. and Bulpitt, C. J. (1978). How obstetricians manage hypertension in pregnancy. *Br. Med. J.*, **1**, 626
V. Eiff, A. W. (1974). Zentralnervöse und psychosomatische Aspekte der Hypertonie. *Med. Welt*, **25**, 2077
Leighton, P. W. and Tighe, H. (1974). A critical survey of drugs used in the treatment of hypertensive crises in pregnancy. *Med. J. Aust.*, **61/II**, 680
Michael, C. A. (1978). Treatment of hypertension arising in pregnancy. *Drugs*, **15**, 317
Pozenel, H., Bückert, A. and Amrein, R. (1975). The antihypertensive effect of bromazepam (Lexotan). – A new benzodiazepine derivative. Presented at *3. Internationaler Kongress für psychosomatische Medizin*, September 16–20, Rome.
Ueno, K., Kitanaka, I., Mizushima, N., Miyabo, S., Hisada, T., Kishida, S., Ogawa, N. *et al.* (1977). The alleviating effects of medazepam on psychologically induced rise in the blood pressure of essential hypertensives. *Jpn. J. Clin. Pharmacol.*, **8**, 17
Wheatley, D. (1977). Circulatory manifestations of soma and psyche. In Antonelli, F. (ed.). *Therapy in Psychosomatic Medicine, Proc. 3rd Congr. Intern. College of Psychosomatic Medicine*, September 1975, Vol. 2, pp. 163–167. (Rome: Pozzi)
Wheatley, D. (1977). Antianxiety drug trials in hypertension. *Psychopharmacol. Bull.*, **13**, 27
Whitehead, W. E., Blackwell, B. and Robinson, A. (1977). Why physicians prescribe benzodiazepines in essential hypertension. – A phase IV study. *Biol. Psychiatry*, **12**, 597
Masso, M. and Pérez, H. (1979). Double-blind clinical trial of bromazepam and alpha-methyldopa in arterial hypertension. *Pharm. Ther.*, **2**, 195

Myocardial infarction

Abjörn, C., Karlsson, E. and Sonnhag, C. (1977). Ventricular arrhythmias in acute myocardial infarction. *Acta Med. Scand.*, **201**, 119
Apps, M. C. and Tinker, J. (1978). The measurement and control of myocardial infarct size. *Intens. Care Med.*, **4**, 21
Calvert, A., Mitchell, A. S. and Sinclair, G. (1974). A double-blind evaluation of diazepam and amylobarbitone in acute myocardial infarction. *Med. J. Aust.*, **61/II**, 624

Chaptal, P. A., Grolleau-Raoux, D., Millet, F. and Grolleau-Raoux, R. (1975). Les crises hypertensives dans la chirurgie de l'insuffisance coronarienne. Prévention par le diazépam. *Ann. Chir. Thorac. Cardio-vasc.*, **14,** 255

Falk, R. B., Denlinger, J. K., Nahrwold, M. L. and Todd, R. A. (1978). Acute vasodilation following induction of anesthesia with intravenous diazepam and nitrous oxide. *Anesthesiology*, **49,** 149

Gedeon, A. and Varkonyi, S. (1973). Myokardinfarkt und akutes Psychosyndrom. Symptomatische Behandlung mit Seduxeninjektion. *Ther. Hung.*, **21,** 45

Hayward, R. P. (1977). Emergency care of the cardiac patient. *Nursing Mirror*, **144,** 45

Julian, D. G. (1975). Cardiac infarction. *Med.*, **1975,** 1348

Kucharski, A. (1978). Psychologic stress in myocardial infarction. *Am. Fam. Physician*, **17,** 154

Landa, C. R., Palacios, G. N., Avellaneda, M. and Gareca, C. R. (1975). Ensayo terapéutico del clonazepam en la inestabilidad eléctrica ventricular. Comunicación preliminar. *Prensa Universitaria*, **504,** 8358

Leickert, K. H. (1977). Valium Roche en el infarto de miocardio. *Med. Welt*, **10,** 263

Lenzner, A. S. (1974). Psychiatry in the coronary care unit. *Psychosomatics*, **15,** 70

Markiewicz, W., Hunt, S., Harrison, D. C. and Alderman, E. L. (1976). Circulatory effects of diazepam in heart disease. *J. Clin. Pharmacol.*, **16,** 637

Melsom, M., Andreassen, P., Melsom, H., Hansen, T., Grendahl, H. and Hillestad, L. K. (1976). Diazepam in acute myocardial infarction. Clinical effects and effects on catecholamines, free fatty acids, and cortisol. *Br. Heart. J.*, **38,** 804

Prokudin, V. N., Raiskii, V. A., Romanov, Y. D., Paramonova, E. G., Bolshakova, T. D. and Lukicheva, T. I. (1974). Differential utilization of Elenium and Seduxen in young adults in the post-infarct period. *Zh. Nevropat. Psikhiat.*, **74,** 282

Raiski, V., Rozonov, Y. and Chichkanov, G. (1972). Diazepam and the cardiovascular system. *Soviet Sci. Rev.*, **3,** 215

Rozonov, Y. B., Chichkanov, G. G. and Raiski, V. A. (1973). The effect of Seduxen (diazepam) on the regulation of the vasomotor tone regulation. *Farmakol. Toksikol.*, **36,** 225

Steelman, R. B. (1978). 20 questions physicians most often ask. – About the diagnosis and treatment of myocardial infarction. *Consultant*, **18,** 29

Wieluch, W., Lang, E. and Niedermaier, K. (1977). Sofortbehandlung des akuten Myokardinfarktes. *Notfallmed.*, **3,** 311

Respiratory disorders

Abel, H. and Trendelenburg, F. (1978). Leitsymptom – Atemnot. Der Notfall. Atemnot bei respiratorischer Insuffizienz II. – Ohne Bronchialobstruktion. *Beil. Bayerischen Aerzteblatt*, **33,** 47

Casali, L., Pozzi, E., Rampulla, C. and Serra, R. (1977). Psychotropic drugs. Influence on respiratory function. *Int. J. Clin. Pharmacol.*, **15,** 480

Kronenberg, R. S., Cosio, M. G., Stevenson, J. E. and Drage, C. W. (1975). The use of oral diazepam in patients with obstructive lung disease and hypercapnia. *Ann. Int. Med.*, **83,** 83

Puritz, R., Henderson, M. A., Baker, S. N. and Chamberlain, D. A. (1977). Ventricular arrhythmias caused by prenylamine. *Br. Med. J.*, **1977/II**, 608
Satter, P. (1978). Die Embolektomie bei Lungenembolie. In Schlegel, B. (ed.), *Verhandlungen 84. Kongress Deutsche Gesellschaft für Innere Medizin, Wiesbaden, Apr. 1978*, pp. 356–366. (München: Bergmann)
Wesley, A. G., Thambiran, A. K., Pather, M. and Cronje, C. J. (1978). Continuous positive pressure ventilation in children with broncho-pneumonia. *Anaesthesia*, **33**, 466

Rheumatic disorders

Anonymous (1974). Therapy for stiff shoulder, lumbago, and dorsodynia. *Jpn. Med. J.*, **2642**, 132
Bach, G. L. (1979). Die medikamentöse Therapie der Arthrosen. *Euromedicine*, **19**, 13
Bayley, T. R. and Haslock, I. (1976). Night medication in rheumatoid arthritis. *J. R. Coll. Gen. Pract.*, **26**, 591
Benini, A. and Pinkepank, H. (1976). Lumbago und Ischias. – Umgang mit Patienten bei Bandscheibenerkrankungen der Lendenwirbelsäule. *Praxis*, **65**, 1323
Benini, A. (1977). Behandlungsrichtlinien für Patienten mit Bandscheibenerkrankungen der Lendenwirbelsäule. *Med. Mschr.*, **31**, 487
Bremer, C. and Leickert, K. H. (1976). Therapeutische Aspekte bei akuter Lumbago. *Med. Welt.*, **27**, 1351
Downie, W. W. and Wright, V. (1977). Choice of anti-inflammatory drugs in the rheumatic diseases. *Practitioner*, **219**, 463
Hart, F. D. (1976). The use of psychotropic drugs in rheumatology. *J. Int. Med. Res.*, **4, Suppl. 2**, 15
Hart, F. D. (1976). Which antirheumatic drug. *Drugs*, **11**, 451
Haslock, I. (1978). Keep it safe and simple when treating rheumatoid arthritis. *Mod. Med.*, **23**, 7
Hiedl, P. and Struppler, A. (1978). Therapie des Kreuzschmerzes und der Ischialgie. *Pharmakother.*, **1**, 27
Hobkirk, D., Rhodes, M. and Haslock, I. (1977). Night medication in rheumatoid arthritis. – II. Combined therapy with indomethacin and diazepam. *Rheum. Rehab.*, **16**, 125
Jacquot, F. (1977). Utilisation de l'effet myorelaxant du diazépam en pratique rhumatologique. *Gaz. Méd. Fr.*, **84**, 2747
Josenhans, G., Netter, K. J., Schmidt, K. L. and Wittenborg, A. (1977). Chronisch rheumatische Erkrankungen. Wer behandelt heute wie? *Med. Trib.*, **10**, 20
Kay, N. R. (1976). Clinical diagnosis and management of pain in the neck and arms. *Update*, **13**, 1019
Kugler, J. (1977). Therapie des Lumbago-Syndroms. 5. *Fortbildungsveranstaltung in Neurologie und Psychiatrie für niedergelassene Aerzte aller Fachgebiete*, Erlangen, 26–27. März. *Medizin*, **5**, 680
Lequesne, M. (1978). Le traitement de la lombalgie et de la lombo-sciatique communes. *Méd. Hyg.*, **36**, 1313, 4245
Loretan, G. (1975). Ergebnisse der klinischen Prüfung von Matalgon. *Diss.*, Bern, pp. 28
Müller, W. (1975). Therapie psychosomatischer Schmerzsyndrome des Bewegungs-

apparates. Pharmakotherapie und Physiotherapie. In Weintraub, A., Battegay, R., Beck, D., Kaganas, G., Labhardt, F. and Müller, W. (eds.). *Symp. Psyche und Rheuma*, Basel, Mai 1974, pp. 208–210 (Basel: Schwabe)
Paul, F. (1977). Medikamentöse Behandlung und Physiotherapie der lumbalen Nervenwurzel-Irritation. *Berl. Aerztek.*, **14,** 381
Popert, A. J. (1977). Drugs used in rheumatic diseases. *Physiotherapy*, **63,** 124
Rampon, S. and Leroy, V. (1975). Etude clinique du Valium en rhumatologie. *Rev. Méd. Clerm.-Ferr.*, **5,** 361
Satoyoshi, E., Murakami, K., Kokubu, T., Morita, S., Oinuma, S., Nozue, H., Nakanishi, T., Sugaha, A., Yoshitake, S., Kowa, H., Takagi, Y. and Adachibara, K. (1975). Comparative efficacy of muscalm (tolperisone hydrochloride) and diazepam in scapulohumeral periarthritis. *Strides Med.*, **93,** 78
Schaer, J. (1979). Medikamentöse Behandlung von Lumboischialgien. *Praxis*, **68,** 141
Schneider, H. (1976). Die psycho-pharmakotherapeutischen Möglichkeiten für das Wohlbefinden am Arbeitsplatz aus der Sicht des Allgemeinarztes. *Arbeitsmed. Soz. Med. Präv. Med.*, **11,** 271
Schrott, A. (1976). Diazepam bei akuter Lumbago. Vorteile einer Kombinationstherapie. *Aerztl. Prax.*, **28,** 741
Sharma, B. K. and Haslock, I. (1978). Night medication in rheumatoid arthritis. III. The use of Sulindac. *Curr. Med. Res. Opin.*, **5,** 472
Snader, T. C. (1974). Inflammatory disorders. III. Clinical management. *Am. J. Pharm.*, **146,** 169
Straube, W. (1976). Der Rheumakranke als Problem des Neuropsychiaters. *Therapiewoche*, **26,** 3260
Weintraub, A. (1977). Zur Psychosomatik der Epikondylitis. *Ther. Umsch.*, **34,** 96
Wieck, H. H. (1977). Diagnose und Therapie lumbaler Schmerzsyndrome in Praxis und Klinik. *Med. Welt*, **28,** 1365
Zeidler, H., Ritter, J. and Freyberger, H. (1977). Zur Psychosomatik des Weichteilrheumatismus. *Notabene Medici*, **7,** 23

Sexual disorders

Cooper, A. (1978). Drugs in the treatment of sexual inadequacy. Part I. *Br. J. Sex. Med.*, **5,** 32
Duddle, M. (1978). A GP's guide to the management of psychosexual problems. *Mims Mag.*, **2,** 351
Haslam, M. T. (1978). Depression and anxiety in relation to psychosexual disorder. *Br. J. Sex. Med.*, **5,** 29
Joel, C. A. (1978). The pathogenesis and therapy of impotentia coeundi with particular regard to diazepine derivatives. In Hasegawa, T., Hayashi, M. *et al.* (eds.), *Fertility and Sterility. Proc. 7th World Congr. Oct. 1972*, (*Tokyo and Kyoto*), pp. 206–209. (Amsterdam: Excerpta Med. and New York: Elsevier)
Pasini, E. (1978). Traitements psychothérapeutique et pharmacothérapeutique associés dans la thérapie de l'impuissance psychogène. *Praxis*, **67,** 1185
Reckless, J. and Geiger, N. (1975). Impotence as a practical problem. *Disease-A-Month*, **1975,** 1

10

Clinical Experience with Benzodiazepines in Neurological Disorders

T. R. Browne and R. G. Feldman

A large number of benzodiazepines have undergone clinical trials for a wide variety of neurological disorders. This chapter is confined to the three principal uses of benzodiazepines for neurological disorders in the United States. These are: (1) clonazepam as a chronic oral antiepileptic drug, (2) intravenous diazepam for status epilepticus, and (3) diazepam for spasticity.

Clonazepam for epilepsy

Mechanism of action

Benzodiazepines suppress most forms of paroxysmal activity on the electroencephalogram (EEG)[5, 8]. Generalized EEG abnormalities are more readily suppressed than are focal EEG abnormalities[5, 8]. These observations are presumably due to the ability of benzodiazepines to enhance polysynaptic inhibitory processes at all levels of the central nervous system[24].

The ultimate mechanism of the antiepileptic action of benzodiazepines presumably involves action upon neurotransmitters and/or cell membranes. The most likely hypothesis at the present time is that benzodiazepines facilitate the action of postsynaptic GABA receptors[16] (see Chapter 4).

Indications

Absence (petit mal) seizures

In a large double-blind randomized collaborative study coordinated by the US National Institutes of Health, clonazepam was compared with ethosuximide in the longterm treatment of absence seizures[22]. Both drugs were found to be extremely effective. In another double-blind study, Chandra[9] randomly assigned 39 patients to receive clonazepam or diazepam as the sole anti-epileptic drug for absence seizures. The clonazepam group had significantly ($p<0.0001$) greater reduction in seizure frequency and in 3 Hz spike-wave discharges on follow-up EEGs. A single-blind crossover study with sequential analysis comparing clonazepam with placebo showed clonazepam to be significantly ($p<0.05$) better than placebo in 10 trials[18]. In addition, there are at least 34 published uncontrolled studies of clonazepam for absence seizures, and they almost invariably report a favourable response.

Atypical absence (atypical petit mal) seizures

Two small double-blind studies and a large (21 patients) uncontrolled study where clonazepam was used as an adjunct to other anti-epileptic drug therapy reported that atypical absence seizures were completely controlled in 38 to 100% of patients and were reduced in frequency by 50% or more in 75–100% of patients[7].

Myoclonic seizures

In a double-blind cross-over study of clonazepam versus placebo as adjunctive anti-epileptic drugs, 12 of 15 patients receiving clonazepam had complete abolition of myoclonic seizures, and the other 3 had some improvement[20]. None of the 15 patients improved while on placebo. Four uncontrolled studies of clonazepam as an adjunctive anti-epileptic drug with 9 or more patients reported that myoclonic seizures were completely controlled in 20 to 33% of patients and were reduced in frequency by 50% or more in 57 to 100% of patients[6].

Infantile spasms (infantile myoclonic, massive spasms, salaam seizures)

Five uncontrolled studies with 12 or more patients using clonazepam as an adjunct to other anti-epileptic therapy reported that infantile spasms were completely controlled in 12 to 37% of patients and that a 50% or greater reduction in seizure frequency was obtained in 21–75% of patients[6].

Atonic (akinetic, drop attack) seizures

Three uncontrolled studies with 10 or more patients taking clonazepam as an adjunctive anti-epileptic drug reported atonic seizures were completely controlled in 0 to 30% of patients and were reduced in frequency by 50% or more in 49–90% of patients[7].

Elementary partial (focal motor) seizures

In a single-blind study using sequential analysis, clonazepam proved significantly ($p<0.05$) more effective than placebo for treatment of elementary partial seizures[18]. In 7 uncontrolled studies with 10 or more patients who took clonazepam as an adjunctive anti-epileptic drug, elementary partial seizures were completely controlled in 9 to 100% of patients and were reduced in frequency by 50% or more in 63 to 100% of patients[6].

Complex partial (psychomotor, temporal lobe) seizures

In a small (7 patients) double-blind study[1] of clonazepam versus placebo as adjunctive anti-epileptic drugs for complex partial seizures, 3 patients had 100% seizure control and 5 patients had 50% or greater seizure control while on clonazepam. Two patients had complete seizure control and 5 patients had no significant improvement while on placebo. In a single-blind cross-over study with sequential analysis, clonazepam proved preferable to placebo ($p<0.05$) as an adjunctive therapy for complex partial seizures after 21 patients[2]. Seven large (17 or more patients) uncontrolled studies of clonazepam as an anti-epileptic adjunct have reported complete suppression of complex partial seizures in 26 to 47% (median 34%) of patients and a 50% or greater reduction in 35 to 89% (median 65%) of patients[5].

Tonic–clonic (grand mal) seizures

Studies of the efficacy of clonazepam for tonic–clonic seizures have yielded conflicting results. In two double-blind comparisons of clonazepam with placebo as adjunctive anti-epileptic drugs, the clonazepam group had a greater reduction in seizure frequency in one study[20], and the placebo group had a greater reduction in the other study[12] (R. G. Feldman, written communication, March 26, 1977). Sixteen large uncontrolled studies have yielded varying results[5].

Toxicity

Common side-effects

Six studies with 50 or more patients report side-effects with clonazepam in 13 to 91% (median 46%) of patients, requiring discontinuance of the drug in 9 to 26%[5]. The three most common side-effects are drowsiness, ataxia, and behaviour changes. Twelve studies with 50 or more patients report drowsiness in 3 to 85% (median 33%) of patients and ataxia in 4 to 79% (median 13%) of patients[6]. Co-administration of a barbiturate may add to patient drowsiness[6]. The drowsiness and ataxia caused by clonazepam tend to be dose-related, to occur early in the course of administration, and to subside with chronic administration. Drowsiness and ataxia can usually be reduced to tolerable levels by decreasing the dosage of clonazepam.

Behavioural disturbances caused by clonazepam occur in a minority of patients, usually children. Affected children are described as hyperactive[5]. The frequency of this complication ranges from 2 to 52% (median 15%) of patients[6]. Behavioural disturbances can be reduced to tolerable levels in some patients by reducing the dosage of clonazepam. Clonazepam is a potent sedative and can improve the behaviour of some patients[6].

Other not uncommon side-effects of clonazepam include hypotonia, dizziness and thick speech. Hypersalivation and bronchial hypersecretion can create respiratory difficulties in children[5]. Both anorexia and increased appetite have been reported with clonazepam[6]. Uncommon side-effects of clonazepam include increased seizure frequency and thrombocytopenia[6].

Clinical pharmacology

Clinical pharmacokinetics

Peak serum concentrations of clonazepam occur 1 to 3 hours after oral administration[7]. Clonazepam is 47% protein-bound in man[6]. The elimination halflife of clonazepam is 20–40 hours in most persons[7]. The serum concentration produced by a given dose of clonazepam is quite variable, and one cannot accurately predict serum clonazepam concentration from dosage[6].

Therapeutic and toxic serum concentration

Most patients whose seizure are controlled with clonazepam have serum concentrations of 5–70 ng/ml[6]. Unfortunately, the serum concentrations of patients who do not respond to clonazepam and/or have side-effects with clonazepam also usually fall in the same range[7]. Thus there is no clear-cut minimum therapeutic serum concentration or usual toxic serum concentration.

Dosage and administration

The initial dose for infants and children (up to 10 years of age or 30 kg of body weight) should be 0.01 to 0.03 but not in excess of 0.05 mg kg^{-1} day^{-1} given in two or three divided doses. Dosage should be increased by no more than 0.25 to 0.5 mg every three to seven days until a daily maintenance dose of 0.1 to 0.2 mg/kg of body weight has been reached, unless seizures are controlled or side-effects preclude further increase. The initial dose for adults should not exceed 1.5 mg/day divided into three doses. Dosage may be increased in increments of 0.5 mg every three to seven days until seizures are adequately controlled or side-effects preclude any further increase. Maximum daily dose in adults is 20 mg. It is usually best to wait at least 7 days between increases in dosage of clonazepam in order to allow steady-state serum concentrations to be reached and the full therapeutic and toxic effects of the increase to be appreciated. More rapid increase in clonazepam dosage is possible in emergency situations, but carries a greater risk of side-effects. Tonic–clonic status epilepticus can occur when clonazepam is abruptly discontinued[5], and it is prudent to withdraw the drug slowly.

Diazepam for status epilepticus

Indications

The objectives in treating status epilepticus are to support vital functions, to treat the precipitating factors, and to administer a loading dose of a long-acting anti-epileptic drug. Intravenous diazepam has a relatively brief duration of action, is not a definitive therapy for status epilepticus, and can cause side-effects. However, because intravenous diazepam transiently produces high plasma and brain concentrations of the drug, diazepam can be a helpful adjunct in the treatment of status epilepticus. Intravenous diazepam is indicated for status epilepticus: (1) if generalized tonic–clonic activity has been going on without interruption for more than a few minutes, (2) if a tonic–clonic seizure occurs in a postictal patient who is being evaluated and is receiving a loading dose of a long-acting anti-epileptic drug, and (3) if continuing non-convulsive seizure activity (e.g. absence, complex partial) represents a serious threat to the patient. The effectiveness of diazepam in controlling various types of status epilepticus is documented in Table 10.1.

Table 10.1 Summary of reported effectiveness of diazepam in various types of status epilepticus*

			Effects on status epilepticus		
Type of status epilepticus	*No. of reports*	*No. of patients*	*No effect*	*Temporary control*	*Lasting control*
Tonic–clonic	19	188	23 (12%)	37 (20%)	128 (68%)
Secondarily generalized tonic–clonic	6	38	4 (10%)	6 (16%)	28 (74%)
Focal motor (including unilateral and Jacksonian)	17	103	13 (13%)	15 (15%)	75 (73%)
Absence (petit mal)	10	30	2 (7%)	3 (10%)	25 (83%)
Myoclonic	9	28	4 (14%)	4 (14%)	20 (71%)
Complex partial (psychomotor, temporal lobe)	4	8	2 (25%)	1 (13%)	5 (62%)
Tonic	4	8	3 (38%)	0	5 (62%)
Clonic	3	9	1 (11%)	0	8 (89%)
Hemiclonic	2	22	2 (9%)	6 (27%)	14 (64%)
Infantile myoclonic	2	5	0	4 (80%)	1 (20%)

*Reproduced from reference 8 with the kind permission of the publishers

Contra-indications and warnings

Diazepam is contra-indicated in patients with known hypersensitivity to the drug, acute angle glaucoma and open angle glaucoma. Because of possible cardiorespiratory depression, extreme care must be taken in administering intravenous diazepam to the elderly, the very ill, patients with limited pulmonary reserve, patients in shock, and patients who have received sedative drugs (including alcohol).

Probably the most common, and most dangerous, error made in the management of status epilepticus is to treat repeated seizures with repeated doses of intravenous diazepam without definitively treating the precipitating factors and without administering an adequate loading dose of a long-acting anti-epileptic drug. In this situation, the patient will continue to seize, toxic concentrations of diazepam and/or diazepam metabolites will accumulate, and serious morbidity may result from diazepam overdosage.

Pharmacokinetics

EEG studies indicate that serum diazepam concentrations of at least 0.5μg/ml are needed to control interictal paroxysmal activity on the EEG[3]. Injection of 10mg of diazepam intravenously in adults produced peak serum concentrations of 0.3 to 2.0 (mean 0.9)μg/ml in the study of Booker and Celesia[3]. Injection of 20mg of diazepam intravenously in adults produced a mean serum concentration of 1.6μg/ml in the study of Hillestad *et al.*[14]. The clearance of diazepam from the serum follows a biphasic curve. Immediately after an intravenous injection of diazepam the 'distribution phase' ($\alpha - t_{\frac{1}{2}}$) halflife of the serum concentration is 16 to 90 minutes[3,17]. The later 'elimination phase' ($\beta - t_{\frac{1}{2}}$) halflife of diazepam is much slower[3,17]. Serum diazepam concentrations decrease by 34 to 50% during the first 20 minutes after intravenous injection and decrease by 62 to 72% during the first 2 hours after an intravenous injection[3,14,15]. This rapid clearance of diazepam from the serum after an intravenous injection during the distribution phase probably accounts for the frequent recurrence of seizure activity when diazepam alone is used to control status epilepticus[8].

Animal work indicates that maximum brain parenchyma diazepam concentration is reached 1 minute after the end of an intravenous infusion and that the brain parenchyma concentration of diazepam falls rapidly at a rate which closely parallels the fall of serum diazepam concentration[7]. The brain parenchyma concentrations of phenytoin and phenobarbital rise more slowly after an intravenous injection of drug, but the brain concentrations tend to remain relatively constant despite falling serum concentrations[7]. These observations provide a pharmacokinetic basis for the frequently employed therapeutic strategy of initial use of intravenous diazepam to effect immediate seizure control followed by prompt administration of a loading dose of phenytoin or phenobarbital to maintain seizure control when the serum and brain concentrations of diazepam fall below the therapeutic range[7].

Intramuscular diazepam should not be used to treat status epilepticus because the onset of action is too slow and because even large doses may not produce serum concentrations of diazepam which are effective against epilepsy[7].

Dosage and administration

The usual initial adult dosage of diazepam for tonic–clonic status epilepticus is 5 to 10 mg intravenously at a rate of no more than 5 mg per minute. In children 5 years of age or older the recommended dose is 1 mg every 2 to 5 minutes up to a maximum of 10 mg. In infants over 30 days of age and children under 5 years of age the recommended dosage is 0.2 to 0.5 mg slowly every 2 to 5 minutes up to a maximum of 5 mg. The efficacy and safety of parenteral diazepam has not been established in infants 30 days or less of age.

Because diazepam for injection is an irritative substance, it should not be administered into small veins and care should be taken to avoid extravasation or intra-arterial injection. Diazepam should not be mixed with intravenous fluids.

Toxicity

The most worrisome complications of intravenous diazepam are respiratory depression and hypotension. In an earlier review[8] the author found 26 cases of respiratory depression and/or cardiac depression among 401 cases of various types of status epilepticus treated with diazepam. The incidence of cardiorespiratory depression is probably greater when diazepam is given in combination with other depressant drugs[8]. Animal work indicates that some of the adverse cardiorespiratory effects of intravenous diazepam (and also intravenous phenytoin) may be due to the propylene glycol solvent used in preparing the drug. Other less serious side-effects of intravenous diazepam include: drowsiness, ataxia, dysarthria, confusion, paradoxical excitement, and diplopia.

Diazepam for spasticity

Mechanism of action

The proposed mechanism of action of diazepam for spasticity for which there is the most evidence involves the inhibitory neurotransmitter GABA[12,16]. Benzodiazepines appear to interact with a specific benzodiazepine receptor. This interaction in turn increases the effect of GABA receptors (i.e. increases chloride permeability of membrane with GABA receptors). This in turn increases the presynaptic inhibition effects of GABA. Such an increase in presynaptic inhibition would decrease the excitatory inputs to spinal motor neurones.

Diazepam is postulated to have sites of therapeutic action in the limbic system[4]. Diazepam may thus reduce muscle tension due to anxiety.

Diazepam has been reputed to diminish electrically elicited mono- and polysynaptic reflexes[11]. There is also evidence that diazepam may depress fusimotor activity[11].

Indications

There is evidence that diazepam is effective for spasticity due to a variety of causes including: cerebral lesions (e.g. cerebral palsy), complete and incomplete spinal cord transections, multiple sclerosis, and reflex spasm due to local pathology (e.g. inflammation or trauma of muscles or joints)[10,11,13,21,23]. Diazepam is also useful in several other disorders associated with increased muscle tone including athetosis, stiff-man syndrome, and tetanus.

Dosage

The usual starting dose is 5 to 10mg. This is followed by 5 to 10mg every 4 hours as necessary. Larger doses may be required for tetanus.

Toxicity

Drowsiness, fatigue and ataxia are the side-effects that are commonly encountered with chronic diazepam therapy for spasticity. A hyperexcitable state occasionally occurs, especially in children. A confusional state sometimes occurs in older persons taking diazepam chronically. These side-effects may limit the dose of diazepam which can be given and may limit the usefulness of the drug.

Acknowledgement

Supported in part by the Veterans Administration.

References

1. Bensch, J., Blennow, G., Ferngren, H., Gamstorp, I., Herrlin, K. M., Kubista, J., Arvidsson, A. and Dahlström, H. (1977). A double blind study of clonazepam in the treatment of therapy-resistant epilepsy in children. *Dev.Med. Child Neurol.*, **19**, 355
2. Birket-Smith, E., Lund, M., Mikkelsen, B., Vestermark, S., Zander Olsen, P.

and Holm, P. (1973). A controlled trial of Ro 5-4023 (clonazepam) in the treatment of psychomotor epilepsy. *Acta Neurol. Scand.*, **49** (Suppl. 53) 18
3. Booker, H. E. and Celesia, G. G. (1973). Serum concentration of diazepam in subjects with epilepsy. *Arch. Neurol.*, **29**, 191
4. Brazier, M. A., Crandall, P. H. and Walsh, G. O. (1976). Enhancement of EEG lateralizing signs in temporal lobe epilepsy: A trial of diazepam. *Exp. Neurol.*, **51**, 241
5. Browne, T. R. (1976). Clonazepam: A review of a new anticonvulsant drug. *Arch. Neurol.*, **33**, 326
6. Browne, T. R. (1978). Clonazepam. *N. Engl. J. Med.*, **299**, 812
7. Browne, T. R. (1979). Drug therapy of status epilepticus. *Drug Ther. Rev.*, **2**, 449
8. Browne, T. R. and Penry, J. K. (1973). Benzodiazepines in the treatment of epilepsy: A review. *Epilepsia (Amsterdam)*, **14**, 277
9. Chandra, B. (1973). Clonazepam in the treatment of petit mal. *Asian J. Med.*, **9**, 433
10. Cook, J. B. and Nathan, P. W. (1967). On the site of action of diazepam in spasticity in man. *J. Neurol. Sci.*, **5**, 33
11. Davidoff, R. A. (1978). Pharmacology of spasticity. *Neurology*, **28**, 46
12. Feldman, R. G. (1976). Chlorazepate in temporal lobe epilepsy. *J. Am. Med. Assoc.*, **236**, 2603
13. Greenblatt, D. J. and Shader, R. I. (1974). *Benzodiazepines in Clinical Practice*. (New York: Raven Press)
14. Hillestad, L., Hansen, T., Melsom, H. and Drivenes, A. (1974). Diazepam metabolism in normal man: 1. Serum concentrations and clinical effects after intravenous, intramuscular, and oral administration. *Clin. Pharmacol. Ther.*, **16**, 479
15. Kaplan, S. A., Jack, M. L., Alexander, K. and Weinfeld, R. E. (1973). Pharmacokinetic profile of diazepam following single intravenous and chronic oral administrations. *J. Pharm. Sci.*, **62**, 1789
16. Karobath, M. (1979). Molecular basis of benzodiazepine action. *Trends Neurosci.*, **2**, 166
17. Klotz, V., Antoinin, K. H. and Bieck, P. R. (1976). Pharmacokinetics and plasma binding of diazepam in man, dog, rabbit, guinea pig, and rat. *J. Pharmacol. Exp. Ther.*, **199**, 67
18. Mikkelsen, B., Birket-Smith, E., Holm, P., Lund, M., Vestermark, S. and Olsen, P. Z. (1975). A controlled trial of clonazepam (Ro 5-4023, Rivotril (R)) in the treatment of focal epilepsy and secondarily generalized grand mal epilepsy. *Acta Neurol. Scand.*, **Suppl. 60**, 55
19. Mikkelsen, B., Birket-Smith, E., Brandt, S., Holm, P., Lund, M., Thorn, I., Vestermark, S. and Olsen, P. Z. (1976). Clonazepam in the treatment of epilepsy: A controlled clinical trial in simple absence, bilateral massive epileptic myoclonus and atonic seizures. *Arch. Neurol.*, **33**, 322
20. Nanda, R., Keogh, H. D., Lambie, D., Johnson, R. H., Melville, I. D. and Morrice, G. D. (1976). The effects of clonazepam upon epilepsy control and plasma levels of other anticonvulsants. In Janz, D. (ed.), *Epileptology: Proceedings of the Seventh International Symposium on Epilepsy*, pp. 145–151. (Stuttgart: Thieme)
21. Neill, R. W. K. (1964). Diazepam in the relief of muscle spasm resulting from spinal-cord lesions. *Ann. Phys. Med.* (Suppl.), 33

22. Sato, S., Penry, J. K., Dreifuss, F. E. and Dyken, P. R. (1977). Clonazepam in the treatment of absence seizures: A double-blind clinical trial. *Neurology (Minneap.)*, **27**, 371
23. Verrier, M., MacLeod, S. and Ashby, P. (1975). The effects of diazepam on presynaptic inhibition in patients with complete and incomplete spinal cord lesions. *Can. J. Neurol. Sci.*, **2**, 179
24. Young, A. B., Zukin, S. R. and Snyder, S. H. (1974). Interaction of benzodiazepines with central glycine receptors: Possible mechanism of action. *Proc. Natl. Acad. Sci. USA*, **71**, 2246

11

The Use of Clonazepam on Patients with Generalized Epilepsy

M. P. Lison and J. G. Speciali

This paper is a report on experience in the use of clonazepam (Rivotril) in the treatment of primary and secondary generalized epilepsies in children.

Summary

Improvement was observed in twelve patients with daily epileptic manifestations of absence seizures (five with simple absences, two with automatic absences and five with myoclonic absences). Two patients had not been treated with the usual drugs prior to the investigation (one with simple absences and the other with automatic absences). In the case of eleven patients observed from two to ten months, there was a decrease or control of seizures.

At the start of the therapeutic study, seizures were controlled in seven patients (four with simple absences, two with automatic absences and one with myoclonic absences). By the end of the observation period, four patients (two with simple absences and two with automatic absences) remained free from seizures. Of the eight remaining patients, the condition of one patient with myoclonic absences remained unchanged, two (one with simple absences and the other with myoclonic absences) showed a reduction of 50 to 75% in the frequency of seizures, and five showed a reduction greater than 75%.

As part of the study of the treatment of epileptic manifestations of the Lennox–Gastaut syndrome, the action of clonazepam was evaluated in the case of tonic, clonic, myoclono-atonic and atonic seizures and atypical absences.

Control of tonic seizures was achieved in five cases, improvement in six cases, deterioration in two cases, and in three cases the incidence of seizures remained unaltered. Control or improvement of clonic seizures was obtained in two cases, but the condition of another patient remained unaffected. Myoclono-atonic and atonic seizures were controlled in five cases, improved in four, remained unchanged in four and deteriorated in two. Such seizures appeared for the first time during treatment with clonazepam in three cases.

Atypical absences were reduced in frequency in one case, increased in frequency in another case, remained unchanged in two cases and appeared for the first time during treatment with clonazepam in another two cases.

These effects were compared empirically with those obtained with diazepam, nitrazepam, barbiturates and diphenylhydantoin.

Methods

Primary generalized epilepsy

We investigated *12 patients* (eight male with a diagnosis of absences), suffering daily seizures. Eleven were aged from 5 to 15, and one was aged 30. Five suffered from simple absences, while seven were affected by complex absences. Of the latter, two showed automatic absences and the other five myoclonic absences. The inclusion of each of these patients was made only after personal observation of at least one seizure.

Before treatment with clonazepam, ten patients (four with simple absences, one with automatic absences and five with myoclonic absences) had been treated with other drugs (ethosuximide, diones, barbiturates, diazepam and nitrazepam) without showing improvement. Diazepam or nitrazepam, in particular, had been administered to two patients with simple absences and three with myoclonic absences. The effects of the antiepileptic medication that had been used previously were evaluated after at least one month of observation. When the ineffectiveness of the previous treatment had been confirmed, clonazepam was added in association and the former medication either maintained at the same dosage or reduced.

The daily dosage of benzodiazepine compound did not exceed 0.10 mg per kg body weight and was given in divided dose at 8-hour intervals.

The evaluation of the number of seizures before and after the different phases of treatment was performed using a diary kept by family members. Special emphasis was laid on the need for continuous vigilance.

The duration of the study was seven to ten months in the case of patients with simple absences, two to eight months for those with automatic absences, five to ten months for four patients with myoclonic absences, and only three weeks in the case of a patient with myoclonic absences.

Secondary generalized epilepsy

We also investigated the action of clonazepam in the treatment of epileptic manifestations (tonic, clonic, myoclono-atonic, atonic seizures, or atypical absence) in *29 patients* with Lennox–Gastaut syndrome (22 of whom were without a previous history of the West syndrome). This report was part of a broader clinical electroencephalographic study.

All patients had at least two types of epileptic seizures daily. All, except one, were taking anti-epileptic medication (at least one benzodiazepine derivative and phenobarbital) when the investigation began. When a patient was being treated with more than two anti-epileptic drugs, one drug at a time was withdrawn over a period of not less than two weeks to observe changes in frequency and/or intensity of the different types of seizures. If the patient's condition deteriorated, the drug was reintroduced. Subsequently, one of the drugs being investigated was added and changes in the epileptic symptoms were recorded. When the patient did not show satisfactory improvement, the studied drug was replaced by another. A minimum interval of one week was observed between the withdrawal of one drug and the administration of another to avoid summation of therapeutic effects.

Only the changes that occurred during the first month following each change of treatment were considered because of the possibility of spontaneous changes in the patient's condition.

Clonazepam was administered in a divided daily dose of about 0.1 mg per kg body weight (every eight hours). The dose was kept within each individual's tolerance limits to avoid excessive sleepiness which would make it difficult to evaluate the number and intensity of the seizures. In the case of patients with night-time tonic seizures, higher doses were administered at night. In addition to clonazepam, the drugs used were phenobarbital, primidone, diphenylhydantoin, diazepam, nitrazepam, sodium dipropylacetate and ACTH.

Results

Primary generalized epilepsy

After the start of treatment with clonazepam we found: control of seizures in four of the five patients with simple absences, in the two with automatic absences, and in one of the five with myoclonic absences. One patient with simple absences and two with myoclonic absences showed a reduction of more than 75%. One patient with myoclonic absences showed a reduction from 50 to 75%, and another patient showed no change in his condition as a result of which the drug was suspended at the end of three weeks.

At the end of the investigation, the seizures were controlled in two patients with simple absences, the two with automatic absences, but not in those with myoclonic absences. A reduction of more than 75% was observed in two patients with simple absences and three with myoclonic absences.

One patient with simple absences and another with myoclonic absences experienced a reduction of 50 to 75% in the number of seizures.

Secondary generalized epilepsy

(1) *Tonic seizures.* Seizure control was obtained in five patients and an improvement of more than 50% in another six patients. The condition of three patients remained unchanged, while that of two deteriorated.

(2) *Clonic seizures.* Seizure control was obtained in one patient, improvement in another patient, and there was no change in a third patient.

(3) *Myoclono-atonic seizures.* Seizure control was obtained in two patients and an improvement of more than 50% in two others. Seizures remained unchanged in another two patients and appeared for the first time during treatment with clonazepam in another patient.

(4) *Atonic seizures.* Seizure control was achieved in three cases and there was an improvement of more than 50% in two further cases. There was no change in the incidence of seizures in two patients; the number increased in two cases, and seizures appeared for the first time during treatment in another two cases.

(5) *Atypical absences.* One patient showed an improvement of more than 50%. Incidence of seizures remained unchanged in two cases, increased in one case and occurred for the first time during the treatment in another two patients.

Evaluation of the results obtained with the 11 most mentally retarded patients, with no previous history of West syndrome, disclosed a greater frequency of unchanged condition: two patients with tonic seizures, one with myoclono-atonic seizures, two with atonic seizures, and one with atypical absences. The other results obtained were control of tonic seizures in one case and improvement of myoclono-atonic seizures in another case. Atypical absences appeared for the first time in one case.

Comments

Our findings show that the onset of therapeutic effect of clonazepam is prompt with significant reduction in the frequency of simple and complex absences despite the failure of previous treatments, not including valproic acid. There occurred, at the end of the investigation, a slight drop in the therapeutic effectiveness, unaffected by adjustment of dosage. Nevertheless, nine of the twelve patients remained controlled or had a reduction of more than 75% in their seizures. The effects observed in the case of patients with complex absences are very significant in view of the fact that ethosuximide does not, as a rule, cause any changes in the frequency of these seizures. Myoclonic absences are particularly resistant to the usual treatments.

The major disadvantage of clonazepam is the sleepiness that was observed in four cases. However, this side-effect, which was problematic in cases of children of school age, tends to subside with time. We observed no changes in liver and kidney functions, or in blood content.

Unlike diazepam and nitrazepam, clonazepam has a significant effect on all forms of epileptic seizures that occur in the Lennox–Gastaut syndrome. However, the results are generally better in the case of patients with a lesser degree of mental retardation or suffering from less 'primitive' types of epilepsy. Similar observations have been recorded by different authors[1–3,5,6].

The effect on atonic seizures is not uniform and different results occur in practically the same proportion: improvement, no change, deterioration or the appearance of seizures for the first time during treatment with clonazepam. This variation in effect has been mentioned by Oller-Daurella[4]. The extreme difficulty of control and the frequently traumatic consequence of these seizures make the use of clonazepam advisable despite the impossibility of foreseeing its effectiveness in individual cases. Deterioration of the patient's condition or the first appearance of atonic seizures are less frequent in the case of diazepam and nitrazepam usage.

The action of clonazepam is equivalent to that of diphenylhydantoin and superior to that of phenobarbital in the case of tonic seizures. The latter two drugs, however, cause a high frequency of deteriorating condition or occurrence of atonic seizures. Diazepam and nitrazepam can cause the number of tonic seizures to increase in many patients and diazepam can cause clonic seizures.

References

1. D'Onghia C., A., Luccas, F. J. C., Marques-Assis, L. and Lefèvre, A. B. (1973). Estudo clínico do Ro 5-4023 no tratamento de epilepsias. *Arq. Neuro-Psiq. (São Paulo)*, **31**, 21
2. Hanson, R. A. and Menkes, J. H. (1972). A new anticonvulsant in the management of minor motor seizures. *Dev. Med. Child Neurol.*, **14**, 3
3. Martin, D. and Hirt, H. R. (1973). Clinical experience with clonazepam (Rivotril) in the treatment of epilepsies in infancy and childhood. *Neuropédiatrie*, **4**, 245
4. Oller-Daurella, L. (1972). Experiencia con Ro 5-4023 en el tratamiento agudo y crónico de las diferentes crises epilépticas. Presented at the *Symposium Rivotril*, April, Marseille.
5. Rebollo, M. A. (1971). El Ro 5-4023 en el tratamiento de la epilepsia del niño. Presented at *III Panamerican Congress on Neurology*, 10–14th October, São Paulo.
6. Schlack, L., Clericus, J. and Novoa, F. (1971). Ensayo clínico con el preparado antiepiléptico Ro 5-4023 en niños. Presented at *III Panamerican Congress on Neurology*, 10–14th October, São Paulo.

Bibliography

Clonazepam in epilepsy

Bergamini, L., Mutani, R., Benna, P. and Dal Fiume, F. (1973). Ro 5-4023 – Un nuovo importante farmaco antiepilettico. *Acta Neurologica*, **31**, 4

Bielmann, P., Levac, T. and Gagnon, M. A. (1978). Clonazepam. Its efficacy in association with phenytoin and phenobarbital in mental patients with generalized major motor seizures. *Int. J. Clin. Pharmacol. Biopharm.*, **16**, 268

Browne, T. R. (1976). Clonazepam. A review of new anticonvulsant drug. *Arch. Neurol.*, **33**, 326

Browne, T. R. and Penry, J. K. (1973). Benzodiazepines in the treatment of epilepsy. *Epilepsia*, **14**, 277

Buecking, P. H. (1977). Elektroklinische Korrelationen während der antikonvulsiven Behandlung des Status epilepticus und chronischer Epilepsien fokaler Genese mit Clonazepam. *Schw. Arch. Neurol. Neurochir. Psychiat.*, **121**, 187

Buehr, P. A. (1970). A new benzodiazepine for epilepsy. In Lubis, D. B. (ed.), *Proc. of 1st Regional Seminar on Psychotropic Medication, Djakarta/Indonesia, March 23–28, 1970*, pp. 260–261, *Indones. Psychiat. Q.*, **3**, No. 3–4

Daurella, L. O. (1971). The present state of the treatment of absences. Presented at the *13th International Congress of Pediatrics*, August 29–September 4, Vienna.

Gastaut, H. (1973). Rapports sur l'activité antiépileptique d'une nouvelle benzodiazépine, le Ro 5-4023. Symposium de Marseille, 28 avril 1972. *Thérapeutique (Supplément de la Semaine des Hôpitaux)*, 49, No hors série, 5–6

Goldberger, E. (1975). Benzodiazépines et épilepsie. *Actual. Psychiat.*, **6**, 87

Groh, C. and Blankenhorn, V. (1971). Weitere Mitteilungen über die klinische Wirksamkeit von Clonazepam. In Kruse, R. (ed.), *Epilepsie*, pp. 37–40. (Stuttgart: Georg Thieme Verlag)

Groh, C. and Rosenmayr, F. (1975). Clonazepam in der Epilepsietherapie – eine Standortbestimmung. Presented at the *3rd International Symposium on Child Neurology*, June 18–20, Prague.

Ketz, E. (1971). Neueste Entwicklungen auf dem Gebiet der antiepileptischen Pharmakotherapie. In Kruse, R. (ed.), *Epilepsie*, pp. 20–30. (Stuttgart: Georg Thieme Verlag)

Kruse, R. (1971). Zusammenfassung und Diskussion der klinischen Erfahrungsberichte über Clonazepam Ro 5-4023. In Kruse, R. (ed.), *Epilepsie*, pp. 40–46. (Stuttgart: Georg Thieme Verlag)

Lagenstein, I. and Iffland, E. (1977). Die intravenöse Behandlung des Petit-Mal-Status mit Diazepam und Clonazepam. *Z. Elektroenzephalogr. Elektromyogr.*, **8**, 82

Leboulanger, J. (1973). Un nouvel anti-épileptique d'action polyvalente. Le Ro 5-4023 ou clonazépam. *Nouv. Presse Méd.*, **2**, 377

Lefevre, A. B. (1971). Perspectivas animadoras – clonazepam é a mais recente droga em experiência no tratamento do epiléptico. *Am. Rev. Atual. Med.*, **7**, 32

Leickert, K. H. (1979). Rivotril. – Das neue Antiepileptikum. Eine Uebersicht. *Therapiewoche*, **29**, 3408

Levratti, M. G. and Pastena, L. (1977). Studio comparativo dell'azione di alcune benzodiazepine (clonazepam, diazepam, nitrazepam). *Riv. Neurologia*, **47**, 282

Madalena, J. C. (1972). As benzodiazepinas no tratamento dos disturbios epilépticos. Presented at the *II Brazilian Congress of Psychiatry* October 1–7, Belo Horizonte.

Marinello, R. (1974). Considerazioni su un nuovo farmaco antiepilettico – clonazepam Ro 5-4023 Rivotril / Studio clinico e sperimentale Diss., Padova/ It. 1973–74, pp. 85

Moene, Y. and Courjon, J. (1972). Place des benzodiazépines dans le traitement des épilepsies. *Cahiers Médicaux Lyonnais*, **48,** 4271

Pinder, R. M., Brogden, R. N., Speight, T. M. and Avery, G. S. (1976). Clonazepam. A review of its pharmacological properties and therapeutic efficacy in epilepsy. *Drugs*, **12,** 321

Reuter, H. (1977). Rivotril (Clonazepam), ein neues Antiepileptikum. *Allg. Med.*, **53,** 463

Taylor, W. J., Mutchie, K. D., Meinhold, J. M. and Bowers, D. C. (1976). Clonazepam (Clonopin-Roche). *Drug Intelligence Clin. Pharm.*, **10,** 216

Van Huffelen, A. C. and Magnus, O. (1976). De behandeling van de status epilepticus met clonazepam. *Med. T. Geneesk.*, **120,** 1734

12

Benzodiazepines and Depression

J. A. Costa e Silva

Introduction

The use of anxiety-reducing drugs in the treatment of anxiety syndromes accompanied by depression or of depressive illness with an anxiety component has been extensively debated in recent times. Many workers in this field have written about the efficacy of treatment of patients with symptoms of neurosis characterized by anxiety and depression. According to some of these authors, neither the anxiety-reducing drugs nor the hypnosedatives have been very successful in the treatment of depression–anxiety syndromes. On the other hand, it has been shown that these drugs can lead to the development of acquired tolerance and habit formation, a problem involving the barbiturates especially and, to a lesser degree, the minor tranquillizers.

Emphasis has been placed on the fact that anxiety and depression tend to occur simultaneously in an anxiety–depression syndrome. Taking this frequent coincidence of anxiety and depression as our base, we will discuss the advantages and drawbacks of using tranquillizers when depression is seen in an anxious patient. Before proceeding with this, however, we would like to establish some basic concepts to provide a better understanding of this complex matter.

Concept of depression

According to Pierre Pichot, concepts of depression have undergone important modifications in recent years. Introduction of various types of antidepressant drugs, as well as research in cerebral biochemistry, stressing the role of the biogenic amines, have contributed to a better understanding of the phenomenon of depression. A rethinking of diagnostic criteria on a clinical and psychopathological basis has led to important innovations in concepts and terminology without abandoning the traditional foundation. The term depression has come to be used to mean either a symptom or a syndrome.

Diagnosis of the depressive syndrome is based principally on the presence of the depression symptom, that is, an alteration of mood or, in US terminology, an affective disturbance characterized by a pathological sadness, a pessimism, in which are found together a number of symptoms of different form; among these, the most characteristic are an impairment of thought (slowness, fixed idea of grief, etc.), changes in the motor behaviour patterns (usually a reduction but, sometimes, a sterile agitation), affective disturbances and anxiety, all these symptoms being accompanied generally by physiological modifications such as changes in sleep patterns, in appetite, loss of weight, cardiovascular disturbances.

Thus, in making a differential diagnosis, normal sadness and anxiety syndromes must also be taken into consideration.

Clinical types of depression

Robins, Guze, Winokur and associates have drawn a distinction between primary and secondary depression. They see the diagnosis of primary depression as depending, firstly, on the existence of a depressive syndrome, secondly on the absence in the antecedents of any psychic alteration except for depressive or manic occurrences and, thirdly, on the absence of any life-threatening or seriously disabling somatic disease.

Any other depressive syndrome not fulfilling these criteria would be called secondary depression, although secondary is not to be regarded as being synonymous with symptomatic.

Primary depressive syndrome can be either endogenous (manic-depressive psychosis, affective disease) or exogenous (psychogenic). Leonhard has described unipolar and bipolar forms of endogenous depression, and Angst and Perris have demonstrated that the symptomatology, evolution and biological and genetic characteristics of the two forms are different. The depressive phases of these two types, however, have the same characteristics. Primary exogenous depressive syndrome is subdivided into neurotic and reactive types of depression.

Different classifications of depression are given in the Diagnostic and Statistical Manual (DSM-III) of the American Psychiatric Association (1978) and in the ICD-9 of the World Health Organization, ninth revision.

Biochemical types of depression

Besides a clinically-based classification of depressions, some authors have proposed a biochemical classification based on the hypothesis of the central monoamines. Two types have been described: one is related to the depletion of noradrenaline and the second to a serotonin deficiency. The former is more suitably treated with desipramine or imipramine, whereas the latter is more appropriately treated with amitriptyline.

Thus, in recent times, we have witnessed an attempt to define the concept of depression on the basis of psychopathology, clinical experience, biochemistry, genetics and reaction to treatment.

Anxiety and depression

Recently, the question of whether anxiety and depression are two distinct entities or only different aspects of the same disease has been the subject of lengthy discussions.

In the past, one of the arguments most commonly used to support the contention that anxiety and depression are separate entities was the conviction that the reaction to treatment of the two disorders differed; in other words, that there existed anxiety-reducing and depression-reducing drugs.

This attitude has changed recently because it has come to be recognized that the drugs formerly prescribed for a single indication are capable of performing a double function, acting on both anxiety and depression. Even earlier, Claghorn had proposed the concept of a depression–anxiety syndrome based partly on these arguments stemming from therapeutic response.

A number of significant authors like Zung, Dorfman, Lindner, Kielholz, Pichot, Lewis and de Lerma came to the conclusion that, as long as anxiety is associated with a significant degree of depression, it can be classified as an anxiety–depression symptom complex; depression, however, in their view, can exist as a unique entity.

This contention has been disputed by other workers. Loo has put forward the view that psychotic depression without anxiety does not exist, while admitting that, in neuroses and other syndromes, anxiety can exist without depression.

For Lambert, the diagnosis of anxiety and depression should be independent but not differential; anxiety, in his opinion, is rarely found alone.

Another view is presented by Ragot who believes that the frequent confusion of anxiety and depression often results in inappropriate therapy. He is of the opinion that, while the majority of depressive conditions display an anxiety component, anxiety and depression are essentially different disorders.

Thus, it is clear that, even today, opinions are far from unanimous, even though it is generally agreed that anxiety often coincides with depression.

It was mentioned earlier that serotonin and noradrenaline play a role in depression and anxiety. It has been shown that certain centres of the GABAergic system are also involved. We know that the benzodiazepines act on GABAergic transmission. However, the presence of specific benzodiazepine receptors in the cortex, hippocampus and amygdalae has also been demonstrated with high concentrations having been shown to occur in the hippocampus. This would tend to support the argument in favour of an effect of benzodiazepines on depression by means of a GABAergic mechanism. The equally high concentrations of these receptors found in the cortex and in the diencephalic and mesencephalic structures suggest a direct role of these structures in the anxiety-reducing, sedative and anticonvulsant effects of the benzodiazepines.

Recently, Shulman and associates described the activity of erythrocyte catechol-*O*-methyl-transferase in patients with depressive disorders and states of anxiety.

The use of anxiety-reducing drugs in depression

The use of anxiety-reducing drugs in depression is a subject generating even more split in opinion than the question of the relation between anxiety and depression. For many authors, the use of anxiety-reducing drugs is contraindicated when depression is the dominant symptom of the actual disease. Other authors allow the use of some types of anxiety-reducing drugs in the treatment of the depression–anxiety syndrome. Kuhn, on the other hand, objects to the use of benzodiazepines in this case, and recommends the use of beta-blockers. Other authors, like Shammas, believe it to be perfectly possible to use the benzodiazepine anxiety-reducing drugs in depression–anxiety syndromes and that, furthermore, one of these benzodiazepines, bromazepam, may have an effect on depression as well as acting to reduce anxiety. Henry and colleagues, studying hospitalized patients, came to the conclusion that benzodiazepine tranquillizers are more effective than antidepressant drugs in relieving the depression–anxiety syndrome in short-term therapy.

From the work of Klein on the use of imipramine and chlorimipramine in the treatment of phobic and obsessive compulsive states, we also know that some tricyclic antidepressants exercise an effect on anxiety and in phenomena corresponding to the displacement of anxiety, as in situations of panic, phobias and obsessions. We also know of the anxiety-reducing effects produced by amitriptyline and maprotiline; this dual-action mechanism of the antidepressants can raise the question of a possible dual action of the anxiety-reducing drugs and invite speculation about the relation between those two phenomena.

From the foregoing, however, we can prepare some line of action:

(1) We do not believe that the use of anxiety-reducing drugs is absolutely contraindicated in cases where the patient presents depression;

(2) Anxiety-reducing drugs should be used in the depression–anxiety

syndromes when anxiety represents a certain importance in the clinical picture;

(3) The choice of anxiety-reducing drug may vary in accordance with the patient's reaction to the medication: in patients who become drowsy when taking benzodiazepines, it may be preferable to use meprobamate; for patients in whom it is difficult to induce sleep, we prefer the benzodiazepines; patients whose anxiety is translated into complaints of palpitations and tachycardia offer a sound indication for the use of beta-blockers;

(4) Dosage of the anxiety-reducing drugs should be individualized for each patient;

(5) We do not believe that the adequate use of anxiety-reducing drugs can accentuate thoughts of suicide;

(6) In depression–anxiety syndromes, the anxiety-reducing drug should always be used in combination with antidepressants because, in our opinion, an anxiolytic alone exerts insufficient antidepressant effect;

(7) Such a combined therapy can comprise a fixed combination (like Limbitrol), or free combination of anxiety-reducing and antidepressant agents. In the more serious cases of depression, the latter form should be preferred because it permits a more balanced use of one drug in relation to the other, whereas the fixed combination should be preferred in cases of anxious depression, neuroses or so-called 'masked depressions'.

Benzodiazepines and depression

The benzodiazepines, a group of drugs with a potent anxiety-reducing effect, are being prescribed in the treatment of anxiety syndromes, epilepsy, sleep disturbances, psychosomatic disorders, etc. Their use in the depression syndromes with elements of anxiety, however, is more recent. One of these drugs, bromazepam (Lexotanil), has been shown to possess an antidepressant component. A placebo-controlled study was conducted by Shammas to compare bromazepam and amitriptyline, a tricyclic antidepressant of proven efficacy.

The study was carried out with 72 patients diagnosed as anxious–depressive to moderate or severe degree. Assessment was made by means of the Brief Psychiatry Rating Scales (BPRS) and the Hamilton Psychiatric Rating Scale for Depression, conducted at the beginning of treatment and at weekly intervals thereafter. The conclusion of the investigator was that more patients improved with bromazepam than with amitriptyline. Bromazepam was also superior to amitriptyline in the degree of improvement obtained and in causing fewer side-effects. The statistical difference of 0.05

of the alterations observed after one week was even greater after four weeks, especially with regard to the BPRS items of somatic aspect, depression, anxiety and tension, as well as in almost all of the representative psychic and somatic symptoms of the depression scale which, combined, provided an overall evaluation.

Thus, bromazepam can, from now on, very appropriately be prescribed for depression in which there is an element of anxiety. As a combined dosage form, we have Lexpiride, a combination of bromazepam and sulpiride, a neuroleptic agent with antidepressant, anxiety-reducing and antiemetic properties. The two substances are complementary in effect and are well tolerated, even in high dosage.

We now also know that the benzodiazepines can be combined with the tricyclics as they do not induce metabolic interference. According to Silvermann and Braithwaite: 'The benzodiazepines do not interfere with the plasma levels of the antidepressants of the tricyclic groups and, for that reason, should be preferred when there is need of an anxiety-reducing drug during the treatment of depressives.'

Since the depressive disorders are rarely observed without severe insomnia and are also frequently accompanied by anxiety and hyperactivity, it is common to prescribe hypnotics and sedatives together with the antidepressant drugs. According to the studies carried out by Alexander, Hammer and other researchers, barbiturates interfere with the metabolism of the drugs of the tricyclic group. Barbiturates are potent inducers of the enzymes of the microsomes responsible for the metabolism of many drugs and can thus shorten the halflife of the tricyclics. The phenothiazines, on the other hand, can have just the opposite effect, for example, maintaining above-normal levels of imipramine. As there is evidence that the action of the tricyclics is related to the serum levels, it is strongly recommended to avoid the use of these drugs in combination with others that can modify their pharmacokinetics.

Today it is possible to affirm that the benzodiazepines have assumed a place in the treatment of the anxiety–depression syndromes and that, by mitigating anxiety, they contribute indirectly to an improvement of the depression. The new benzodiazepine bromazepam may also possibly exert a certain direct effect on depression and, combined with sulpiride (Lexpiride), it provides satisfactory results in a number of different indications.

Lexpiride has been investigated by a number of workers in Brazil. Here we might mention the following authors: de Barros, 'Lexpiride in the treatment of personality behaviour disturbances in children and adolescents'; Moreira and de Almeida, 'Clinical evaluation of Lexpiride in patients with depression–anxiety syndromes'; Lins *et al.*, 'The treatment of depressive symptoms during the menopause'; Penteado *et al.*, 'Gastroenterology in patients suffering from anxiety and depression'; Ganance and associates, 'Anti-dizziness activity'; Gomide in 'Cardiology in patients suffering from anxiety and depression'. We have investigated the use of

Lexpiride in patients suffering from anxiety–depression syndromes of diverse aetiology and obtained satisfactory results.

Summary

The concept of depression with regard to its evolution, classification and delimitation, as well as the present biochemical classifications of depression, are discussed.

Consideration is given to the relations between anxiety and depression, and to the question of whether they are different phenomena which can coincide. The nosological, biochemical, neurophysiological and therapeutical aspects, as discussed by various authors, are reviewed.

Arguments regarding the validity of the use of anxiety–reducing drugs in depression are presented.

Reference is made to the anxiety-reducing properties of certain antidepressants and an attempt is made to relate them to the possible effect on depression of specified benzodiazepines. The role of these drugs in the treatment of depression is discussed.

Finally, there is a review of some recent work and studies carried out with bromazepam, used alone or in combination with sulpiride, in the treatment of anxiety–depression syndrome of any aetiology. There is also reference to other benzodiazepines used for similar indications but in combination with antidepressants.

Bibliography

Benzodiazepines in depression

Adolphe, A. B., Dorsey, E. R. and Napoliello, M. J. (1977). Neuropharmacology of depression. *Dis. Nerv. Syst.*, **38,** 841

Alexanderson, B., Price Evans, D. A. and Sjöqvist, F. (1969). Steady-state plasma levels of nortriptyline in twins: influence of genetic factors and drug therapy. *Br. Med. J.*, **4,** 764

Angst, J. (1964). Antidepressiver Effekt und genetische Faktoren. *Arzneim.-Forsch.*, **14,** 496

Åsberg, M., Thorén, P., Träskman, L., Bertilsson, L. and Ringberger, V. (1977). Serotonin, depression. – A biochemical subgroup within the affective disorders? *Science*, **191,** 478

Braestrup, C. and Squires, R. F. (1978). Brain specific benzodiazepine receptors. *Br. J. Psychiatry*, **133,** 249

Brauzer, B., Goldstein, B. J., Steinbook, R. M. and Jacobson, A. F. (1974). The treatment of mixed anxiety and depression with Loxapine. – A controlled comparative study. *J. Clin. Pharmacol.*, **14,** 455

Chase, T. N. and Murphy, D. L. (1973). Serotonin and central nervous system. *Ann. Rev. Pharmacol.*, **13,** 181

Choi, D. W., Farb, D. H. and Fischbach, C. D. (1977). Chlordiazepoxide selectively augments GABA action in spinal cord cell cultures. *Nature* (*Lond.*), **269,** 342

Cleckley, H. M. (1965). Use of diazepam as adjunctive therapy in psychiatric disorders. *J. S. Carolina Med. Assoc.*, **61**, 1

Costa, E., Guidotti, A. and Telfano, G. (1978). Molecular mechanisms mediating the action of diazepam on GABA receptors. *Br. J. Psychiatry*, **133**, 239

Covi, L., Lipman, R.S. and Derogatis, L.R. (1973). Imipramine, diazepam and group psychotherapy in long-term treatment of depressive neurotics. *Psychopharmacol. Bull.*, **9**, 57

Covi, L., Lipman, R.S. and Guzman, R.A. (1975). Drug psychotherapy interactions in depression. In *128th Ann. Meet. of the American Psychiatric Association, Anaheim*, May 5–9, pp. 89–90

Cromwell, H.A. (1973). Management of anxiety, depression in geriatric patients. *Med. Tms* (Lond.), **101**, 47

Daneman, E.A. (1970). A comparative trial of medazepam (Nobrium) in anxiety–depressive states. *Psychosomatics*, **10**, 366

Daskalopoulos, N.T. and Maruani, G. (1976). Neurophysiologie et neurochimie de l'angoisse. *Perspect. Psychiatriques*, **56**, 155

Deniker, P. (1977). Le traitement biologique des dérèglements de l'humeur. *Confront. Psychiatriques*, **14**, 229

Diethelm, O. (1976). The evolution of the concept of depression. In *The Nature and Treatment of Depression*, pp. 11–29. (New York: John Wiley)

Ditman, K.S. and Benor, D. (1966). Diazepam (Valium) very high dosage. Longitudinal and single case study. *West. Med.*, **7**, 109

Downing, R.W. and Rickels, K. (1974). Mixed anxiety–depression. Fact or myth. *Arch. Gen. Psychiatry*, **30**, 312

DSM III Draft – Third Edition (1978). *Diagnostic and Statistical Manual of Mental Disorders.* (The American Psychiatric Association)

Fann, W.E. and Wheless, J.C. (1977). Pharmacological treatment of the moderately anxious and depressed patient. In Fann, W.E. *et al.* (eds.), *Phenomenology and Treatment of Depression.* (New York: Spectrum Publication)

Feighner, J.P., Robins, E., Guze, S.B., Woodruff, R.A., Winokur, G. and Munoz, R. (1972). Diagnostic criteria for use in psychiatric research. *Arch. Gen. Psychiatry*, **26**, 57

Fieve, R.R. and Dunner, D.L. (1976). Unipolar and bipolar affective states. In *The Nature and Treatment of Depressions*, pp. 145–161. (New York: John Wiley)

Fournier, A., Crocq, L., Rigal, J. and Aubin, J.P. (1964). L'association d'iproclozide et de chlordiazépoxide dans le traitement des états dépressifs. (A propos de 61 observations) *Ann. Méd.-Psychol.*, **122**, 625

Frazier, S.H. (1976). Changing patterns in the management of depression. *Dis. Nerv. Syst.*, **37**, 25

Freeman, H.L., Bourne, M.S. and Schiff, A.A. (1974). The treatment of anxious/depressive states. – A double-blind comparison of medazepam with fluphenazine/nortriptyline. *J. Int. Med. Res.*, **2**, 197

Gillespie, F.A. (1971). The use of intravenous diazepam in stupor. *Can. Psychiat. Assoc. J.*, **16**, 445

Gold, R.L. and Dribben, I.S. (1964). Diazepam therapy of depressed patients. *J. Neuropsychiatry*, **5**, 366

Guidotti, A. (1978). Synoptic mechanisms in the action of benzodiazepines. In Liptons, M.A., Di Mascio, A. and Killan, K.F. (eds.), *Psychopharmacology: A Generation of Progress*, pp. 1349–1357. (New York: Raven Press)

Haefely, W. E. (1977). Synaptic pharmacology of barbiturates and benzodiazepines. *Ag. Act.*, **7**, 353

Haefely, W. E. (1978). Central actions of benzodiazepines: General introduction. *Br. J. Psychiatry*, **133**, 231

Hawkins, D. R. and Mendels, J. (1968). The psychophysiologic investigation of sleep in patients with depression. In Lopez-Ibor, J. J. (ed.), *Psychiatry, Proc. of 4th World Congr. of Psychiatry. Part 3, Madrid, September 5–11, 1966*, pp. 1893–1897. (Amsterdam: Excerpta Med.)

Heiberg, A. and Lingjaerde, O. (1977). A controlled study on the possible effect of dihydroergotamine against dryness of the mouth in patients treated with tricyclic antidepressants. *Acta Psychiat. Scand.*, **48**, 353

Higuchi, M., Nagahama, F., Inanaga, K., Kobatake, S., Murakami, E., Kawakita, Y., Kotorii, M., Kobayashi, J. *et al.* (1975). The clinical evaluation of a new minor tranquilizer clorazepate dipotassium (Mendon) in the treatment of patients with psychosomatic disease, neurosis and depressive state in a double-blind clinical study. *J. Jpn. Psychosom. Soc.*, **15**, 236

Hollister, L. E., Overall, J. E., Pokorny, A. D. and Shelton, J. (1971). Acetophenazine and diazepam in anxious depressions. *Arch. Gen. Psychiatry*, **24**, 273

ICD 9 (1979). (Geneva: WHO)

Itil, T. M. (1974). Report of early clinical drug evaluation unit no. 11. *Psychopharmacol. Bull.*, **10**, 5

Johnson, F., Sacco, F. A. and Yellowley, T. W. (1973). Chlordiazepoxide and dothiepin compared in anxiety. Depression in general practice. *Practitioner*, **211**, 362

Kay, D. W. K., Fahy, T. and Garside, R. F. (1970). A seven-month double-blind trial of amitriptyline and diazepam in ECT-treated depressed patients. *Br. J. Psychiatry*, **117**, 667

Kearney, T. R. (1964). Treatment of atypical depression with Librium and Parnate. *Dis. Nerv. Syst.*, **25**, 443

Kellner, R. (1973). Chlordiazepoxide in depressive neurosis. An open label crossover study wth amitriptyline. *Can. Psychiat. Assoc. J.*, **18**, 393

Kielholz, P. (1972). *Etats Dépressifs*. (Bern: Huber)

King, L. J. (1970). Chemotherapy of mental depression. *Ann. Rev. Med.*, **21**, 367

King, L. J. (1975). The depressive syndrome. – A follow-up study of 130 professionals working overseas. *Am. J. Psychiatry*, **132**, 636

Klein, D. F. (1976). Differential diagnosis and treatment of the dysphorias. In Gallant, M. and Simpson, G. M. (eds.), *Depression: Behavioral, Biochemical, Diagnostic and Treatment Concepts*, pp. 127–154. (New York: Spectrum Publications)

Kraepelin, E. (1921). *Manic Depressive Insanity and Paranoia*. (Edinburgh: Livingstone)

Krainin, J. M. (1972). Psychotherapy by counter-manipulation. *Am. J. Psychiatry*, **129**, 749

Kuhn, R. (1974). Ambulante Depressionsbehandlung. In Kielholz, P. (ed.). *Die Depression in der täglichen Praxis*. Intern. Symp. January 1974, St. Moritz, pp. 98–101. (Bern: Huber)

Kuhn, R. (1978). Estado actual del tratamiento de los depresivos. *Rev. Psiq. Psicol. Med. Europ. Am. Lat.*, **III**, 427

Lader, M.H. (1977). Keeping up with advances in clinical psychopharmacology. *Mod. Med.*, **22,** 6

Lader, M. (1978). Current psychophysiological theories of anxiety. In Lipton, M.A., DiMascio, A. and Long, P.L. (eds.), *Psychopharmacology: A Generation of Progress*, pp. 1375–1380. (New York: Raven Press)

Lambert, P. (1972). *Actualités de Thérapeutique Psychiatrique*. (Paris: Masson)

Leedy, J.J. (1970). What we learned from a double-blind study of Librium. *Med. Tms* (Lond.), **98,** 72

Leickert, K.H. (1977). Lexotanil. – Ein neuer Benzodiazepin-Tranquilizer mit stimmungsaufhellenden Eigenschaften. *Med. Welt*, **28,** 1317

Lemperière, T., Feline, A. and Gutmann, A. (1972). Le dépamide. – Problèmes posés par son association à d'autres psychotropes. *Ann. Méd. Interne*, **123,** 783

Leonhard, K., Korff, I. and Schulz, H. (1962). Die Temperamente in den Familien der monopolaren und bipolaren phasischen Psychosen. *Psychiat. et Neurol.* (Basel), **143,** 416

Lewis, A. (1971). 'Endogenous' and 'exogenous' a useful dichotomy? *Psychol. Med.*, **1,** 191

Lipman, R.S., Covi, L. and Smith, V.K. (1975). Prediction of response to drug and group psychotherapy in depressed outpatients. *Psychopharmacol. Bull.*, **11,** 38

Lopes de Lerma, J. (1962). *Problemas en Torno de la Depresión*. (Madrid)

Maas, J.W. (1975). Biogenic amines and depression. Biochemical and pharmacological separation of two types of depression. *Arch. Gen. Psychiatry*, **26,** 256

Maas, J.W., Dekirmenjian, H. and Fawcett, J.A. (1974). MHPG excretion by patients with affective disorders. *Int. Pharmacopsychiatry*, **9,** 14

Madalena, J.C. (1967). Observações clínicas preliminares com um novo derivado benzodiazepínico – o Ro 5-4556. *Folha Méd.*, **55,** 77

Magnus, R.V. (1975). A placebo controlled trial of viloxazine with and without tranquillizers in depressive illness. *J. Int. Med. Res.*, **3,** 207

Marino, A. (1966). Treatment with amitriptyline and chlordiazepoxide. In Lopez-Ibor, J.J. and Plogsties, H.R. (eds.). *IV Congreso Mundial de Psiquiatría, Madrid, September 5–11, 1966*, pp. 294–295. (Amsterdam: Excerpta Med.)

Maruani, G. (1976). Anxiety Clinic. *Psychiat. Persp.*, **2,** No. 56

Mendels, J. and Hawkins, D.R. (1971). Sleep and depression. IV. Longitudinal studies. *J. Nerv. Ment. Dis.*, **153,** 351

Möhler, H. and Okada, T. (1978). The benzodiazepine receptor in normal and pathological human brain. *Br. J. Psychiatry*, **133,** 261

Namba, T., Nishida, K., Nozawa, A., Kato, G., Saito, T. and Tsutsui, S. (1973). Double-blind cross-over comparison of bromazepam and diazepam in psychosomatic disease. Neurosis and depression. *J. Med. Soc. Toho Univ.*, **20,** 445

Nardini, M. and Barba, C. (1975). Sugli effetti clinici di una nuova benzodiazepina (bromazepam) sulla sindrome depressivo-ansiosa. *Minerva Med.*, **66,** 1198

Ohara, T., Kojima, H. and Kasahara, H. (1973). Investigation of anti-depressive effects of Ro-4556 (Nobrium) in the field of psychiatry. *Jpn. J. Clin. Exp. Med.*, **50,** 2409

Ohara, M., Isogai, S., Ohashi, K. and Yoshinaga, S. (1972). Clinical investigation of bromazepam for neurotic or depressive patients with manifest anxiety and irritability. *Jpn. J. Clin. Exp. Med.*, **49,** 3184

Okasha, A., Ghaleb, H. A. and Sadek, A. (1973). A double-blind trial for the clinical management of psychogenic headache. *Br. J. Psychiatry*, **122,** 181

Okuma, T., Nakao, T., Ogura, C., Kishimoto, A. and Majima, K. (1971). Effect of 7-bromo-5-(2-pyridyl)-3H-1,4-benzodiazepine-2 (1H)-one, bromazepam (Ro 5-3350), a new minor tranquilizer, on psychoneurosis and psychosis with special reference to the obsessive-compulsive symptoms. *Folia Psychiat. Neurol. Jpn.*, **25,** 199

Paim, I. and De Moraes, T. M. (1968). Sôbre um caso de 'depressio sine depressione' *Folha Méd.*, **56,** 137

Pavan, R., Bezoari, M. and Vender, S. (1974). Profil d'effet du bromazépam (Ro 5-3350) relevé pendant trois années d'étude clinique 'ouverte'. Presented at the *9. Congresso di Neuropsicofarmacologia*, Juli 7–12, Paris.

Perris, C. and d'Elia, G. (1966). A study of bipolar (manic-depressive) and unipolar recurrents depressive psychosis. *Acta Psychiat. Scand.*, **42,** (Suppl.), **194,** 1

Pichot, P. (1978). *Les Voies Nouvelles de la Dépression.* (Paris: Masson)

Plauchu, M., Malluret, J., Lachieze-Rey, E., Piquet, G., Eyraud, M.T., Orgiazzi, J. and Gauthier, J. (1968). Intérêt du diazépam dans un service de médecine générale. *Lyon. Méd.*, **219,** 1127

Ragot, M. (1978). Depression, new physiopathogenetic concepts. *Actual. Psychiat.*, **No. 2**

Raskin, A. (1973). Depressives diazepam aids anxiety. *U.S. Med.*, **9,** 18

Raskin, A., Schulterbrandt, J. G., Reatig, N., Crook, T. H. and Odle, D. (1974). Depression subtypes and response to phenelzine, diazepam, and a placebo. Results of a nine hospital collaborative study. *Arch. Gen. Psychiatry*, **30,** 66

Richou, H. and Hug, R. (1970). Essais cliniques du Nobrium, une nouvelle benzodiazépine. – Le Nobrium, sa place en psychiatrie tant à l'hôpital qu'en cure ambulatoire. *Vie Méd.*, **51,** 4121

Rickels, K. (1971). Diazepam vs phenobarbital vs amitriptyline. *Psychopharmacol. Bull.*, **7,** 85

Rickels, K. (1977). Résumés of research projects in psychopharmacology. NIMH-PRB pharmacotherapy of anxiety and depression. *Psychopharmacol. Bull.*, **13,** 56

Rickels, K., Hesbacher, P. and Downing, R. W. (1970). Differential drug effects in neurotic depression. *Dis. Nerv. Syst.*, **31,** 468

Rickels, K., Raab, E., De Silverio, R. and Etemad, B. (1967). Drug treatment in depression. Antidepressant or tranquilizer? *J. Am. Med. Assoc.*, **201,** 675

Rickels, K., Gordon, P. E., Jenkins, B. W., Perloff, M., Sachs, T. and Stepansky, W. (1970). Drug treatment in depressive illness. (Amitriptyline and chlordiazepoxide in two neurotic populations). *Dis. Nerv. Syst.*, **31,** 30

Rickels, K., Chung, H. R., Feldman, H. S., Gordon, P.E., Kelly, E. A. and Weise, C. C. (1973). Amitriptyline, diazepam, and phenobarbital sodium in depressed outpatients. *J. Nerv. Ment. Dis.*, **157,** 442

Robinson, D. S., Nies, A., Ravaris, C. L. and Lamborn, K. R. (1973). The monoamine oxidase inhibitor, phenelzine, in the treatment of depressive–anxiety states. *Arch. Gen. Psychiatry*, **29,** 407

Roger, G. (1972). Traitement des états dépressifs par le prolintane. Bilan de deux années d'expérience en pratique hospitalière et privée. *Cah. Méd. Lyon.*, **48,** 3867

Rosenthal, S.H. and Bowden, C.L. (1973). A double-blind comparison of thioridazine (Mellaril) versus diazepam (Valium) in patients with chronic mixed anxiety and depressive symptomes. *Curr. Ther. Res.*, **15**, 261

Ross, S.B. and Renyi, A.L. (1975). Tricyclic antidepressant agents. *Acta Pharmacol. Toxicol.*, **36**, 382

Schildkraut, J.J. (1979). Norepinephrine metabolites as biochemical criteria for classifying depressive disorders and predicting responses to treatment: Preliminary findings. *Am. J. Psychiatry*, **130**, 695

Schopbach, R.R. (1967). A pilot study with Ro 5-4556 in the treatment of anxiety and depression. *Int. J. Neuropsychiatry*, **3**, 494

Schuster, T.S., Winslow, W.W. and Kellner, R. (1972). A comparison of thioridazine and diazepam in non-psychotic anxiety-depression. – A pilot study. *Curr. Ther. Res.*, **14**, 131

Shammas, E. (1977). Controlled comparison of bromazepam, amitripyline and placebo in anxiety-depressive neurosis. *Dis. Nerv. Syst.*, **38**, 201

Shulman, R., Griffiths, J. and Diewold, P. (1978). Catechol-*O*-methyl transferase activity in patients with depressive illness and anxiety states. *Br. J. Psychiatry*, **132**, 133

Spitzer, R.C. (1975). *Research Diagnostic Criteria.* (New York: N.Y. State Psychiat. Institute)

Sprogis, G.R. (1966). Control of anxiety/depression reactions in general practice. *Curr. Ther. Res.*, **8**, 490

Stein, L., Belluzzi, J.D. and Ritter, S. (1974). Self-stimulation reward pathways: norepinephrine vs dopamine. *J. Psychiatr. Res.*, **11**, 115

Strotzka, H. (1970). Zur medikamentösen Behandlung neurotisch larvierter Depressionen. *Wien. Med. Wschr.*, **120**, 401

Swenson, J., Hackett, E. and Kline, N.S. (1968). The use of Valium in the treatment of depression. In Lopez-Ibor, J.J. (ed.), *Psychiatry, Proc. of 4th World Congr. of Psychiatry, Part 3, Madrid, Sept. 5–11, 1966*, pp. 2030–2033. (Amsterdam: Excerpta Med.)

Taylor, K.M. and Laverty, R. (1969). The effect of chlordiazepoxide, diazepam and nitrazepam on catecholamine metabolism in regions of the rat brain. *Eur. J. Pharmacol.*, **8**, 296

Volmat, R., Allers, G., Vittouris, N. and Dufoy, F. (1973). Note préliminaire sur l'activité thérapeutique et la tolérance clinique et biologique du 34.276 BA en cures endo-veineuses dans les mélancolies et les états dépressifs. *Schweiz. Arch. Neurol. Neurochir. Psychiatry*, **113**, 410

Winokur, G. (1974). The division of depressive illness into depression spectrum disease and pure depressive disease. *Int. Pharmacopsychiatry*, **9**, 5

Wise, C.D., Berger, B.D. and Stein, L. (1972). Benzodiazepines: anxiety-reducing activity by reduction of serotonin turnover in the brain. *Science*, **177**, 180

Yamamoto, J., Kline, F.M. and Burgoyne, R.W. (1972). Double-blind drug study in depressed outpatients. *Rocky Mtn. Med. J.*, **69**, 71

Zapletalek, M., Strnad, M., Komenda, S., Vačková, M., Barboraková, B., Stepanová, M., Hrbek, J., Beran, I. and Široka, A. (1966). Alimenazine, chlordiazepoxide, meprobamate and placebo in anxious depression therapy. *Activ. Nerv. Super.*, **8**, 437

Zung, W.W. (1971). The differentiation of anxiety and depressive disorders: a biometric approach. *Psychosomatics*, **12**, 380

13

Benzodiazepines in Masked Depressions

E. Azzi

Introduction

Depressive illness is gradually becoming the pathology-symbol of our era of crisis, showing ever-growing epidemic proportions in its several forms and clinical manifestations: endogenous (MDP and involutional melancholia), reactive (depressive reactive psychosis), neurotic (neurotic depressions), symptomatic (in other psychiatric disturbances) and many organic diseases. In 1977, in São Paulo, Brazil, the prevalence of depressive illness was considered by all the physicians (more than 7000, mostly non-psychiatrists) interviewed by our group, to have increased by 83%.

In the past decades, besides an increase in the prevalence of depressive illness, a kind of 'mutation' has been noted in depressive symptomatology translated as a more frequent phenomenon of 'depressive somatization'. This brings patients to seek repeated somatic examination, searching in vain for physical changes that lead to expensive and varied clinical and surgical treatments.

Although thymopathic masking can appear in different forms (obsessions, aggressiveness, alcoholism, toxicomania, etc.), the term 'masked depression' usually refers to a depressive illness in which classic psychopathological symptoms of depression do exist, but are masked or hidden by a dominating somatic symptomatology. The non-psychiatrist is usually poorly prepared to deal with the emotional state underlying somatic complaints; on the other hand, he is called by most patients of this kind on account of the nature of the dominating symptomatology.

Masked depression in daily practice

Non-psychiatrist physicians should be aware of hidden depression and be trained in detecting hidden or masked depressive symptoms, such as: reduced initiative, decreased interest in other people and things, diminished capacity to enjoy life, reduced performance, creativity and working capacity, unexplained increase of worries, sleep disturbances with rumination, death ideation, feelings of worthlessness, exaggerated anxiety and diurnal variation, alternation and emergence of somatic symptoms.

If we can exclude somatic and toxic causes with relative certainty, if we detect disturbances in the three essential elementary and fundamental necessities of the human being, which are love (implying the existence of object relationships and interests), general enjoyment of life and active engagement in work, it is likely that we are dealing with a masked depression. In case of suspicion or doubt, it is worthwhile trying antidepressants simultaneously with symptomatic and tranquillizing therapy. The antidepressant therapy is recognized by all authors, including ourselves, as good or even excellent in these cases for inducing feelings of well-being and optimism. This is acknowledged even by patients who have never before complained of depression.

Masked depression is by no means a new disease and this term has only a relative and purely pragmatic significance.

The diagnosis of what is behind the 'mask' depends mainly on the competence and experience of the physician who examines the situation. Once physicians, mainly the non-psychiatrists, have learned how to diagnose a depression correctly, the term 'masked depression' will disappear.

Nevertheless, this concept is still valid and very useful, mainly for the non-psychiatrists who have to deal daily and with increasing frequency with this kind of patients, whose depressive dysthymic background they do not or only rarely recognize and who have devoted a great deal of time, without success, to treating somatic disturbances because a thymopathic somatization (whether endothymic, reactive or symptomatic) has not been thought of.

The *somatic symptomatology* that can mask a depression varies from person to person, and in the same person during his lifetime. Practically all organic systems (gastro-intestinal, cardiovascular, urogenital, respiratory, cutaneous, neurological, etc.) can participate in the process, either on a purely functional level or when injury is involved, where often it becomes difficult if not impossible to distinguish clearly between 'thymopathic, psychosomatic and hypochondriac', mainly on account of the absence of biological, biochemical or bioelectrical criteria.

The following aspects speak in favour of the thymopathic character: periodic character, phasic or undulating evolution of symptoms, premorbid personality, family background, discovery of microphenomenology of some nuclear psychic symptoms, and sometimes psychological tests[3].

Treatment of masked depression

The *treatment* of masked depression demands intelligent and critical coordination of pharmacotherapeutic and psychotherapeutic measures.

Psychotherapy is of great value in depressive states. The type of psychotherapy is adapted to the circumstances and clinical characteristics of each case. In masked depression it is important to reassure the patient by explaining his symptoms to him.

The *biological and pharmacotherapeutic* measures are aimed either at dominant somatic symptoms (headaches, lumbago, paresthesia, gastrointestinal or cardiovascular disturbances, etc.) or at the *depression* 'masked' by these somatic symptoms.

Different products (such as derivatives of the type of imipramine, nomifensin, amitriptyline, maprotiline, sulpiride) are available today to treat depressive states.

The antidepressant therapy for masked depressions has the same clinical and dynamic effect as that for other forms of depressions:

Progressive improvement, day by day;
Relapse when the therapy is suspended too early;
Need for prolonged treatment continued by maintenance dosage even when depressive symptoms have disappeared.

The physician's own uncertainty should not be allowed to influence him to give too high a dosage in the hope of obtaining a more rapid response or to make other unnecessary changes in treatment.

Use of benzodiazepines

In masked depressions, in addition to sleep disturbances, there is always a significant anxiety component which is an indication for the prescription of a minor tranquillizer in associaton with antidepressants, which remain the basic and essential medication for depressive mood.

Among the minor tranquillizers, the benzodiazepines are the most widely used: surveys carried out in Europe[4] (West Germany, Austria, France, Italy, Switzerland) and at São Paulo[1,2] show them to be the drugs most frequently prescribed in combination with antidepressants, followed in second place by hypnotics.

In any case, the benzodiazepines appear to be specifically indicated in most instances of masked depression because they mainly act on emotional tension and anxiety, exert an euhypnic effect and have very low toxicity.

In connection with this, one must pay attention to the perils of *exclusive use* of anxiolytic drugs (benzodiazepines or others) in thymopathic somatic masking cases, as seems to occur in the practice of some general practitioners, or when the patient is admitted to a general medical hospital.

There is a risk that these substances may cause affective indifference, general loss of interest and motor hypotony, which is often very inconvenient, and sometimes may induce forms of 'atypical depression'[5] or contribute even more to concealing the underlying depression.

However, it seems to me that in masked depressions treated by non-psychiatrists, combination of benzodiazepines with antidepressants is the best way to avoid the inconvenient effects mentioned above.

An open clinical study was recently carried out in our clinic with a small group of patients with a greater or lesser degree of somatized depression using Ro 10–7122 (Lexpiride) which combines bromazepam and sulpiride in a daily average dosage of 3 capsules, corresponding to 3 mg and 75 mg respectively of these substances. Although this study is still under statistical evaluation, we can already say that the investigator considered the results good or fair in about 82% of the cases and unsatisfactory in 18%, while, *in the opinion of the patients*, these figures were 73% and 27% respectively.

Conclusion

In recent decades, non-psychiatrist physicians have been confronted more and more with the so-called 'masked' depressions, in which the somatic symptomatology masks the depressive illness. When once recognized, it is essentially treated with antidepressant drugs. Optimal treatment consists in a combination of benzodiazepines with an antidepressant. Exclusive use of antidepressants or benzodiazepines may not be very helpful in general practice.

References

1. Azzi, E. (1978). Inquérito sobre depressão, depressão mascarada e sintomas psicossomáticos em um grupo de médicos não psiquiatras e psiquiatras da cidade de São Paulo. *Ciên. Méd.*, **11,** 20
2. Azzi, E. (1979). Clínica e terapêutica da depressão mascarada. *Rev. Bras. Clín. Terap.*, **8** (special edition), 34
3. Goolishian, H. A. (1975). Some psychometric characteristics of depression. In Freedman, A. M. and Kaplan, H. I. (eds.). *Comprehensive Textbook of Psychiatry.* (Baltimore: William Wilkins Co.)
4. Kielholz, P. (ed.) (1974). *Depression in Everyday Practice.* (Bern: Huber)
5. Kuhn, R. (1979). Estado actual del tratamiento de las depresiones. *Rev. Psiq. Ur.*, **261,** 130

14

Some Salient Clinical Findings from the Use of Benzodiazepines in Childhood and Adolescence

G. M. Jacobides

Several factors have given impetus to the great advances that we have witnessed in the field of psychopharmacology. As Silverstone wrote, 'one of the most significant factors which have promoted recent progress, has been the continuing dialogue conducted between laboratory-based research workers, probing into the ways psychotropic drugs interact with neurotransmitter systems in the brain, and clinical psychiatrists evaluating in patients the way these same drugs alter the symptoms and signs of mental illness'[17].

We believe the interested psychiatrist should not confine himself to the clinical studies of these drugs, but should try to meet the laboratory researcher half-way and should come to know a little more about his conceptualizations and about the experimental animal models of abnormal behaviour he so frequently uses.

It is generally conceded, of course, that experimental animal models, fundamental as they may be for the neuropharmacologist, possess (mainly because of their simplicity and neatness) an allure for the clinician who might thus hasten to inadmissible extrapolations from mouse to man!

However, such experimental data regarding mainly *affective* behavioural responses retain their suggestive value and, we feel, the clinical psychiatrist should, albeit circumspectly, come to know them and weigh up their significance for his own work with patients. For, in the clinical field, affective symptomatology is probably *the* widest area of psychological disturbance that a psychiatrist has to deal with; and its treatment has, indeed, been revolutionized by modern neuropharmacology.

Again, in affective symptomatology, *anxiety* is a pivotal phenomenon.

In clinical practice it is found as an all-pervasive manifestation, often transcending the borderland of primary affective illness and crossing into practically every area of mental disturbance.

Benzodiazepines and aggression

Benzodiazepines, the most extensively used psychotropic drugs to-day, appear to have a *selective* action on anxiety, and their tranquillizing effect is often found useful in cases of aggression. On the other hand, benzodiazepines were said to diminish, also selectively, the abundance of serotonin in the mesolimbic region and to affect various brain sites that are believed to modulate aggression (such as the amygdala); this has been associated by many researchers with the inhibition of aggressive behaviour, which is usually described as 'taming effect' in animals.

The 'taming' effect of drugs was specifically mentioned first by Berger[1], and after the first days of Librium it was convincingly shown in animals by Randall and co-workers[15] who found it 8.6 times as potent as meprobamate. Also Boff and Scheckel in Basel and others in many laboratories confirmed and extended the anti-aggressive action. Yet, unlike the 'anxiolytic effect' of practically all benzodiazepines, proven by operant conditioning in the so-called 'punishment' (conflict) tests, extrapolation from animals to humans in the case of 'taming effect' has not been successful, as we shall indicate later.

In experimental animals, several models of aggressive behaviour have been studied (foot-shock or brain-lesion induced aggression, the isolation and frustration models, the muricide model and the stimulus-bound attack) before and after the use of drugs, with the aim of finding chemical agents that selectively reduce aggression without affecting locomotion and alertness, i.e. without producing heavy sedation which then dampens *all* activity – including aggression[8].

In particular, the ratio of aggression score over the score of general motor activity is calculated, and obviously drugs with a low such ratio are taken to be more *selectively* anti-aggressive.

With regard to the anti-aggressive effect of benzodiazepines, studies on a normally aggressive monkey, the *Cynomolgus*, by the Basel group have shown that Lexotanil (bromazepam) is twice as 'taming' as Librium (Table 14.1) while oxazepam (like chlorpromazine) reduces aggressive manifestations only when the general activity of the animal is reduced.

This attempt to produce a *selective* action on particular 'target symptoms' is most certainly a prominent trend in modern psychopharmacology and goes parallel to the general hopes recently voiced by Professor Linford Rees and co-workers that through further research we may be able to select patients with specific disorders that are specifically susceptible to a particular pharmacological agent.

Table 14.1 The 'taming effect' of various benzodiazepines vs chlorpromazine (based on reports on *Cynomolgus* monkey[15])

Compound	*Route*	*Depressant* M.A.D.	*Taming dose* (mg/kg)	*Taming effect* (a/a ratio 0.5)	*Aggr./act. ratio*
Chlordiazepoxide	p.o.	1.0	2.5–5.0	++	0.3
Diazepam	p.o.	1.0	2.0–2.5	++	0.3
Bromazepam	p.o.	1.0	2.5	+++	0.16
Oxazepam	p.o.	40.0	40.0	nil	1.0
Chlorpromazine	s.c.	0.3	0.6	nil	1.9
Chlorpromazine	p.o.	10.0	20.0	nil	1.0

Total $n = 24$

In such a quest of a particular benzodiazepine drug with a true 'taming effect' we administered bromazepam in aggressive morons (children and adolescents). (The results of this research are presented in the 2nd International Child Neurology Congress in Sydney.)

During the study of this material some salient clinical findings emerged which, in connection with our wider experience with bromazepam, we thought would be of interest as having a bearing on the use of benzodiazepines in general (especially in childhood), on the endeavour to avoid misapplication of psychotropic drugs and to promote a better selection of patients for the 'specific' target treatment and on pathogenetic formulations of certain psychiatric conditions.

Clinical material

In our Out-Patient Department at St. Sophia Children's Hospital, which is the largest Teaching Paediatric Hospital in Greece and has an annual turnover exceeding 1000 patients of mixed neurological and psychiatric conditions, the 'aggressive oligophrenics' feature rather highly: they constitute a serious problem, especially in the provinces, whence these patients are brought to the capital for therapeutic advice after the local GP or paediatrician has 'doped' them (mainly with neuroleptics) in an attempt to make their existence at home tolerable and avoid institutional care. The result is, of course, disastrous, as heavy sedation (leading to confusion) reduces their limited mental power; and the need for a genuine anti-aggressive medicament in this group of patients becomes imperative.

On the evidence concerning the allegedly specific and strong anti-aggressive effect of bromazepam we proceeded to carry out a clinical trial and aggressive dullards were first treated according to a project design, which will be reported elsewhere in detail. In the course of this open trial it emerged that some of the patients whose retardation was due to organic brain damage and who had psychotic admixtures in the clinical picture did worse while on bromazepam, which seemed to exacerbate the psychotic features.

This required the inclusion in the study of two clinical control groups, i.e. psychotic aggressives and non-psychotic aggressives with normal intelligence (the latter were neurotics and aggressive psychopaths).

At the conclusion of this prospective study and evaluative investigation, results from 30 aggressive children and adolescents, aged mostly 10–14 (extreme range 5–16), were finally compared with the effect of bromazepam on 30 non-aggressive outpatients treated mainly for anxiety and phobic–obsessional states.

Main findings

In full agreement with our previous experience, prominent in our results was the anxiolytic effect which, in the absence of sedation, ran parallel to an 'activation' of the patients treated with bromazepam. In our work with benzodiazepines, we have also observed this phenomenon with chlordiazepoxide, medazepam and diazepam, in that order.

Tension and frustration was helped less and then variably, and agitation tended to be aggravated by bromazepam in our material. Aggression proper (both assaultive behaviour and verbal aggression) was helped in the neurotic group of patients where it usually occurs as an expression of anxiety or as the 'acting out' of hostile feelings.

When given to this type of patients, bromazepam often had the striking effect of bringing about a 'ventilation' of repressed feelings which were then strongly verbalized. This effect of bromazepam necessitated *prompt* psychotherapeutic handling and a careful management of the 'acting out'. The instability and the impulsiveness of aggressive psychopaths was in a few cases greatly helped by bromazepam treatment.

Aggression in psychotic patients was very frequently made much worse. Interestingly, in such patients even non-aggressive psychotic symptomatology was made worse as if bromazepam enhanced the psychotic process. This unexpected (and outwardly paradoxical) effect is not easy to explain on the basis of the current theory of psychosis.

Aggression in morons was helped to varying degrees. When the retardation is due (as is fairly usually the case) to organic brain damage, there is an admixture of psychotic manifestations and then bromazepam may have a negative effect. When the mental deficiency is 'idiopathic', the aggression follows the pattern seen in normal intelligence and bromazepam may prove a useful tool for the psychotherapist.

Aggression as a result of frustration, proven by elegant animal experiments, is also seen in patients and especially in cases of mild oligophrenia. Bromazepam seemed to help this type of aggression, too, as it helped aggression due to fear, but, again, only when the patients had no organicity or psychotic features.

The type of clinical material which is usually helped by bromazepam and the assessment of personality structure in our patients seem to indicate that best results are to be expected among the unstable extraverts rather than the unstable introverts, who are helped by other members of the benzodiazepine group.

Discussion

A discussion such as this should, we believe, start with some basic facts. We, clinicians, are striving for drug-*efficacy* and drug *specificity* but we may overlook (or ignore) the general principles governing psycho-active agents, benzodiazepines included.

Drugs can redress the abnormalities of behaviour (i.e. they restore a '*balance*' of excitatory/inhibitory circuits in the neuronal subsystems of the CNS, in response to external stimuli) by acting on the biochemistry and thence on the electrophysiology of the brain (mainly the reticular formation and the limbic system). Their *specificity* depends: (a) on the biochemical/electrophysiological correlates of the particular behavioural/affective abnormality, in discrete brain sites, (b) on the selective action of the drug in the brain sites concerned. It so happens that brain sites subserving basic emotional states are functionally complex and in a most delicate and intricate balance; for example the amygdala–hypothalamus circuitry.

Now, the newcomer from clinical psychiatry to the study of psychopharmacology is inescapably plagued by 'selective perception' in his endeavour to reconcile a disparate literature and unify scattered findings into a working concept. Despite the risk of being 'simplistic' in the face of very complex phenomena he usually manages, often with procrustean methods, to reach some 'conclusion' which, of course, may be both erroneous and clinically hazardous.

In part, this is because neuropharmacological papers reporting on isolated pieces of research avoid (and quite legitimately so!) extrapolating from their results or making formulations that are relevant to patients. Furthermore, reports on a particular biogenic amine in humans that fail to emphasize that in man there is a *constant* homoeostatic *balance* governing the whole gamut of neurotransmitters could be worthless from a pathogenetic point of view.

But even at a somewhat more advanced level of experience the clinician may have difficulty with drug 'efficacy' and drug 'specificity', with which the former is inextricably interwoven. And this usually follows on diagnostic over-inclusion (i.e. poor patient selection) or misapplication of the drug (i.e. poor psychopharmacological know-how).

Clinical associations

In search of clues for the recognition of a more 'specific' drug, the practising psychiatrist turns, of course, to clinical characteristics[14].

Our findings concerning personality structure of the patients and the 'stimulating' effect of some benzodiazepines could be of assistance firstly in the choice of a more specific (and effective) drug and, secondly, in the avoidance of an activating benzodiazepine when organic and psychotic patients are treated.

Also by analogy with various animal models of aggressive behaviour having *different* biochemical correlates (muricide, stimulus-bound attack, isolation and rival fighting)[8] we have observed at least three different clinical types of aggression in humans (neurotic, psychotic and organic brain damage) that require different handling and medication. This should suggest that one should treat 'psychiatric patients with aggression' rather than aggression *per se*, as a target-symptom.

With regard to the taming effect of some benzodiazepines which is proven to be quite specific in animals (Table 14.1), extrapolation to man has not been possible. Interestingly, oxazepam, which in animals has no true taming effect at all, is described by Essman[5], and also by Valzelli[18] with the very same phrase, as 'eminently useful in the control of aggressive outbursts in patients'. Yet this preference for oxazepam is not a measure of its anti-aggressive power but, rather, of its non-stimulating nature which promises safety from misapplication. In our experience, however, although bromazepam has a vastly smaller aggressivity ratio than oxazepam and is twice as potent as Librium in animals, there is no reflection of such differential effectiveness in the treatment of aggressive patients.

Extravert personality

The other clinical finding in our investigation, namely that best results are mostly seen in the unstable extraverts, if confirmed, will promote better patient selection covering the wide age brackets of childhood and adolescence where both instability and extraversion preponderate.

It is already half a century since McDougall stressed the special susceptibility of the extravert to the influence of a psychoactive agent known to man for thousands of years, namely alcohol! Differently phrased, he emphasized the '*specific effect*' of ethanol in extraverts and this notion was probably the leading idea in Eysenckian research and theorization about dimensions of personality and drug effects[7]. At the beginning of the psychopharmacology era, from 1954 to 1960 I joined the Maudsley and Bethlem Royal under Professor Linford Rees and had the good fortune to listen to Eysenck's compelling arguments and take an interest in the research that led to his first 'drug-postulate', in 1957, about Drugs and Personality[6].

Irrespective of strong controversy, Eysenckian views made their mark on at least three decades of research worldwide and greatly influenced important work (which was substantiated by factor analysis), such as Gray's in Oxford[9] about distinct emotional systems dealing with punishment and reward and with fight or flight. The view that these three systems may respond in predictable ways to psychoactive drugs[11] and the possible associations with certain biogenic amines at specific brain sites that subserve these systems play a crucial role in today's research on arousal and 'activation theory'[12]. The type of drug and personality structure in Eysenckian terms were studied by many investigators[10]; what seems relevant in our context is the introverting effect of drugs which have a stimulant action (Table 14.2).

Table 14.2 Relation between type of drug and personality structure

Type of drug	*Effect on personality traits towards extravers./introvers.*		*Effect on arousal excitat./inhibit.*		*Paradoxical effect*
Stimulant	−	+	+	−	+
Depressant	+	−	−	+	+

Modifications of Eysenck's dimensions of personality were produced, by (among others) Gray who, rotating Eysenck's factors through 45°, contrasts anxiety and impulsivity syndromes and associates his Approach System with extraversion; and by Claridge[2] who extends the notion of excitability to cover sympathetic nervous system responsiveness.

Paradoxical excitation and psychosis

One aspect which is not adequately covered by Eysenckian theory is variability of drug response in the same individual and cyclothymia. Accumulating evidence since 1958, when Shagass and Jones[16] first reported their work on *sedation thresholds* along the extraversion vector, which was in line with Eysenck's theory, has indicated that the state of cortical arousal at any given time is a decisive factor for drug response and that unstable extraverts who are 'cortically inhibited' respond more promptly to sedatives than normals. In his important PhD research at the University of London, Costello[3] used meprobamate to test the duration of the Archimedean spiral after-effect; this, as inhibition deepened, decreased but only to a point and then started increasing again. Costello construed this as the result of 'homoeostatic excitation' and he propounded the theory[4] that 'if the degree of cortical inhibition exceeds a certain *critical level* a state of homoeostatic or paradoxical excitation sets in'.

This theory, we believe, amply explains the reported 'paradoxical' effect of the 'activating' benzodiazepines especially in the extravert, whose cortical inhibition tends more easily to go beyond this 'critical' level of inhibition, particularly in the presence of other predisposing factors.

It is interesting to note that in some of our patients who showed such an unexpected or 'paradoxical' response to bromazepam, previous treatment with sodium valproate (which also enhances GABA in the brain) had produced exactly the same exacerbation of psychotic features.

The possibility that bromazepam may cause an increase of the psychotic process is very difficult to explain on the basis of catecholamine or GABA theory in schizophrenia. One could, conceivably, speculate that childhood autism, for which a raised serotonin level has been reported, is pathogenetically distinct from adult schizophrenia where dopamine and dopamine receptor sensitivity have been incriminated, but such speculation cannot be upheld without further research – especially as the methodology of the existing reports has been heavily criticized.

Another train of thought, also highly speculative, could perhaps connect the psychotic deterioration with a displacement by bromazepam of the endogenous benzodiazepine ligand, which some believe may be nicotinamide[13], so that faulty co-enzyme action may lead to excessive *N*-methylation of noradrenaline and, finally, to excessive amounts of adrenochrome. However, the evidence in support of such speculation is extremely frail.

A final point in this discussion should be that bromazepam (like chlordiazepoxide and diazepam), despite their 'activating' or 'stimulant' effect, have not been known to cause addiction in childhood. It should be remembered that even proper stimulants like methylphenidate and the amphetamines are not addictive in children either.

Summary and conclusions

Extensive experience with benzodiazepines since 1962 at Saint Sophia, a large Teaching Paediatric Hospital in Athens, has amassed cogent evidence that this important group of psychotropic drugs make an invaluable and safe adjunct in the psychiatric (and the neurological) management of children and adolescents.

With regard to psychiatric patients, although all drugs used have shown a clear anxiolytic action, a *differential effect* is seen in the clinical application of benzodiazepines. Two usual such points of divergence regarding clinical material are: on the one hand the 'tension/frustration' constellation of symptoms which are differentially affected by benzodiazepines and, on the other, the 'agitation' symptom-complex which may even be aggravated (Table 14.3).

Probably the most significant within-group psychopharmacological difference of benzodiazepines (with an obvious bearing on specificity) is the 'stimulating' effect observed in some (bromazepam, chlordiazepoxide,

Table 14.3 Usual associations of personality structure and affective symptom-complexes

	Personality Structure	
Symptom-complex	*Extraversion sens. inhibition*	*Introversion sens. excitation*
Anxiety–fear	−	+
Tension	−	+
Agitation	−	+
Phobic–obsessional	+	−
Aggression	+	−
Dissociative	+	−

medazepam and diazepam, in that order) and not in others (e.g. oxazepam, clorazepate). This activating effect, possibly associated with absorption rates often ignored in practice, may lead to misapplication of the drug and probably accounts, together with the patients' individual differences, for cases of therapeutic failure and so-called 'paradoxical effect' reported in the literature.

Basically, the differential action of benzodiazepines could be seen as the end result of the 'activation', depending on the state of arousal of the particular individual, his balance of excitation/inhibition and his inherent ability to control effectively any disturbance of this balance.

Although it is important to recognize this clinical division of benzodiazepines into stimulating and non-stimulating members (Table 14.4),

Table 14.4 Clinical differentiation of two groups of benzodiazepines exemplified by bromazepam and oxazepam

	Type of clinical effect			
Type of benzodiazepine	*Anti-tension*	*Anti-aggression*	*Anti-agitation*	*Activating*
Bromazepam	±	+	−	+
Oxazepam	+	−	+	−

it should be remembered that the response of any individual patient is determined not only by arousal levels and personality structure in general but, also, by his *baseline* activity ('initial value law'), by dosage and by environmental factors (Table 14.5).

Apart from tension and agitation, the clinical manifestations termed 'aggression' have been described as selectively influenced by certain benzodiazepines. Although the allegedly specific 'taming' or anti-aggression effect is shown for most benzodiazepines in animals, results

Table 14.5 Factors associated with differential response to the same drug

Origin of factors	*Type of factors*
A. Relating to the drug	Dosage schedules Reinforcement schedules Route of administration
B. Relating to the recipient	Species, strain, sex etc. Physical state and nutrition CNS tissue maturity (age, lesions etc.) State of arousal Drive systems Individual differences (structural/functional) Reflecting on thresholds etc.
C. Relating to the environment	Social stability Isolation Past experience (including drugs)

with patients are not uniform. Using bromazepam, which is found to produce the smallest 'aggressivity ratio' (Table 14.1), the anti-aggression effect of this drug was investigated by us on 30 aggressive patients.

The results of this investigation (which are reported elsewhere) have convincingly indicated that *aggression* in general, unlike 'free-floating anxiety' usually dealt with by the GP, requires the *expert* handling of a psychiatrist, for it may mean much to the patient's ego-defences – or else it may be a symptom of psychosis and/or temporal lobe dysfunction, in which case a different medication is needed to curb it; therefore insistence on the use of a benzodiazepine is a misapplication and does injustice to the drug employed.

Our findings also showed that psychotic aggression is very often made worse by bromazepam. Speculation that the psychotic process in autistic children is mainly serotonin-dependent, whereas in schizophrenic adults it is mainly dopamine-dependent, requires extensive research and cannot be substantiated with the available evidence. The same is true with regard to speculation about the involvement of the endogenous benzodiazepine ligand.

In the non-organic and non-psychotic aggressive patient, bromazepam was very effective but required the expertise of a psychiatric specialist and is not recommended to be used by the general practitioner so far as aggression is concerned.

From our general experience with bromazepam, which singularly lacks sedation as a side-effect, satisfactory results were observed in most anxiety states of childhood and adolescence; particularly patients with 'somatization' and the phobic–obsessionals who are usually resistant to treatment.

The areas of psychiatric disturbance in which bromazepam was found most effective, and the clinical assessment of personality structure of our patients, have led us to believe that the unstable extravert rather than the unstable introvert is more likely to show better results during the drug treatment. When confirmed, this finding should suggest that bromazepam is more suited than other benzodiazepines in childhood and adolescence, where both instability and extraversion are a prominent feature.

References

1. Berger, F. M. (1954). The pharmacological properties of 2-methyl-2-*n*-propyl-1,3-propanediol dicarbamate (Miltown), a new interneuronal blocking agent. *J. Pharmacol. Exp. Ther.*, **112,** 413
2. Claridge, G.S., Wawman, R.J. and Davies, M.H. (1963). Sedation threshold, autonomic lability and the excitation inhibition theory of personality. *Br. J. Psychiatry*, **109,** 548
3. Costello, C.G. (1960). The effect of a depressant drug on certain perceptual tests. *PhD Thesis*, University of London
4. Costello, C.G. and Smith, C.M. (1963). The relationships between personality, sleep and the effects of sedatives. *Br. J. Psychiatry*, **109,** 568
5. Essman, W.B. (1978). Benzodiazepines and aggressive behavior. *Mod. Probl. Pharmacopsych.* Vol. 13, pp. 13–28. (Basel: Karger)
6. Eysenck, H.J. (1957). Drugs and personality. I. Theory and methodology. *J. Ment. Sci.*, **103,** 119
7. Eysenck, H.J. (ed.) (1963). *Experiments with Drugs. Studies in the relation between Personality, Learning Theory and Drug action.* (London: Pergamon Press)
8. Goldberg, M.E. and Horovitz, Z.P. (1978). Antidepressants and aggressive behavior. *Mod. Probl. Pharmacopsych.* Vol. 13, pp. 29–52. (Basel: Karger)
9. Gray, J.A. (1972). The structure of the emotions and the limbic system. In *Physiology, Emotion and Psychosomatic Illness.* Ciba Foundation Symposium 8, pp. 87–120. (Amsterdam: Elsevier)
10. Heninger, G., DiMascio, A. and Klerman, G.L. (1965). Personality factors in variability of response to phenothiazines. *Am. J. Psychiatry*, **121,** 1091
11. Hinde, R.A. (1972). Concepts of emotion. In *Physiology, Emotion and Psychosomatic Illness.* Ciba Foundation Symposium 8, pp. 3–13. (Amsterdam: Elsevier)
12. Janke, W., Debus, G. and Longo N. (1979). Differential psychopharmacology of tranquilizing and sedating drugs. *Mod. Probl. Pharmacopsych.* Vol. 14, pp. 13–98. (Basel: Karger)
13. Moehler, H. and Okada, T. (1979). The benzodiazepine receptor in human brain. In Priest, R.G., Pletscher, A. and Ward, J. (eds.) *Sleep Research*, pp. 3–12. (Lancaster: MTP Press)
14. Pare, C.M.B., Rees, Linford and Sainsbury, M.J. (1962). Differentiation of two genetically specific types of depression by the response to antidepressants. *Lancet*, **2,** 1340
15. Randall, L.O., Schallek, W., Heise, G.A., Keith, E.F. and Bagdon, R.E. (1960). The psychosedative properties of methaminodiazepoxide. *J. Pharmacol. Exp. Ther.*, **129,** 163

16. Shagass, C. and Jones, A.L. (1958). A neurophysiological test for psychiatric diagnosis: results in 750 patients. *Am. J. Psychiatry*, **114,** 1002
17. Silverstone, T. (1979). Psychopharmacology. *Br. J. Psychiatry*, **134,** 640
18. Valzelli, L. (1979). Effects of sedatives and axiolytics on aggressivity. *Mod. Probl. Pharmacopsych.* Vol. 14, pp. 143–56. (Basel: Karger)

Bibliography

Benzodiazepines in paediatrics

Anders, T.F. (1976). What we now know about sleep disorders in children. *Med. Times (Lond)*, **104,** 75, 80

Anders, T.F. and Ciaranello,R.D. (1977). Psychopharmacology of childhood disorders. In Barchas, J.D., Berger, T.A., Ciaranello, R.D. and Elliott, G.R. (eds.). *Psychopharmacology from Theory to Practice*, pp. 407–24. (New York: University Press)

Bain, D.J. (1975). Prescribing psychotropic drugs for children. *J. Roy. Coll. Gen. Pract.*, **25,** 49

Bolton, A. (1972). The anxious child. *Br. Med. J.*, **3,** 690

Campbell, M. (1973). Biological interventions in psychoses of childhood. *J. Aut. Child. Schizo.*, **3,** 347

Campbell, M. and Small, A.M. (1976). The use of psychotherapeutic drugs in pediatrics. In Simpson, L.L. (ed.). *Drug Treatment of Mental Disorders*, pp. 209–36. (New York: Raven Press)

Conners, C.K. (1976). Classification and treatment of childhood depression and depressive equivalents. In Gallant, D.M. and Simpson, G.M. (eds.). *Depression, Behavioral, Biochemical Diagnostic and Treatment Concepts*, pp. 181–204. (New York: Spectrum Publications)

Cooper, S.F., Leach, C., Storer, D. and Tonge, W.L. (1977). The children of psychiatric patients.—Clinical findings. *Br. J. Psychiatry*, **131,** 514

Delong, A.R. (1972). What have we learned from psychoactive drug research on hyperactives? *Am. J. Dis. Child*, **123,** 177

Diesing, J. (1972). Psychopharmakologische Therapie der Enuresis. *Saar. Aerztebl.*, **25,** 361

Duche, D.J. and Castagnet, F. (1972). Le diazépam en psychiatrie infantile. *Rev. Neuropsychiat. Infant. Hyg. Ment. Enfance*, **20,** 81

Eggers, C. (1977). Psychopharmaka-Therapie im Kindesalter. *Fortschr. Med.*, **95,** 2028

Ehrhardt, K.J. (1975). Leitsymptom – Konzentrationsstörungen bei Schulkindern *Dtsch. Aerztebl.*, **72,** 3179

Engelhardt, D.M. (1969). Outpatient use of psychotropic drugs. – Guidelines for the non-expert. In Black P. (ed.). *Drugs and the Brain*, pp. 223–38. (Baltimore: Johns Hopkins Press)

Eveloff, H.H. (1970). Pediatric psychopharmacology. In Clark, W.G. and del Giudice, J. (eds.). *Principles of Psychopharmacology*, pp. 683–94. (New York: Academic Press)

Fish, B. (1968). Drug therapy in children's psychiatric disorders. *Mod. Probl. Pharmacopsych.* Vol. 1, pp. 60–72. (Basel: Karger)

Fish, B. (1970). Children's psychopharmacology unit. *Psychopharmacol. Bull.*, **6,** 27

Foerster, C. (1976). Anwendung von Psychopharmaka in der Kinderheilkunde. *Therapiewoche*, **26,** 3808, 3811, 3814, 3817

Franková, S. and Jakoubek, B. (1974). Long-term behavioural effects of diazepam and ACTH, administered early in life. *Activ. Nerv. Sup.* (*Praha*), **16,** 247

Fujii, I. (1973). Tranquilizers in pediatrics. *J. Pediatr.*, **36,** 1206

Graham, P. (1976). Management in child psychiatry. – Recent trends. *Br. J. Psychiatry*, **129,** 97

Green, M. and Zelson, C. (1976). The effect of psychotherapeutic drugs on the neonate. In Usdin, E. and Forrest, I.S. (eds.). *Psychotherapeutic Drugs, Principles. Psychopharmacol. Series*, Vol. 2, part 1, pp. 521–43. (New York: Dekker)

Guensberger, E. and Fedor, P. (1967). Psychosedierung bei Kindern mit organischen Hirnläsionen. *Internationales Symposium über Psychosedierung in Geriatrie und Paediatrie am 24–25.2.1967* in Wien. *Oesterr. Monatsh. Aerztl. Fortbild.*, special issue, pp. 129–35

Harbauer, H. (1974). Kinderpsychiatrische Aspekte bei der Betreuung des behinderten Kindes. *Therapiewoche*, **24,** 1254, 1256, 1259

Harms, D. (1973). Psychopharmaka im Kindesalter. Indikationen, Kontraindikationen und Nebenwirkugen. *Paediatr. Prax.*, **12,** 505

Helwig, H. (1972). Psychopharmaka im Kindesalter. *Kinderarzt*, **20,** 353

Helwig, H. (1973). Psychopharmaka im Kindesalter. *Mschr. Kinderheilk.*, **121,** 114

Herxheimer, H. (1970). Sedativa und Tranquilizer in der Kinderheilkunde. *Kinderarzt*, **18,** 13

Ishibashi, Y. (1972). Usage of antianxiety and antidepressant drugs with regard to psychosomatic and neurotic diseases of children. *J. Ther.*, **54,** 2379

Itil, T.M. and Mukhopadhyay, S. (1978). Pharmacological management of human violence. *Mod. Probl. Pharmacopsych.* Vol. 13, pp. 139–58. (Basel: Karger)

Koupernik, C. (1972). Chemotherapy in child psychiatry. *Br. Med. J.*, **3,** 345

Masanes, P., Touchard, F.M., Kohler, M. and Barret, T. (1975). Bilan de 3 ans d'utilisation du diazépam en pédopsychiatrie ambulatoire. *Rev. Neuropsychiat. Infant. Hyg. Ment. Enfance*, **23,** 465

Neuhaeuser, G. (1972). Psychopharmakotherapie bei Kindern. *Hippokrates*, **43,** 449

Neuhaeuser, G. (1974). Indikationen zur Psychopharmakotherapie bei Kindern. Die Behandlung muss vorher mit Eltern und Kind besprochen werden. *Aerzt. Prax.*, **26,** 1311, 1313

Nissen, G. (1975). Leitsymptome einer psychopharmakologischen Therapie im Kindesalter. *Kinderarzt*, **6,** 1171, 1175

Nissen, G. (1975). Verhaltensanomalien. Pharmaka helfen. Psycho-Medikation Bestandteil, nicht Mittelpunkt der Therapie. *Prax. Kur.*, **13,** 11

Nissen, G. (1977). Bei Verhaltensstörungen Medikamente kritisch einsetzen. *Euromed*, **17,** 824, 826

Nissen, G. (1978). Behandlungsmöglichkeiten kindlicher Verhaltensstörungen. *Med. Welt*, **29,** 1358

Oda, Y. and Uchiyama, S. (1975). Clinical study of bromazepam (Lexotan) in pediatrics. *Clin. Med.*, **17,** 387

Purvis, R. J. (1978). The management of the hyperkinetic child. *Br. J. Psychiatry*, **132**, 201

Rosenmayr, F. and Groh, C. (1974). Unerwünschte Effekte durch Psychopharmaka bei Kindern. *Paediat. Paedol.*, **9**, 144

Safer, D.J. (1978). Drug treatment in child psychiatry. In Iversen, L.L., Iversen, S.D. and Snyder, S.H. (eds.). *Handbook of Psychopharmacology, sect. 3, Human Psychopharmacology, vol. 11, Stimulants*, pp. 167–217. (New York: Plenum Press)

Sefrin, P. (1975). Erstversorgung bei Notfällen im Kindesalter. *Anaesth. Intensivmed. Prax.*, **10**, 17

Simeon, J. and Itil, T.M. (1973). Pediatric psychopharmacology outside the United States. *Psychopharmacol. Bull.*, **9**, 50

Simeon, J., Huque, M., Davis, S. and Itil, T.M. (1976). Sleep in children with psychiatric disorders. In Baronet-Lacroix, D. (ed.). *Résumés/Abstracts 10th Congress* Collegium Intern. Neuro-Psychopharmacologicum, Quebec, July 1976, p. 178, abstr. no. 264. (Quebec: Univ. Laval)

Srinath, M.G. and Suvarna, G.C. (1976). Trial of diazepam (Calmpose) syrup in behaviour disorders of children. *Antiseptic*, **73**, 486

Steinhausen, H.C. (1976). Das hyperkinetische Syndrom. *Klin. Paediatr.*, **188**, 396

Strunk, P. (1972). Therapie mit Psychopharmaka bei Kindern und Jugendlichen. *Internist*, **13**, 197

Teicher, J.D. (1978). Kinder, die sterben wollen. *Tempo Med.*, **2**, 24

Weingaertner, L. (1976). Arzneimittel in der Kinderheilkunde. *Mod. Arzneim. Ther.*, **1**, 171

Wiesener, H. (1975). Psychopharmaka im Kindesalter. *Z. Allgemeinmed.*, **51**, 436

Willner, M.M. and Gordon, L.E. (1969). Psychotropic drugs in children. Pharmacotherapy as an adjunct to counseling or psychotherapy. *Clin. Pediatr.*, **8**, 193

15

Some Data on Parenteral Bromazepam

J. de Souza Campos

Patients and methods

In our trial, bromazepam 10 mg ampoule was administered by i.m. or i.v. routes to 80 patients with emotional disorders, compulsions, phobias, several types of neurosis, and functional and encephalopathic psychosis. The intramuscular route was used in 72 patients and the intravenous route in eight. The number of ampoules administered and duration of the treatment varied according to the intensity of the symptoms. In the first days, a higher dosage was used at shorter intervals; as the symptoms declined, the dosage was reduced or administered at longer intervals. In most cases, a single ampoule was injected at a time, and the dose repeated some hours later. In more severe cases, we administered 2 ampoules every 6 hours for 24 hours. The average observation period was 6 days.

The medical prescriptions that the patient had been taking, especially the antiepileptics, were not discontinued in any case.

The following parameters have been investigated: clinical effect on psychiatric symptomatology, vital functions (blood pressure, pulse, axillary and cutaneous temperature, respiratory movements), ergographic tests, muscular strength and ophthalmological examinations.

Results

Overall effect

In all patients with *anxious neurotic symptoms*, excitement and compulsion, bromazepam after parenteral administration showed a clear anxiolytic action and it was therapeutically effective in the state of psychic hyper-excitement, 'ruminative thoughts', psychomotor tiredness and mental fatigue, emotional tension and consequent somatization, aggressiveness, inhibition–excitement conflicts, confused neurotic states, obsessive rituals and incapacity and ambivalence of decisions.

In psychiatric disorders due to either psychogenic or organic causes, bromazepam showed rapid onset of action in reducing or eliminating symptoms of agitation and on the corresponding productive activity.

It was observed that 70 out of the 80 patients maintained a normal alertness state throughout the day and 8 experienced prolonged sleepiness. The alert patients carried on normal activity or went to the occupational therapy sessions.

Blood pressure, pulse, axillary temperature, respiratory movements and cutaneous electrothermometry of the extremities before and after administration, both in orthostatic and supine positions were controlled; no abnormal change in these parameters was noted.

Role of the different routes of administration

In acute hypnotic states induced by *intravenous injection* of bromazepam (10 mg), a state similar to the crepuscular one, with discrete disturbance of the hemispheric dominance, and haptic sensitivity changes, were observed in some patients upon awakening. These changes were evidenced by the proportional screw test, by the Bloomenfeldt test and by electric tremblemeter.

In this awakening phase, some aspects of the Gerstmann's syndrome were also observed, such as finger agnosia, right and left disorientation, agraphia, dyslexia and acalculia.

Upon reversion to the normal alert state (two hours afterwards, on average), neither these changes nor the simultaneous agnosia of Wolpert were to be observed; the haptic sensitivity, the Weber zones of epicritic sensitivity and the acmesthesia were also normal.

Some minutes *after the i.m. injection* of bromazepam, a state of sleepiness, hyporeflexia and discrete dysmetria occurs, hardly ever exceeding half an hour. In 14 cases after the administration of 2 ampoules (20 mg) a pronounced palpebral ptosis was observed, sometimes preceded by diplopia.

The dynamometric tests performed on all patients given 20 mg i.m. doses showed a clear reduction of muscular strength, in both right and left hands, thirty and sixty minutes after administration.

Special investigations

Ergographic tests were performed on 20 patients with anxious neurotic crises. Before the treatment, the tracings obtained were considered very deficient in a global analysis: muscular contractions of small width, irregular rhythm, early tiring. After the treatment, the new tests exhibited great width of muscular contractions, constant rhythm and prolonged work without fatigue.

Ophthalmological investigations were performed in 12 patients. Since some increase in intraocular pressure has been reported in the literature on benzodiazepines, in six patients treated with bromazepam by i.m. route, tonometry tests were performed before, during and at the end of the treatment. No tonometric changes occurred. In these six patients the visual acuity, chromatic sense and manual perimetry were also controlled. At the last pressure reading all results found were normal. In six patients the physiological parameters were controlled 10 minutes after the administration of 20mg bromazepam i.m. and in six other patients 5 minutes after the administration of 10mg bromazepam i.v. No abnormal change was noted.

Comments

Among the benzodiazepines, bromazepam has been showing a clear therapeutic effect without toxic manifestations, even with high dosage. The suppression of anxiety symptoms without great changes in the state of alertness or any disturbance of the watchful and elaborative functions must be emphasized. When bromazepam is administered by the oral route, it is possible to attain a calm state without sedation allowing the patient to maintain his normal pragmatic activity.

After intramuscular and, especially after intravenous administration, sleepiness appears after injection. While recovering some patients show aspects of Gerstmann's syndrome, agraphia and simultaneous agnosia of Wolpert. These disturbances of the 'corporal schema', space–time concept and directional orientation did not last long (20–30 minutes). These changes in sensitivity suggest parieto-occipital dysfunction of a transitory nature.

The anxiolytic, sedative, hypnotic and muscle-relaxant effect of bromazepam (shown clearly in the reduction of postural tonus and the palpebral ptosis after i.m. administration) must be emphasized.

In fatigue and psychic tiredness, bromazepam had a good effect by normalizing the emotional state and allowing return to work with good efficiency. The motor performance tests confirmed the reduction in fatiguability in anxious patients.

It appears that parenteral use of bromazepam is indicated in acute psychiatric states with agitation, aggressiveness, restlessness and insomnia. It is also efficient for controlling acute manic states. In schizophrenic and encephalopathic patients, the effects of bromazepam on psychomotor agitation, excitability and dromic crises were less favourable: usually good results at first, but of short duration. In epileptic agitation the results were also only moderate.

Conclusion

Our clinical observations have confirmed the advantageous effect of parenteral use of bromazepam as a symptomatic medication in acute psychic states. The results have been good also in anxious somatizations, nervous fatigue, neurotic anxiety and muscular tension.

Bibliography

Bromazepam

Auf der Maur, A., Huber, H., Thüer, R., Vogel, M. and Wetterwald, O. (1974). Lexotanil, ein neues Benzodiazepinderivat in der ambulanten Praxis. *Ars Medici*, **64,** 437

Barclay, C. A. (1975). Flunitrazepam. – Aspectos farmacológicos. Presented at the *Symposium 'Flunitrazepam en Anestesiología y Clínica Médica'*, November 26, Buenos Aires.

Burrell, R. H., Culpan, R. H., Newton, K. J., Ogg, G. J. and Short, J. H. (1974). Use of bromazepam in obsessional, phobic and related states. *Curr. Med. Res. Opin.*, **2,** 430

Carlier, L., Delattre, A. and Demanet, G. (1974). Etude clinique ouverte et à double insu d'une nouvelle benzodiazépine dans les troubles névrotiques. *Ars Med.* (Brux.), **29,** 935

Deberdt, R. (1974). Treatment of obsessional and phobic neurosis with Ro 5-3350. *Medikon*, **3,** 27

De Silva, J. A. F., Bekersky, I., Brooks, M. A., Weinfeld, R. E., Glover, K. and Puglisi, C. (1974). Determination of bromazepam in blood by electron-capture GLC and of its major urinary metabolites by differential pulse polarography. *J. Pharm. Sci.*, **63,** 1440

Fink, M., Irwin, P. and Gastpar, M. (1976). Pharmacokinetic analysis of quantitative EEG data. In Lucchelli, P. E. *et al.* (eds.), *Rationality of Drug Development. Proc. 2nd Int. Meet. of Med. Advisers in the Pharm. Industry, Florence, Oct. 13–15, 1975*, pp. 177–180. (Amsterdam: Excerpta Med.)

Gayral, L. F. (1975). Qualifications thérapeutiques des 1,4 (et 1,5) benzodiazépines psychotropes. *Actual. Psychiat.*, **6,** 26

Goldstein, N. (1973). Klinische Prüfung des Präparates Ro 5-3350 ('Lexotanil') bei psychosomatischen Krankheitsbildern. (Uebersetzung) *Rev. Argent. Psicofarmacol.*, **1973,** 10

Guerrero-Figueroa, R., Guerrero-Figueroa, E., Sneed, G. A. and Kennedy, H. J. (1974). Effects of lorazepam on CNS structures: Neurophysiological and behavioral correlations. *Curr. Ther. Res.*, **16,** 137

Kaplan, S. A., Jack, M. L., Weinfeld, R. E., Glover, W., Weissman, L. and Cotler, S. (1976). Biopharmaceutical and clinical pharmacokinetic profile of bromazepam. *Pharmacokin. Biopharm.*, **4,** 1

Ladame, F. G. (1974). Essai comparatif ambulatoire du Ro 5-3350 (Lexotanil) et de l'oxazépam. *Praxis*, **63,** 1005

Laffranchini, S. (1975). Expérience de cinq années en pratique psychiatrique ambulatoire avec un tranquillisant nouveau, le Lexotanil (Ro 5-3350). *Ther. Umschau*, **32,** 741

Modestin, J. and Hodel, J. (1976). Lorazepam (Temesta) versus bromazepam (Lexotanil). – Kontrollierter Kreuzversuch. *Münch. Med. Wschr.*, **118,** 1335

Plavec, J. (1977). Long-term treatment of patients with psychosomatic ailments with bromazepam (LEXOTANIL[R]). Presented at the *4th Congress of the International College of Psychosomatic Medicine*, September 5–9, Kyoto.

Porot, M., Perol, J. Y. and Coudert, A. J. (1975). Le bromazépam en médecine psychosomatique. Presented at '*3. Congrès du Collège Intern. de Méd. Psychosomatique*', September, Rome.

Raaflaub, J. (1975). On the pharmacokinetics of bromazepam in man. In Antonelli, F. (ed.), *Psychopharmacology of Somatization, Biological and Psychological Assessments, 3. Congr. Mondiale dell'International College of Psychosomatic Med.*, pp. 57–60. (Rome: Pozzi)

Schwartz, M. A., Postma, E., Kolis, S. and Leon, A. S. (1973). Metabolites of bromazepam, a benzodiazepine, in the human, dog, rat and mouse. *J. Pharm. Sci.*, **62,** 1776

Solomon, K. (1976). Benzodiazepines and neurotic anxiety. Critique. *NY State J. Med.*, **76,** 2156

Vianello, M. (1974). Lunga sperimentazione clinica di un nuovo psicofarmaco. *Pubb. Med. Ticinesi*, **21,** 33

Bromazepam ampoules

Chung, W. H., Choi, J. Y. and Suh, B. S. (1974). Clinical trial of a new benzodiazepine derivate – Ro 5-3350. *Korean Centr. J. Med.*, **26,** 433

Deffeminis Rospide, H. A. (1974). Acción de algunos benzodiazepínicos en la hipertonía piramidal. Evaluación durante 5 años. Presented at the *VII Simposio Neurológico José María Ramosmejia – Progresos en Neurología*, December 2–3, Buenos Aires.

De Giacomo, P. and Pierri, G. (1974). Valutazione clinica del bromazepam con particolare riferimento a sindromi ossessive e fobiche. *Acta Neurol.*, **29,** 307

Gsell, S. (1975). Klinische Erfahrungen mit dem Benzodiazepinderivat Bromazepam bei akuten Unruhe- und Erregungszuständen in der Psychiatrie. *Nervenarzt*, **46,** 463

Pavan, G. and Bezoari, M. (1974). Profilo di azione del bromazepam (Ro 5-3350) rilevato in tre anni di studio clinico 'aperto'. Presented at the *V. Riunione della Società Italiana di Neuropsicofarmacologia*, June 14–15, Bari (Italy).

Pozenel, H., Bückert, A. and Amrein, R. (1977). The antihypertensive effect of bromazepam (Lexotan). – A new benzodiazepine derivative. Further haemodynamic investigations. In Antonelli, F. (ed.), *Psychopharmacology of Somatization, Biological and Psychological Assessments. 3. Congr. Mondiale dell'International College of Psychosomatic Med.*, pp. 48–56. (Rome: Pozzi)

Raaflaub, J. (1977). On the pharmacokinetics of bromazepam in man. In Antonelli, F. (ed.), *Psychopharmacology of Somatization, Biological and Psychological Assessments. 3. Congr. Mondiale dell'International College of Psychosomatic Med.*, pp. 57–60. (Rome: Pozzi)

Raaflaub, J. and Speiser-Courvoisier, J. (1974). Zur Pharmakokinetik von Bromazepam beim Menschen. *Arzneim. Forsch.*, **24,** 1841

Vincent, O., Deffeminis Rospide, H. A., Scarabino, R. and Medici, M. (1973). A comparative study on the effect of intravenous diazepam and Ro 5-3350 on pyramidal spasticity. *Electroencephalogr. Clin. Neurophysiol.*, **34**, 804, Abstr. No. 35

16

Psychotherapy and Psychopharmacotherapy

W. Pöldinger

In comparing two different methods of therapy, one must be aware that, in considering the individual methods, one starts from different premises and that these may be very dissimilar. This may mean that it is impossible to regard the two therapies from the same viewpoint. An example of this are the different views and theories which are valid for psychosomatics, and which, as Table 16.1 shows, result in different therapeutic approaches. Thus we can apply a psychological view of psychosomatic complaints, leading to practical therapeutic procedures such as autogenic training or psychopharmacotherapy. If we take a casuistic or psychological view of psychosomatic phenomena, however, this will naturally lead us to make use of guidance methods, the content of which will be the various life events. If we regard psychosomatic disorders and diseases from the psychodynamic viewpoint of depth psychology, this results in the various analytical therapeutic approaches. We can, however, regard the development of psychosomatic disturbances from the standpoint of learning theory, and this of course involves behaviour therapy. Finally it is also possible to

Table 16.1 Psychosomatic attitudes and treatment methods

Psychobiological	practical procedures, e.g. autogenic training, drug therapy
Psychological, casuistic	guidance
Psychodynamic	analytical psychotherapy
Learning theory	behaviour therapy
Philosophical, teleological	logotherapy, existential analysis

regard psychosomatic illness from a teleological point of view, and this brings us to more philosophical approaches to treatment such as logotherapy and existential analysis.

If we compare psychotherapy and psychopharmacotherapy, therefore, we must realize that in the one case we are starting from the viewpoint of psychology or depth psychology, and in the other from that of psychobiology. It must be emphasized, however, that these are differences of angle or attitude and not fundamental opposites, since the different aspects and the resulting therapeutic approaches are not mutually exclusive. If we consider, for example, a complicated psychodynamic repressive mechanism, or a learning process, these can only occur if the ganglion cells are functioning properly. Healthy, functioning ganglion cells are essential for any psychological or psychosomatic process. This means that the psychobiological aspect, for instance, cannot be excluded: it is the prerequisite for the other aspects.

Unfortunately, however, the different schools in psychiatry and especially in psychotherapy see matters not from different angles but from completely and fundamentally opposing positions. We must emphasize, nevertheless, that this is really an unmedical attitude, since our aim in diagnosis and therapy is not to confirm existing opinions and theories within the framework of a single therapeutic system; rather, a physician's duty is always, when one therapeutic strategy fails, to apply and if necessary develop new strategies for treating the patient. Even when we do this, and regard psychotherapy in the broadest sense, we have a wide variety of therapeutic possibilities, starting from guidance, via the different forms of analytical psychotherapy and behaviour therapy to the philosophically oriented logotherapeutic and existential analytical treatment methods.

With psychopharmacotherapy, the problem is quite different, and to a certain extent easier, since we know which cerebral substrates are affected by the various drugs and what effects they have in general. The modern psychotropic drugs comprise principally the neuroleptics or major tranquillizers, the (minor) tranquillizers and the antidepressants. As this book is concerned with the benzodiazepines, Table 16.2 shows the main effects of the derivatives of this group of drugs. These properties can be utilized very appropriately in the treatment of emotional and psychosomatic disturbances and diseases. One must realize, however, that the effect is symptomatic and that it is of course not possible to exert a direct influence

Table 16.2 Pharmacodynamics of the benzodiazepines

1. Anxiolytic
2. Autonomic stabilizing
3. Tranquillizing inner and motor restlessness
4. Inducing sleep
5. Muscle-relaxing (possibly)

on intra- or extrapsychic problems or conflicts or even social behaviour. In all truth, however, it must be said that no one has ever claimed otherwise.

Combining psychotherapy and psychopharmocology

This brings us right back again to the antithesis between psychotherapy and psychopharmacotherapy, which can no longer be seen as an antithesis in the light of present-day knowledge; both psychotherapy and psychopharmacotherapy can usefully be applied together. Precisely when we say that intra- and extrapsychic problems and conflicts cannot be solved by psychopharmacotherapy, we must emphasize that only by relieving anxiety, by calming the patient, by raising his spirits, does it sometimes become possible to talk reasonably with him about his problems. Precisely also when we are considering psychosomatic disorders and diseases, it will be necessary at the beginning of what is often a long psychotherapeutic intervention to render the patient's symptoms more bearable. In this connection, the anxiolytic and autonomic stabilizing effects of the benzodiazepines should be particularly mentioned.

In speaking of the combination of psychotherapy and psychopharmacotherapy, however, we must also remember that an addition to the pharmacodynamic action, what Balint called the drug 'doctor', has an important role. We know that, especially with psychotropic drugs, the part played by the so-called 'placebo' effect is considerable, and that very much depends on the form and the words with which we propose or prescribe a drug. We can thus in prescribing a psychotropic drug also to some extent perform a psychotherapeutic gesture in the same way as, in the opposite direction, by giving a psychopharmaceutical which affects not only emotional but also autonomic nervous symptoms, we exert or intensify somatic therapy.

These relationships between psychopharmacotherapy and psychotherapy on the one hand and somatotherapy on the other are shown in Figure 16.1. We see in this way that there is no contradiction between psychotherapy and psychopharmacotherapy, but that these two methods of treatment complement each other and in addition both also influence purely somatic

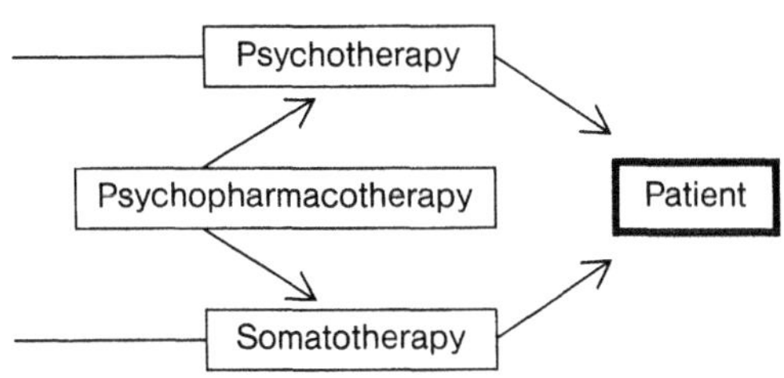

Figure 16.1 Psychosomatically oriented plan of treatment

treatment. Psychopharmacotherapy can in some cases be necessary to create the very possibilities for psychotherapy; conversely, psychotherapy may enable a patient to understand that it is necessary for him to take a psychotropic drug for a certain time, and this drug can then exert direct somatic effects and thereby modify his bodily feelings.

Before concluding, perhaps I may include a critical, historical remark. How did this conflict arise? Historically, there have always been 'psychicists' and 'somaticists' among psychiatrists and the conflict between psychopharmacotherapy and psychotherapy, which has been artificially overinflated, is really nothing more than a repetition of this interesting confrontation in the history of medicine. There is however also a practical factor. Only a physician is allowed to prescribe and use drugs. Yet we know that non-physicians, especially psychologists, can give very valuable psychotherapy. They can neither prescribe nor provide drugs for their patients, and it is therefore understandable that there should be stronger resistance to the psychotropic drugs among the non-medical psychotherapists than among doctors.

Conclusions

In summary, therefore, an antithesis can be constructed between psychotherapy and psychopharmacotherapy, and can be documented from the history of medicine. It begins to crumble, however, as soon as we realize that these are not opposing principles, but merely different aspects. If we do not proceed from schools of thought and theories to be justified and confirmed in the individual patient, but from the patient's need for as comprehensive help as possible, we shall of necessity come to treatment strategies which cannot be one-sided but will contain a variety of therapeutic approaches. In emotional and psychosomatic disorder, the most important, complementary therapeutic measures are psychotherapy and psychopharmacotherapy. In appropriate circumstances, they must of course be further complemented by somatic treatments such as physiotherapy, occupational therapy, creative therapy and music therapy. The wider the range of therapy offered, the better the chance of success and recovery for the individual patient. In this palette, the psychopharmaceuticals have an important place.

Bibliography

Benzodiazepines and psychotherapy

Anonymous (1973). Sperimentazione clinica del bromazepam su pazienti psiconevrotici e psicosomatici in trattamento psicoterapico. *Med. Psicosom.*, **18**, 39

Argyle, M., Bryant, B. and Trower, P. (1974). Social skills training and psychotherapy. – A comparative study. *Psychol. Med.*, **4**, 435

Barahona Fernandes, H. J. (1976). Médicaments psychotropes et relation médecin-malade. Presented at *10e Congrès International de Psychothérapie*, July 4–11, Paris.

Battegay, R. and Rauchfleisch, U. (1973). Pathogenese und Therapie des Alkoholismus. *Z. Allg. Med. Landarzt*, **49**, 945

Beckmann, H., Vogel, P. G. and Braun-Falco, O. (1976). Psychotherapie und Psychopharmakotherapie in der Dermatologie. II. Psychopharmakotherapie in der Dermatologie. *Hautarzt*, **27**, 525

Bellak, L., Chassan, J. B., Gediman, H. K. and Hurvich, M. (1973). Ego function assessment of analytic psychotherapy combined with drug therapy. *J. Nerv. Ment. Dis.*, **157**, 465

Beyme, F. (1965). Das neue Schlafmittel Mogadon und das Traumgeschehen. *Psychiatr. Neurol.*, **149**, 136

Blumberger, S. R. and De Rivera, J. L. (1977). Homosexual dynamics studies with autogenic abreaction and psychotherapy of analytic orientation. In Luthe, W. and Antonelli, F. (eds.), *Therapy in Psychosomatic Medicine, 3. Congr. Mondiale dell'International College of Psychosomatic Medicine, Rome, September* 1975, Vol. 4, Autogenic Therapy, pp. 135–140 (Rome: Pozzi)

Covi, L., Lipman, R. S. and Derogatis, L. R. (1973). Imipramine, diazepam and group psychotherapy in long-term treatment of depressive neurotics. *Psychopharmacol. Bull.*, **9**, 57

Covi, L., Lipman, R. S. and Guzman, R. A. (1975). Drug psychotherapy interactions in depression. In *128th Ann. Meet. of the American Psychiatric Association, May 5–9, Anaheim/Cal.*, pp. 89–90

Covi, L., Lipman, R. S., Alarcon, R. D. and Smith, V. K. (1976). Drug and psychotherapy interactions in depression. *Am. J. Psychiatry*, **133**, 502

Covi, L., Lipman, R. S., Derogatis, L. R., Smith, J. E. and Pattison, J. H. (1974). Drugs and group psychotherapy in neurotic depression. *Am. J. Psychiatry*, **131**, 191

Dean, S. R. (1964). Diazepam as an adjuvant in psychotherapy. *Am. J. Psychiatry*, **121**, 389

Dean, S. R. (1965). Diazepam as an adjuvant in clinical psychotherapy. *Dis. Nerv. Syst.*, **26**, 181

Denham, J. (1963). Psychotherapy of obsessional neurosis assisted by Librium. In Stokvis, B. (ed.), *Topical Problem of Psychotherapy*, Vol. 4, *Selected Lectures, Proc. of the 4th Intern. Congr. of Psychotherapy, Aug. 21–26, 1961, Wien*, pp. 195–198 (Basel: Karger)

Gerz, H. O. (1966). Ueber 7jährige klinische Erfahrungen mit der logotherapeutischen Technik der paradoxen Intention. *Z. Psychother.*, **16**, 25

Gittelman-Klein, R. (1978). Psychopharmacological treatment of anxiety disorders, mood disorders, and Tourette's disorder in children. In Lipton, M. A. DiMascio, A. and Killam, K. F. (eds.), *Psychopharmacology, a Generation of Progress*, pp. 1471–1480. (New York: Raven Press)

Goellner, R. (1978). Medikationen in der psychotherapeutischen Behandlung. *Med. Klin.*, **73**, 539

Hajek, F. and Vojtechovsky, M. (1975). Drug treatment in the first 30 days of hospitalization in the psychiatric hospital in Horny Berkovice. *Activitas Nervosa Superior*, **17**, 299

Hodge, J. R. (1978). Multiple ways to treat anxiety. *Med. Times*, **101**, 148

Holmberg, G. (1974). Bensodiazepiner. Kombination med andra behandlingsformer. In Holmberg, G. (ed.). *Symposium on bensodiazepiner i relation till andra dagsedativa, March 1974, Stockholm*, pp. 97–107. (Stockholm: Roche)

Jores, A. V. and Kerekjarto, M. (1968). Internal medicine and psychosomatic medicine. – Psychotherapy and psychopharmacotherapy. In *Int. Symposium on Psychotropic Drugs in Internal Med., May, 5–8, 1968, Naples*, pp. 7–8. (Hoffmann-La Roche)

Kielholz, P. (1969). The drug treatment of anxiety. In Stoller, A. and Davies, B. (eds.), *Aust. NZJ. Psychiatry*, Vol. 3, No. 3A, Studies Melbourne/Aust., May 1969, pp. 277–281

Kleinsorge, H. (1974). Moderne Hypnotherapie mit medikamentöser Unterstützung. *Therapiewoche*, **24**, 4779

Knoepfel, H. K. (1967). Beispiel einer hausärztlichen Psychotherapie. *Ther. Umsch.*, **24**, 363

Luzes, P. (1966). Psicofarmacos e psicoterapia no tratamento das neuroses. *J. Med. Porto*, **60**, 149

Marks, I. M. (1976). 'Psychopharmacology' – the use of drugs combined with psychological treatment. In Spitzer, R. L. and Klein, D. F. (eds.), *Evaluation of Psychological Therapies, Psychotherapies, Behavior Therapies, Drug Therapies and their Interactions*, pp. 108–126, 150–151. (Baltimore: Johns Hopkins Univ. Press)

Marks, I. M., Cameron, P. M. and Silberfeld, M. (1971). Operant therapy for an abnormal personality. *Br. Med. J.*, **1971/I**, 647

Mikhail, A. R. (1976). Treatment of vaginismus by i.v. diazepam (Valium) abreaction interviews. *Acta Psychiatr. Scand.*, **53**, 328

Pasini, E. (1978). Traitements psychothérapeutique et pharmacothérapeutique associés dans la thérapie de l'impuissance psychogène. *Praxis*, **67**, 1185

Pfefferbaum, A. (1977). Psychotherapy and psychopharmacology. In Barchas, J. D., Berger, P. A., Ciaranello, R. D. and Elliott, G. R. (eds.). *Psychopharmacology, from Theory to Practice*, pp. 481–492. (New York: Oxford Univ. Press)

Podobnikar, I. G. (1971). Implementation of psychotherapy by Librium in a pioneering rural–industrial psychiatry practice. *Psychosomatics*, **12**, 205

Rickels, K. (1964). The use of psychotherapy with drugs in the treatment of anxiety. *Psychosomatics*, **5**, 111

Schonecke, O. W. and Schueffel, W. (1974). Evaluation of combined pharmacological and psychotherapeutic treatment in patients with functional abdominal disorders. Presented at the *10th European Conference on Psychosomatic Research*, September 15–20, Edinburgh.

Schonecke, O. W. and Schueffel, W. (1977). Bromazepam (Lexotanil) in the psychosomatic treatment of patients with functional abdominal disorders. In Antonelli, F. (ed.), *Psychopharmacology of Somatization, Biological and Psychological Assessments, 3. Congr. Mondiale dell'International College of Psychosomatic Med.*, pp. 79–86 (Rome: Pozzi)

Silverstone, T. (1970). The use of drugs in behavior therapy. *Behav. Ther.*, **1**, 485

Spiegelberg, U. (1968). Psychopharmaca in psychoanalysis and hypnotherapy (remarks to the problem of combined therapy). *Int. Pharmacopsychiatry*, **1**, 37

Uhlenhuth, E. H., Lipman, R. S. and Covi, L. (1969). Combined pharmacotherapy and psychotherapy. *J. Nerv. Ment. Dis.*, **148**, 52

Van Rhijn, C. H. (1966). Therapy of psychogenic headaches. A psychosomatic approach. In Lopez Ibor, J. J. and Plogsties, H. R. (eds.), *IV Congreso Mundial de Psiquiatría, Madrid, September 5–11*, p. 421, Abstr. No. 995, int. congr. ser. no. 117 (Amsterdam: Excerpta Med. Found.)

Van Rhijn, C. H. (1967). The therapeutic approach of psychogenic headaches. In Clayton-Jones, E. and Ottley, B. C. M. (eds.), *IV Congreso Mundial de Psiquiatría, Madrid, September 5–11*, pp. 87–88 (Amsterdam: Excerpta Med. Found.)

Vogel, P. G. and Beckmann, H. (1976). I. Psychotherapie und Psychopharmakotherapie in der Dermatologie. Psychotherapeutische Aspekte und Indikationsstellung. *Hautarzt*, **27**, 519

17

Treatment of Alcoholism: Experience with Benzodiazepines

S. C. Kaim

The treatment of alcoholism depends on the phase of the disease which the physician is called on to treat: acute intoxication, acute withdrawal, or chronic alcoholism. When should anti-anxiety drugs be used? Almost never for intoxication, almost always during withdrawal, and sometimes during the treatment of chronic alcoholism.

Acute intoxication

First, acute intoxication, excluding pathological intoxication, but including stupor and coma, should never be treated with any depressant drug. Potentiation of the CNS depression due to the high level of blood alcohol would inevitably lead to a worsening of the condition. Alcohol plus sedative drugs are often a lethal combination. The intoxicated individual should simply be allowed to sleep it off, preferably in the protective environment of his own home. Alcoholic coma may require haemodialysis, although providing a clear airway, fluids, vasopressor drugs, steroids and meticulous nursing care usually will suffice.

The one exception which requires sedative treatment is pathological intoxication. This condition of wild excitement in which the patient is a danger to himself and others probably represents an idiosyncratic reaction

Parts of this paper have appeared elsewhere.

to a relatively small amount of alcohol. Because the blood alcohol level is usually low, it is safe to employ a sedative drug to control the patient's agitation. Intravenous amobarbital, or diazepam (injected very slowly), will usually prove a successful form of treatment.

Chronic alcoholism

Acute intoxication and acute alcohol withdrawal are usually readily diagnosed, and after their treatment the physician should use the opportunity to institute rehabilitative therapy of the underlying alcoholism. But what of the much greater number of patients who present with one of the medical sequelae of alcoholism? The physician may suspect an alcoholic aetiology, but may hesitate to risk offending his patient by enquiring about his drinking habits. Yet, treating the physical consequences while disregarding the cause is akin to treating an epileptic solely by inserting a padded tongue blade in his mouth during a convulsion.

Arriving at the diagnosis of alcoholism in a sober patient is not always easy. I recommend that every physician become acquainted with the Criteria for the Diagnosis of Alcoholism[18], which was published by the National Council on Alcoholism in 1972. Although it encompasses some 90 criteria, it is only eight pages long, and should make the diagnosis of alcoholism relatively easy to rule in or out.

Jacob and Sellers[9] recently pointed out that while drugs are not the major therapy of choice in chronic alcoholism, they can be a very useful therapeutic adjunct in getting anxious and depressed patients involved in treatment and to 'maintain their gains once achieved'. They see drug treatment as valuable in 'alleviation of emotional problems which are involved in both cause and effect of excessive alcohol consumption'. Although drugs cannot substitute for the psychosocial therapies required for successful rehabilitation, short-term (6 to 8 weeks) use of anti-anxiety and/or antidepressant medication can help many alcoholic patients to participate in comprehensive treatment programmes.

The literature reveals conflicting reports of the findings of research devoted to drug therapy in alcoholism, perhaps because many such studies fail to differentiate among the phases of alcoholism being treated, for which the therapeutic modalities may radically differ. Another, and extremely important, variable is the socio-economic and psychological background of the individual patient.

To explore the influence of prognostic factors in the acceptance and outcome of treatment, Kissin *et al.*[15] studied cohorts of male alcoholic patients newly registered at two outpatient clinics. Subjects were randomly assigned to one of four groups: drug therapy, psychotherapy plus adjunctive drug therapy, inpatient rehabilitation, or control – six months without treatment (assigned to a waiting list). Patients assigned to drug therapy could accept or be dropped. Subjects who refused psychotherapy (plus drug treatment) could have the drug therapy alone, or drop out. Patients who rejected the rehabilitation ward could opt for any of the three alternatives.

More than half of the patients assigned to the psychotherapy and rehabilitation groups elected one of the alternative treatments. Outcome was later assessed based on the actual treatment received. Drug therapy usually consisted of a combination of chlordiazepoxide and imipramine. Psychotherapy was in groups conducted by psychologists. The rehabilitation programme involved group psychotherapy, social intervention and drug treatment as indicated. After discharge from the ward, treatment was continued in the after-care clinic.

There were several significant differences between those who accepted or rejected the assigned therapy. Psychotherapy acceptors had significantly higher educational and occupational status than those who rejected the psychotherapy modality. Rehabilitation acceptors had significantly lower occupational status than did acceptors. Socially and psychologically more intact patients accepted psychotherapy and rejected inpatient rehabilitation. The opposite prevailed for socially and psychologically unstable patients. There were no significant differences among the patients randomly assigned to the drug group.

At one year follow-up the patients who had actually been in the psychotherapy (plus drug therapy) group had the highest success rate, followed by the drug only group, then the rehabilitation group, with the controls having the lowest rate of success. Correlating outcome with prognostic factors, the socially and psychologically stable alcoholics tended to do best in psychotherapy; the socially more intact but psychologically less sophisticated patients did best in drug therapy. Surprisingly, the socially unstable but more sophisticated patients did best in the inpatient rehabilitation programme.

These results support the theory that 'different kinds of patients respond differently to different kinds of treatments'. Selecting the most suitable therapeutic modality for the individual alcoholic patient will surely increase the chances for a successful outcome.

Corroborating this conclusion were the results of another drug study by Kissin and Platz[14]. In a double-blind study they found the combination of chlordiazepoxide and imipramine the most effective of the four treatments tested. The patients treated with chlordiazepoxide alone had the next highest success rate, followed by the placebo group, with the imipramine alone group showing the poorest results. The authors suggested that random use of a drug in a heterogeneous alcoholic population might 'be contra-indicated since the benefit derived from the specific effects of these drugs in appropriate patients may be cancelled out by the detrimental effects of these drugs in inappropriate patients (i.e. tranquillizers in retarded patients, or antidepressants in agitated patients)'.

Alcohol withdrawal

Many reports of studies in alcoholism suffer a credibility gap in their failure to differentiate among the various alcohol-related syndromes, which are then treated together, leading to meaningless analyses of a mixed salad of numbers of cases improved, unimproved, worse or dead. The several states associated with excessive use of alcohol may have different aetiologies, courses, signs and symptoms. Some of the therapeutic agents employed in such studies may be contra-indicated in some of the disparate syndromes of the subjects treated. The results of such a 'mixed bag' can provide no real clues as to the comparative merits of the drugs under study.

The acute alcohol withdrawal states result from the discontinuation, or reduction of intake, of alcohol after a prolonged bout of drinking. Although still not universally accepted, several experimental studies have provided scientific proof of the validity of the thesis that abstinence is the cause of these syndromes.

Isbell *et al.*[8] maintained ten human subjects in a chronic state of alcohol intoxication over prolonged periods. Four of these volunteers suffered severe symptoms following discontinuance of alcohol, consisting mainly of nausea, insomnia, excessive perspiration and tremors. The other six subjects, who drank over longer periods, during withdrawal had the same symptoms plus vomiting, diarrhoea, weakness, hyperreflexia, elevated blood pressure and fever. Three of these developed delirium tremens, two had seizures. None of these serious consequences appeared during the periods in which the subjects were ingesting large enough quantities of alcohol to maintain high levels in the blood. Because these ten subjects had a well-balanced diet supplemented with vitamins all through this experiment, it would appear that their symptoms were not due to nutritional or vitamin deficiencies, but rather to the withdrawal of alcohol following prolonged periods of intoxication.

Since that 1955 experiment, Fraser[2] has produced an abstinence syndrome in chronically intoxicated dogs, consisting of tremulousness, seizures, and behavioural changes resembling the delirium seen in man.

Freund[3] has more recently produced a withdrawal model in mice after several days of alcohol intoxication.

Guerrero-Figueroa *et al.*[7] have performed animal experiments to attempt to elucidate the physiological mechanisms which account for the withdrawal syndrome. They produced epileptogenic lesions with aluminium oxide or cobalt stereotaxically implanted into several areas of the brain of cats. Chronic alcohol administration resulted in suppression of cortical and subcortical epileptiform activity. During the stage of withdrawal from alcohol, there occurred activation of cortical and subcortical primary and secondary epileptogenic tissues. The authors postulated that the integrative action of the central nervous system is the result of the balance between inhibition and excitation in normal neuronal populations, and that chronic administration of alcohol produces a potentiation of inhibition. A sudden abstinence from alcohol intoxication then produces a release of CNS inhibition associated with a generalized abnormal increase of excitation, which may produce an increase of motor activity including tremors, initiation of seizures in normal animals and an activation of seizure activity in the epileptic animal or man, as well as disorganized animal and human behaviour (in man mental confusion, often associated with hallucinatory activity).

The usual classification of the several alcohol withdrawal states is given below.

I. Pre-delirium tremens or incipient delirium tremens or 'the shakes'

This, as the name indicates, may be prodromal to a full-blown delirium but in most cases does not progress to delirium tremens. Victor and Adams[20] found only 5% of 266 consecutive alcoholics admitted to the Boston City Hospital developed delirium tremens. In a recent study[12] of 537 alcoholics in 23 Veterans Administration (VA) hospitals only $4\frac{1}{2}$% went on to a full-blown delirium tremens. A report from the Willmar (Minn.) State Hospital[17] cites a delirium tremens incidence of 4.8% in their withdrawn alcoholics. The symptoms of this acute alcohol withdrawal state include anorexia, nausea, restlessness, tremulousness, fitful sleep, hyperhidrosis, anxious depression, hyperreflexia, elevated temperature and hypertension.

Sellers and Kalant[19] recently noted that 'the severity of the reaction varies with both the intensity and the duration of the preceding alcohol exposure. In mild reactions the chief symptoms are tremor, sleeplessness and irritability, appearing within a few hours after withdrawal and usually gone after 48 hours.'

II. Withdrawal seizures

These may represent the only severe symptom of withdrawal or they may be associated with many of the other symptoms and can also occur during delirium tremens. The seizures vary from a single occurrence to multiple convulsions, and even status epilepticus. Victor and Adams[20] found that almost 30% of their patients who had withdrawal seizures developed delirium tremens. In the above-mentioned VA study[12] not quite 20% of the patients with withdrawal seizures also suffered delirium tremens.

III. Alcohol hallucinosis

This syndrome usually follows or is intermingled with the symptoms of the acute alcohol withdrawal state and differs from delirium tremens chiefly in the fact that the patients are not disoriented and that the symptoms are usually not so severe as in the case of delirium tremens.

IV. Delirium tremens

The three cardinal symptoms are tremors, disorientation, and hallucinations. In addition there are many of the same symptoms which have already been enumerated for acute alcohol withdrawal. Delirium tremens usually has a time-limited course of three or four days, although shorter and also longer durations are not uncommon. When the criteria for establishing the diagnosis of delirium tremens are carefully defined, with insistence upon all three of the cardinal symptoms mentioned above, the incidence of this syndrome is rather low. Obviously, many other conditions are misdiagnosed as delirium tremens. It is true there are many atypical varieties of the acute alcohol withdrawal syndrome and one is often hard-pressed to classify the individual case into one or other of the four mentioned above. Because of this, Gross *et al.*[6] and others have suggested classification along a continuum in these conditions, with progressive severity as the factor to be stressed. Although there is some merit to this position, classification into the four states cited above does serve a useful purpose, disciplining the clinician to anticipate the expected course, even though the treatment procedure itself may not be radically different for each of these four states. However, the prognosis is indeed different among these states, and planning the treatment along physiological lines may prevent progression from one state to the next. For research purposes it is certainly essential to differentiate these states, as results of comparative evaluation, for instance, can only be meaningfully analysed if the state of each subject is accurately pre-labelled.

Treatment

Apparently because of the lack of knowledge of the physiological basis for what is now known as the acute alcohol withdrawal syndrome, there has been an enormous variety of therapies advocated and employed in their treatment. All workers know of, and probably many have used: alcohol itself, in tapering-off doses, paraldehyde, adrenal extract, thiamine, insulin, oxygen, nicotinic acid, magnesium sulphate, intravenous fluids, dehydration, etc.

In the mid-1950s, reserpine, and then the phenothiazines, were hailed as the drugs of choice in the treatment of the alcohol withdrawal states. Although early reports were enthusiastic, controlled studies subsequently found these agents less than ideal in this indication. Reserpine, in the large doses required, added to the gastro-intestinal woes of these patients, and often also led to serious hypotensive episodes. Fortunately, it rather quickly lost favour; I have seen no recent references to its use in alcohol withdrawal.

The phenothiazines as a group have been found to lower the convulsive threshold, a severe handicap in the treatment of a condition in which the convulsive threshold is already low. That this is not merely an interesting theoretical consideration is evidenced by the many reports in the literature of increased incidence of seizures in the patients treated with most phenothiazines. Despite this, they are still widely used in alcohol withdrawal.

When chlordiazepoxide was reported to increase the seizure threshold in early animal studies, Kaim and Rosenstein[13] studied this then experimental drug in man in cases of epilepsy and alcohol withdrawal.

We found that it raised the convulsive threshold also in man, and that the drug clinically decreased seizure frequency in epileptics. In the cases of alcohol withdrawal we found that chlordiazepoxide not only reduced the incidence of convulsions, but also of hallucinatory behaviour. We also[16] used this drug intravenously in cases of multiple alcohol withdrawal seizures and reported its effectiveness in terminating them. This was the first report of successful treatment of status epilepticus by a benzodiazepine. Since those early experiments, diazepam, another member of this chemical family, has become the drug of choice in the treatment of status epilepticus.

Fraser[2] has compared alcohol withdrawal to withdrawal from barbiturates. In both indications he suggested treatment with an agent with equivalent effects to prevent the development of seizures and/or delirium tremens.

Jaffe[10] also advocates the treatment of alcohol withdrawal with drugs which show cross-dependence with alcohol, citing in this category paraldehyde, barbiturates, chloral hydrate, meprobamate and chlordiazepoxide.

Several studies have been reported which compared such substances, either with agents which do not show cross-dependence with alcohol, or with each other.

Golbert *et al.*[4] found a combination of paraldehyde and chloral hydrate the most effective in the pre-delirium syndrome, compared with promazine, chlordiazepoxide and alcohol. This study must have been of an unusual patient population. Thirty-nine per cent of the 49 cases developed delirium tremens, which contrasts sharply with the 4 to 5% found in far larger samples reported by Victor and Adams[20], Marvin[17], and Kaim *et al.*[12].

The latter study[12] was a comparative evaluation of chlordiazepoxide, chlorpromazine, hydroxyzine and thiamine, against placebo, in a double-blind, controlled investigation of 537 pre-delirium tremens patients in 23 VA hospitals using the same protocol. Four of the five treatment groups developed an incidence of 10% (or over) of DT and/or convulsions. Of the chlordiazepoxide group only 2% developed either condition. As chlordiazepoxide was the only one of the study drugs which is cross-dependent with alcohol, the findings appear to support the need to employ an adequate pharmacological substitute for alcohol to prevent the development of delirium tremens and convulsions in the treatment of the acute alcohol withdrawal state (Table 17.1).

A subsequent co-operative study[11] was mounted in 17 VA hospitals to determine whether drugs cross-dependent with alcohol would favourably affect the course of already evident delirium tremens. Three such agents – chlordiazepoxide, paraldehyde and pentobarbital – were evaluated in this

Table 17.1 Incidence of delirium tremens and convulsions

	N	*Delirium tremens*	*Convulsions*	*DT and convulsions*	*Total*
Chlordiazepoxide	103	1	1	0	2 (2%)
Chlorpromazine	98	4	9	3	16 (16%)
Hydroxyzine	103	2	6	2	10 (10%)
Thiamine	103	4	7	0	11 (11%)
Placebo	130	7	8	1	16 (12%)
Total	537	18	31	6	55 (10%)

study, against perphenazine, a phenothiazine which has been reported as effective and safe in the treatment of alcohol withdrawal. In this study of 202 cases of uncomplicated delirium tremens, chlordiazepoxide resulted in the shortest duration, paraldehyde in the mildest course. However, none of the differences between drug groups showed statistical significance. The paraldehyde and chlordiazepoxide groups each had one treatment failure, compared with three such in the other two groups. Combining the severity and duration scores also gave the edge to paraldehyde and chlordiazepoxide. But the failure to achieve statistically significant differences might support the thesis that uncomplicated delirium tremens is a time-limited syndrome, whose course is not appreciably affected by these study drugs.

Gross[5] has recently conducted a comparative evaluation of chlordiazepoxide and paraldəhyde in 100 males suffering from alcohol withdrawal states. Thirty-seven were diagnosed as impending delirium tremens, three as hallucinosis; of the remaining cases about half had delirium tremens and half atypical variants. The preliminary analyses of the first 60 patients studied showed no significant differences in terms of the incidence of hallucinations, fever and convulsions. Only one of the 37 patients admitted in impending delirium tremens developed hallucinations. The only significant finding was the shorter duration of severe symptomatology in the chlordiazepoxide group.

In 1974, Favazza and Martin[1] noted that the literature 'revealed markedly different treatment recommendations' for the management of alcohol withdrawal. To ascertain actual practice in assorted hospital settings, these authors sent questionnaires to physicians in hospitals with psychiatry and/or internal medicine residency programmes. Usable replies were received from 101 hospitals, including 15 State mental hospitals, 45 university hospitals, 19 federal hospitals, and 20 community and private hospitals.

Sixty-four physicians listed chlordiazepoxide as their drug of choice, 22 diazepam, 12 paraldehyde, 5 phenothiazines and 4 barbiturates (several physicians listed more than one drug as 'drug of choice'). Thirty-six of these physicians stated that they had changed their drug of choice during the previous five years. The most frequent change was from paraldehyde or a phenothiazine to a benzodiazepine. I am personally gratified that 'the only commonly quoted authority influencing change of primary drug choice' was my report of the 1969 VA collaborative study of the Treatment of Acute Alcohol Withdrawal[12].

As the alcohol withdrawal syndrome is the most serious acute alcohol-related medical problem physicians will frequently be called on to treat, I shall here outline a practical guide to its management.

First, the physician must suspect withdrawal when a patient with a history of heavy drinking presents with several of the following symptoms: anorexia, nausea, vomiting, pruritus, sweating, flushing, insomnia, tremulousness, tachycardia, irritability, apprehension, depression, weakness, fever, clouded sensorium and confusion.

This syndrome is a serious medical condition which, in other than mild cases, usually requires prompt hospitalization.

Approximately 5% of patients suffering acute withdrawal go on to full-blown delirium tremens. Although many of the above cited symptoms may also be present, delirium tremens should be diagnosed only where the following three cardinal symptoms are in evidence: tremors, disorientation, and hallucinations. The latter are usually visual and tactile. The patient may behave as though he were at home or at work, where he imagines himself to be. He may exhibit elaborate delusions in keeping with his imagined setting.

The usual duration of delirium tremens is three or four days, although shorter and longer courses are not uncommon. Untreated, physical exhaustion may occur, with hyperthermia, extreme tachycardia and vascular collapse. The mortality rate is about 15%. Hospitalization should be instituted immediately. With adequate treatment the mortality rate drops to perhaps 5% and is largely related to the presence or absence of serious associated disease.

The recommended management is essentially the same for all patients in withdrawal, whether or not delirium has developed. A careful physical examination, urinalysis, CBC and haematocrit, and chest X-rays should be performed promptly. Additional work-up desirable, to rule out complications and intercurrent conditions, as well as to serve as a guide to therapy, includes: blood alcohol, electrolytes, BUN, blood sugar, bilirubin and skull X-rays. Vital signs should be determined every 3 or 4 hours.

These patients must receive the best nursing care that can be provided. Efforts should be made to allay the patient's fears by reassurance and careful explanation of all procedures. Nightmares, illusions and hallucinations are often reduced if the patient is in a well-lighted room in the presence of others rather than in isolation and/or restraint.

Dehydration and electrolyte imbalance (if present) should be corrected. Fluids should be urged by mouth; if given parenterally, care must be exercised that over-hydration does not result. Examination of the accessible body tissues, specific gravity of the urine and haematocrit serve as clues to patient's state of hydration. A well balanced, nutritious diet should be offered. Antibiotics may be required for infectious conditions. Vitamin B complex may be used if there are signs of a vitamin deficiency. If night-time sedation should be necessary, chloral hydrate, pentobarbital or secobarbital may be employed.

Although some or all of these measures may be a necessary part of treatment, they cannot be considered substitutes for agents which specifically suppress the withdrawal syndrome. The best current therapy is prompt treatment with Librium, 50–100 mg i.v. or i.m. The preferred route thereafter is oral, although the parenteral dose may be repeated in 2 to 4 hours if necessary; not more than 300 mg should be given in a 24-hour period. The initial goal of treatment is to produce light somnolence or sleep. Doses during the next two days should be sufficient to suppress the withdrawal symptoms; usually 25–50 mg will be required at six-hour intervals. During the following three days it will usually be possible to reduce dosage gradually, down to 25 mg once or twice on the last day of treatment. In debilitated and older patients, dosage should be very carefully titrated against symptoms, as these subjects do not tolerate the large doses which may safely be employed in younger alcoholics.

Should a convulsion occur during this regimen, no special additional treatment agent will be required, as Librium has effective anticonvulsant properties. If multiple, recurrent seizures should occur, usually during the first hospital day, Librium (or Valium) should be promptly administered, intravenously. In the case of Librium, 1 mg/kg body weight. The dosage of Valium is usually one fifth that of Librium. Intravenous administration of either drug must be slow, not faster than 20 mg of Librium per minute, or 5 mg of Valium per minute.

References

1. Favazza, A. R. and Martin, P. (1974). Chemotherapy of delirium tremens: a survey of physicians' preferences. *Am. J. Psychiatry*, **131**, 1031
2. Fraser, H. F. (1957). Tolerance to and physical dependence on opiates, barbiturates and alcohol. *Ann. Rev. Med.*, **8**, 427
3. Freund, G. (1969). Alcohol withdrawal syndrome in mice. *Arch. Neurol.*, **21**, 315
4. Golbert, T. M., Sanz, C. J., Rose, H. D. and Leitschuh, T. H. (1967). Comparative evaluation of treatments of alcohol withdrawal syndromes. *J. Am. Med. Assoc.*, **201**, 99
5. Gross, M. (1971). Personal communication.
6. Gross, M., Goodenough, D. R., Bastey, J. M., Rosenblatt, S. M. and Lewis, E. (1971). Sleep disturbances in alcohol intoxication and withdrawal. Recent advances in studies of alcoholism. *HSM Pub.*, **71–9045**, 317
7. Guerrero-Figueroa, R., Rye, M. M., Gallant, D. M. and Bishop, M. P. (1970). Electrographic and behavioral effects of diazepam during alcohol withdrawal stage in cats. *Neuropharmacology*, **9**, 143

8. Isbell, H., Fraser, H. F., Wikler, A., Belleville, M. A. and Eisenman, A. J. (1955). An experimental study of the etiology of 'rum fits' and delirium tremens. *Q. J. Stud. Alc.*, **16,** 1
9. Jacob, M. S. and Sellers, E. M. (1978). The role of drugs in chronic alcoholism. *Drug Therapy*, **Jan. 1978,** 53
10. Jaffe, J. H. (1970). Drug addiction and drug abuse. In Goodman, L. S. and Gilman, A. (eds.), *The Pharmacological Basis of Therapeutics*, 4th Edn., p. 303. (New York: Macmillan)
11. Kaim, S. C. and Klett, C. J. (1972). Treatment of delirium tremens: a comparative evaluation of four drugs. *Q. J. Stud. Alc.*, **33,** 1065
12. Kaim, S. C., Klett, C. J. and Rothfeld, B. (1969). Treatment of the acute alcohol withdrawal state: a comparison of four drugs. *Am. J. Psychiatry*, **125,** 1640
13. Kaim, S. C. and Rosenstein, I. (1961). Experience with chlordiazepoxide in the management of epilepsy. *J. Neuropsychiatry*, **3,** 12
14. Kissin, B. and Platz, A. (1968). The use of drugs in the long term rehabilitation of chronic alcoholics. In Efron, D. H. (ed.), *Psychopharmacology, a Review of Progress*, 1957–1967, pp. 835–851. (Washington: US Govt. Print. Off.)
15. Kissin, B., Platz, A. and Su, W. H. (1971). Selective factors in treatment choice and outcome in alcoholics. Recent advances in studies of alcoholism. *HSM Pub.*, **71–9045,** 781
16. Kurtzke, J. F. and Kaim, S. C. (1962). The acute treatment of convulsive disorders. *Med. Clin.*, **46,** 373
17. Marvin, T. R. (1970). Acute alcoholic withdrawal syndrome. *Minn. Med.*, **1970,** 999
18. National council on alcoholism. Criteria for the diagnosis of alcoholism. (1972). *Am. J. Psychiatry*, **129,** 41
19. Sellers, E. M. and Kalant, H. (1976). Alcohol intoxication and withdrawal. *N. Engl. J. Med.*, **294,** 757
20. Victor, M. and Adams, R. D. (1953). The effect of alcohol on the nervous system. *Proc. Assoc. Res. Nerv. Ment. Dis.*, **32,** 526

18

Longterm Treatment with Diazepam: Clinical and Electroencephalographic Variables

D. Ladewig and E. Schwarz

Introduction

When psychoactive agents were first introduced and their clinical effectiveness was under trial, the question of demonstrating their general action was at first paramount. To this end standardized psychopathological investigational criteria and scales were developed in the sixties. Moreover, well-known psychophysiological methods of examination such as the ECG, EEG, EDA etc. were developed so as to permit the automatic evaluation of these biosignals, thus making it possible to obtain objective evidence of a clinical action.

In recent years growing importance has been attached to problems relating to the longterm effect of psychoactive drugs on patients for whom they have been appropriately prescribed and in particular to questions concerning secondary and tertiary prevention.

The general problem

In our experience it rarely happens – outside the field of epilepsy – that diazepam alone is indicated for longterm treatment. This experience is based on the observation that persistent anxiety appears more especially in the presence of other symptoms of psychiatric disease which call for the use of antidepressants or neuroleptics. On the other hand the general practitioner in particular repeatedly encounters in his practice patients who complain of recurrent acute attacks of anxiety or chronic anxiety in connection with a psychosomatic syndrome or a behavioural disorder (Table 18.1).

Table 18.1 Indications for longterm tranquillizer medication – Target symptom: anxiety

1. Chronically recurrent acute attacks of anxiety with corresponding psychovegetative symptoms
2. Masked anxiety in psychosomatic syndromes
3. Apprehensiveness/sensitivity as a habitual phenomenon in connection with certain stress situations
4. Anxiety as a concomitant symptom in psychiatric/psychosomatic syndromes
   e.g. depression
   schizophrenia
   intoxication syndromes etc.

Against this background the question of abuse and dependence arises in connection with longterm medication. This question is fully warranted. Whereas the phenomenon of tranquillizer abuse is one that is observed today with increasing frequency, actual dependence on drugs of this class is comparatively rare[8, 9, 11].

How is anxiety manifested?

Anxiety is frequently verbalized as fear, restlessness, tension and inhibition; often enough it is not verbalized and is manifested as a somatic symptom, e.g. lump in the throat or pain; that is to say, the psychopathological equivalent is not at first expressed as effect. It is only when the patient has access to therapy that a feeling of ill humour, uneasiness, rage or, verbaliter also of anxiety, is expressed.

Thus anxiety is manifested either more as 'somatic' or more as 'psychic' anxiety (Tables 18.2 and 18.3).

The problem with which we were concerned was the following: how can we obtain objective evidence of the longterm action of diazepam? And in this context a supplementary question arose: are there signs of diminished action after longterm treatment and what happens after longterm medication is discontinued?

Apart from clinical assessment of the course of treatment, we selected as our objective criteria standardized questionnaires, the EEG in the sphere

Table 18.2 Symptoms of 'somatic' anxiety

Cardiovascular	Palpitations, vertigo, blushing, fainting tendency, fear of loss of consciousness, tension headache
Respiratory	Feeling of constriction in the chest, oppression, inability to breathe in the necessary volume of air
Muscular	Tremor Feeling of weakness Uncertain movements Rheumatoid pains
Gastro-intestinal	Queer feelings in the stomach Nausea Vomiting Flatulence Pain

Table 18.3 Symptoms of 'psychic' anxiety

Apprehensiveness
Inner disequilibrium
Irritability
Inner emptiness
Sadness
Rage
Aggressiveness
Self-doubt
  social anxieties
  sexual difficulties
Phobic fears
  heights, bridges, spaces, being in closed spaces, darkness, etc.

Table 18.4 The problem of investigation

1. Definition of the target symptom/criteria for selection of patients
   a. clinical
   b. questionnaire method
2. Choice of therapeutic procedure
   a. psychopharmacological
   b. psychotherapeutic
3. Monitoring of therapy
   a. clinical
   b. electroencephalographic
   c. serum level check
   d. questionnaire

of biosignals, and estimates of the blood level of diazepam and desmethyldiazepam (Table 18.4).

Methods

Criteria for the selection of patients: age, sex, mode of referral, symptomatology

In selecting patients we were guided with regard to sex and age ratios by the conditions obtaining in the doctor's practice. Consequently six women and four men ($n = 10$) aged between 29 and 52 years ($M = 37$; $s = 7.9$) were drafted into the study.

Five patients were referred directly by general practitioners: five others were primarily hospitalized patients. An EEG was made of all patients so as to rule out any neurological disorder. Patients in whose cases there was a prospect of somatic or other pharmacopsychiatric treatment becoming necessary were excluded.

Three patients were excluded as possible 'placebo reactors'. Two of them had shown a diminution of their anxiety symptoms in response to placebo medication: another complained of previously unreported feelings of vertigo and marked muscle relaxation after placebo.

As regards illness, patients with persistent anxiety and psychosomatic syndromes and behavioural disorders were included in the study. These disorders had all without exception an aetiology of several years' standing and consequently a treatment phase lasting a number of months was envisaged.

Medication schedule

Diazepam was prescribed as Ro 5-2807-619: this could on one hand mobilize expectations with regard to a 'new drug'. However, as at the same time a therapeutic longterm plan was formulated with each patient in which the medication was interpreted as an associated therapy and the patient's co-operation was solicited as an essential element in a longterm programme, this aspect can be relativized. The drug was prescribed in an average dose of 15mg/day. Initially a standardized dosage of 10–15mg was aimed at in most cases; the number of tablets taken was entered on a medication card.

In a second phase of treatment the procedure adopted was less restrictive. During this phase, which lasted on average between two and four months, the dosage was kept free inasmuch as the patient was invited to be flexible in his medication, depending on how he felt, always around the recommended dosage of 15mg/day and always with the precautionary measure that medication for 14 days was given by the physician.

Duration of treatments are shown in detail in Figure 18.1.

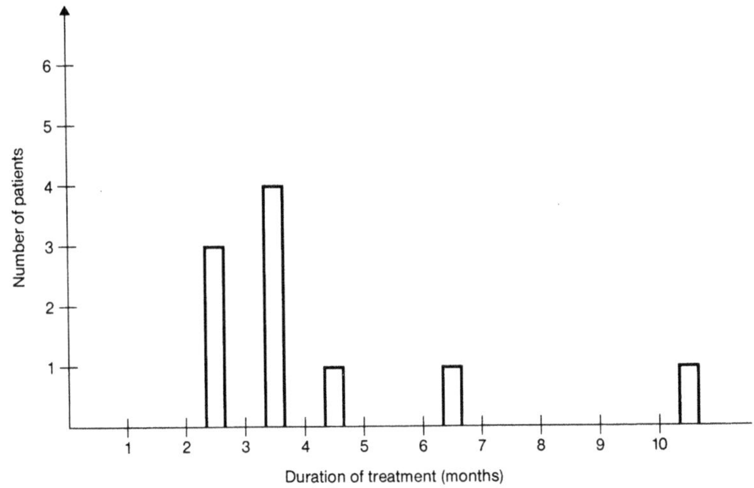

Figure 18.1 Duration of medication

Psychotherapy

During every longterm treatment not only the drug or the psychotherapeutic procedure but also the physician's attitude and the impact of various environmental influences and life events must be seen as important variables influencing the course of treatment for good or ill.

With regard to psychotherapy we were guided by the client-centred therapy of Rogers[14] and the procedures of behaviour therapy[4].

Results

Monitoring of the treatment: Case history illustrating the interaction of pharmacotherapy and psychotherapy

G.B., born in 1942, waitress, divorced, referred by her family doctor: morbus crohn since 1966; she suffered subjectively from pain under the left costal arch; was treated by several doctors for this and had been given antidepressants for several fairly long periods but without clinical success. During several consultations she described her abdominal pain together with 'headache, hair loss and streaks before the eyes' in a monotonous voice. She saw no connections between any feelings or events in her life history and the symptoms complained of. A striking feature was her unrelatedness, the poverty of her inner experience, the banality of her conversation. As therapist one felt in her on the one hand expectations and on the other resistances, extreme sensitivity and vulnerability. In response to diazepam she emerged a little from her 'armoured stance'.

At the same time G.B. participated for several weeks in group therapy sessions where she was at first an outsider. With time she learnt to listen, to show understanding for others, and to establish connections with her own life history. She talked for the first time about the anxiety she had felt in various life situations; she came from a broken home, married an alcoholic, whom she left again after a year. She related that she always met up with brutes who frightened her and described how she sought to defend herself under these circumstances.

As a result of the combined pharmaco- and psychotherapy the patient succeeded in coming to terms with the symptom of pain and also with her 'masked anxiety' and the multitude of hurts she had repeatedly had to endure. Medication was discontinued after 4 months without any withdrawal reaction and without recrudescence of the symptoms treated.

Medication

To find the effective therapeutic dosage at the beginning of the treatment it was clear from the clinical data that in the case of two patients it was necessary to raise the dosage from an initial 10mg/day to 30mg/day.

No real diminution of effect during the longterm treatment was observed in any patient. During the placebo phase of 4 to 6 days after several months of treatment the clinical picture remained unchanged in 5 patients, compared to the state before placebo was given. The medication could be discontinued. In the remaining 5 patients deterioration was observed. Two patients reported sleep disturbances whom we treated after the placebo phase with a combination of a neuroleptic and diazepam; three other patients suffered feelings of anxiety which, in the case of two of them, had a character of a free-floating anxiety. The symptoms reached their climax on the 3rd and 4th day after placebo. One of these patients also exhibited symptoms such as inner restlessness, sweating and tremor as well as a marked desire to continue the medication. It was necessary to switch in 2 of these 3 patients to an anxiolytic–antidepressant medication.

Methods for the employment of the EEG

The EEGs of 6 of the 10 patients were automatically analysed. Of these six, 2 were men and 4 women. No initial examination was made in the case of one female patient and consequently only her EEG records after longterm therapy and discontinuance of the medication are available.

Because of their symptoms, none of our patients managed entirely without medication, and we were therefore unable to examine these subjects before therapy was initiated. There is therefore no baseline. Consequently it is impossible to obtain direct objective evidence of our target symptom – anxiety – from the EEG.

Our question was therefore framed in the following pharmaco-electroencephalographic terms: how does the EEG change after longterm therapy with diazepam, and what happens when medication is discontinued after longterm therapy?

The EEG studies were made at the following times:

(1) 4–6 days after the start of medication,
(2) after 2 to 4 months' treatment (longterm therapy),
(3) 4–6 days after discontinuance of longterm therapy.

After the patients had relaxed with the aid of a standardized set of instructions, we recorded the EEG with the patient at rest with eyes closed for 5 minutes. A further recording was then made at rest for 5 minutes with eyes open. A blood sample was taken at each time of examination.

For the method of recording and the analysis of the analogue EEG signal see reference 16.

For the descriptive statistic evaluation, mean values and standard deviations of the EEG parameters were calculated via the individual patients as a basis for the descriptive part. The chronospectrographic form of representation displays the change in the power values continuously in time. The interhemispheric changes – as indicators of activation or the behavioural state – can also be presented in this form.

Results of the EEG examinations

If we first look at the individual EEG tracings (Figure 18.2), it is noteworthy that in the first examination with 'eyes closed' only one single patient has an alpha percentage value below 40.

In 2 patients the alpha activity dominates in the right hemisphere, in 3 patients in the left. The variability is about equal in both hemispheres and in all patients.

If we now examine the differences in the EEG pattern from the 1st to the 2nd examination, we find in 3 patients a decrease of alpha activity and in 4 patients an increase of beta activity. The slow frequencies (delta and theta activity) also diminish in 4 patients (Figure 18.2).

There is a reversal of alpha dominance in 3 patients.

On *discontinuance of medication* (2nd to 3rd examination) we now see in 4 patients a renewed alpha increase and a beta decrease in all patients. The slow frequencies also show a very small increase (Figure 18.2).

The alpha dominance alters in only 1 patient.

By taking *one patient* as an example we will illustrate these changes with the aid of a graphic plot of a *chronospectrogram*. On the X axis are shown the times of the 3 examinations which have been marked at equal distances (Figures 18.3a and b and 18.4).

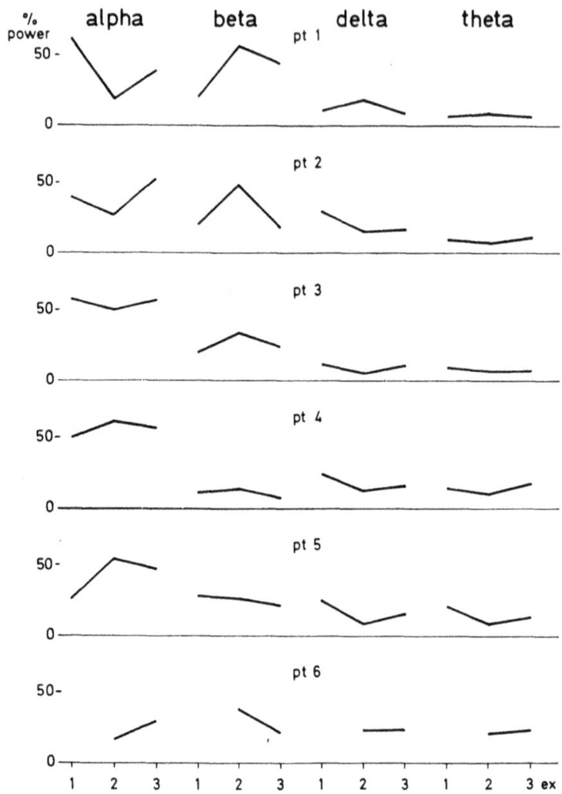

Figure 18.2 Individual time courses of the relative power of the alpha, beta, delta and theta activities; pt = patient. Five-minute resting EEG with *eyes closed*, lead O_1–F_3, was analysed for all three examinations (ex)

On examining the mean value curves (Figure 18.5) we can observe in the *pooled* results a decrease of total power from the first to the second examination and also of alpha, theta and delta activities. At the same time we can see an increase in beta activity. This corresponds to a rise in blood levels.

The reaction on eye-opening becomes smaller, particularly in the case of alpha and beta activity.

After medication had been discontinued for a week, we see, parallel to the diminishing blood level, a renewed increase of the total power and also of the alpha, theta and delta frequencies and a decrease of beta activity. The reactions to eye-opening again become more clearly marked.

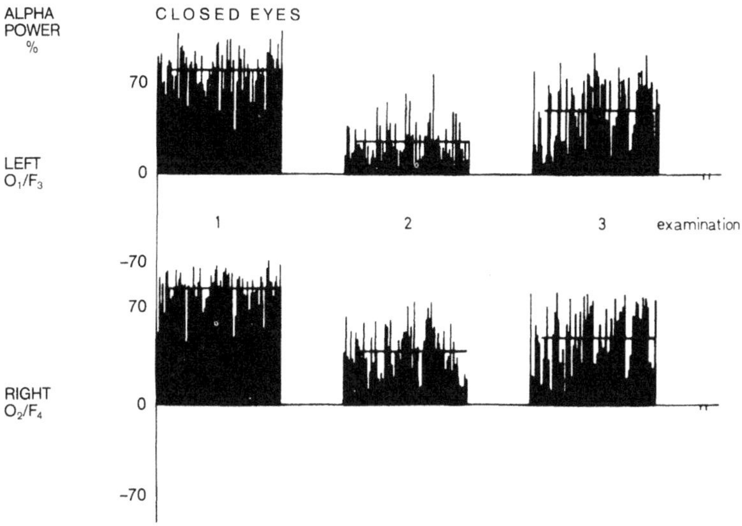

a

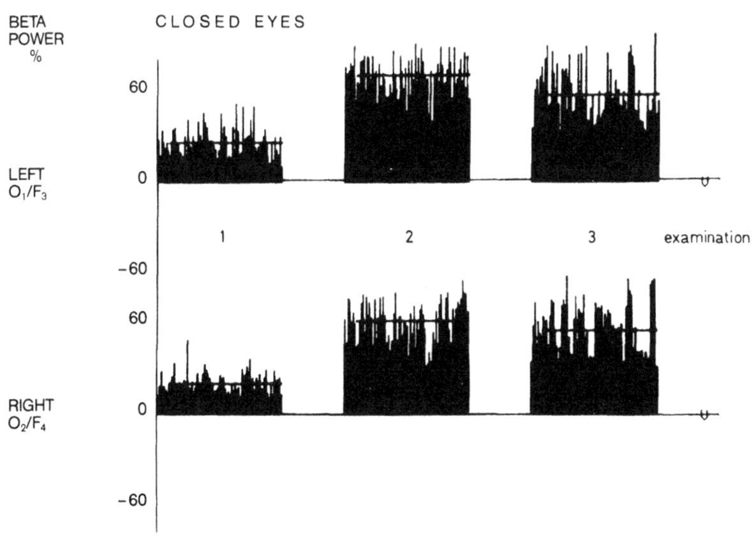

b

Figure 18.3 a and b Chronospectrograms of relative alpha and beta power for all three examinations. The EEG of patient 1 was analysed during 5 minutes with closed eyes, leads O_1–F_3 and O_2–F_4, with 4 seconds resolution

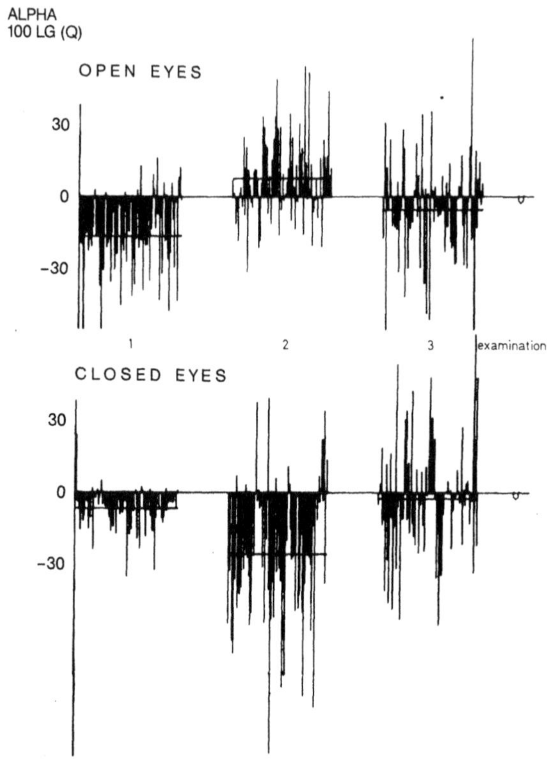

Figure 18.4 Interhemispheric relationships for the relative alpha power of patient 1: chronospectrograms of the ratio Q (left power/right power) were calculated in 4-second epochs over 5 minutes and for the three examinations (resting EEG with closed and opened eyes, leads O_1–F_3 and O_2–F_4)

Serum level check

Because it is obvious today that a majority of patients do not take their medication in the ordered manner, it seems to us very important to make serum level checks during the course of the longterm treatment. As the times of blood sampling varied we cannot make exact conclusions about the time course especially in respect to possible cumulation. At the first examination we observed a mean concentration of 71.75 ng/ml plasma. After longterm treatment the value increased until 260 and decreased again after placebo medication to 50 ng/ml plasma. We observed high inter-individual variations.

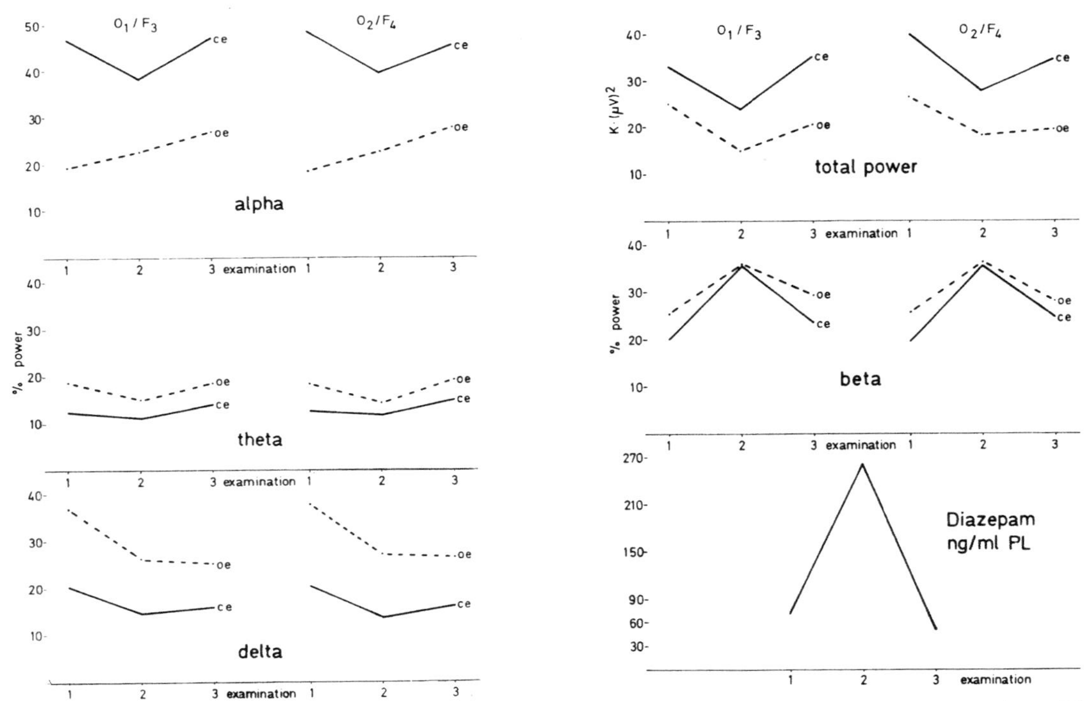

Figure 18.5 Time courses of the mean total power (K(μV)^2), mean relative beta power (%) and concentration of diazepam in the plasma (ng/ml PL) (right) as well as for the mean relative alpha, delta and theta power (%) (left); $n = 6$. These means were calculated from the individual EEGs, analysed for 5 minutes, leads O_1–F_3 and O_2–F_4, under eyes closed (ce) and eyes opened (oe) condition for all three examinations

Results of investigation in FPI (Freiburg Personality Inventory)[3] *after commencement of treatment and after longterm treatment*

The result can be summarized to the effect that there is a decreasing susceptibility to psychosomatic disturbance and an increasing emotional stabilization which gives grounds for enhanced satisfaction and self-confidence. The diminution of scale 3 (depressiveness) is not to be construed as a diminution of clinical depressive symptoms. The increased equanimity, spontaneity and sociability (scales 6, 8 and 9) show that not only psychovegetative symptoms disappear but that there is also an improvement in the whole field of 'social anxieties' (Table 18.5).

Table 18.5 Changes of the FPI (abbreviated form) $n = 10$

Nervousness	S1 (T = 9.04 ss)	diminishing psychosomatic disturbance
Aggressiveness	S2 (T = 1.90 ns)	slight tendency to diminishing aggressiveness
Depressiveness	S3 (T = 6.35 ss)	diminishing depressive mood, increasing satisfaction, self-confidence
Excitability	S4 (T = 2.61 s)	increasing excitability, diminishing dullness
Sociability	S5 (T = 1.44 ns)	slight tendency to sociability, increasing vivacity
Equanimity	S6 (T = 3.20 ss)	increasing relaxedness, self-confidence
Dominance	S7 (T = 1.20ns)	slight tendency to assert oneself better, dominance
Inhibition	S8 (T = 3.11 s)	increasing spontaneity, ability to form relations
Openness	S9 (T = 1.49ns)	slight tendency to greater openness, self-criticism
Extraversion	SE (T = 1.49ns)	slight tendency to introversion
Emotional lability	SN (T = 5.68 ss)	increasing emotional stabilization
Masculinity	SM (T = 1.00ns)	slight tendency to admit feelings more readily

Thus the effectiveness of diazepam is revealed in longterm treatment not only psychovegetatively but also – always in conjunction with simultaneous structurizing psychotherapeutic treatment – in the fields of self-confidence and ability to form social relations.

The findings of scale 2 (aggressivity) should be noted. There is not, as is sometimes reported, an increase of aggressivity but rather a slight tendency to decreasing aggressivity. Clearly, the patients learn in the course of ad hoc treatment to come to terms with their feelings of tension, self-doubt, anxiety or even rage in such a way that they learn to integrate these emotions into their behaviour.

Discussion

Results of clinical examination

In principle it is unusual for longterm treatment with a tranquillizer to be indicated. Treatment combining an antidepressant in order to reinforce its anxiolytic action is much more commonly the aim.

The efficiency of longterm treatment with a tranquillizer is good particularly in the case of acute recurrent symptoms of chronic psychosomatic disturbances. However, it can hold out the prospect of success in the long run only if it is combined with an efficient structurizing of the doctor–patient relationship.

Discussion of the electroencephalographic results of the study

Parallel to the changes in the blood levels we can observe in our patients diazepam-specific changes in the EEG pattern. The diminution of total power and of alpha activity and the increase of beta activity are consistent with the results of other authors who have worked with minor tranquillizers[1,2,5,7,10,13,15].

If we consider our first examination 4 to 6 days after the start of medication, we see a relatively high alpha activity of 40% together with a beta percentage of 20. This pattern does not correspond generally to anxiety. Perhaps a first anxiolytic effect became obvious because of the 'steady state'.

An explanation for the high alpha activity in our patients could be the experience of Siciliani *et al.*[17] who showed an alpha increase after the first and second week of treatment with temazepam, a diazepam metabolite. Perhaps we could have been able to show similar changes if we had had a real baseline measure.

After longterm treatment, however, we found the 'minor tranquillizer'-induced changes with alpha decrease and beta increase.

The positive connection between blood level and beta activity in the acute experiment reported by Fink and Irwin[6] can also be seen in our repeated measurements.

The diminution of both delta and theta activity with a rising blood level is not reported by all authors. Thus Saletu *et al.*[15], for example, emphasize that, with a single dose of 5mg diazepam, it depends on the experimental condition whether there is a rise or fall of the slow frequencies. Contrary to our experiment, these authors found an increase in both slow frequencies with their 8 test subjects at rest with eyes closed. If, on the other hand, the level of vigilance was controlled by the operant, the same frequencies decreased. Bond *et al.*[1,2] likewise did not test their patients under conditions which were truly resting but applied stimuli. After 2 to 4 weeks of therapy these authors also found a lowering of delta and theta rhythms.

Matejcek[13] during a 24-week treatment also observed a diminution of theta activity but there was still an increase of delta activity.

It is possible that after longterm treatment our patients found themselves in a similar state as the patients of the above reported studies, although without external vigilance control. In the 'eyes open' condition this diminution became more apparent. If we consider the fact that 3 of our 5 patients changed their alpha dominance – the hemisphere where alpha predominates – after longterm treatment, this seems to us to be an indication for changes in activation level[12]. In addition, the alpha blocking effect, as a reaction to eye opening, and the beta reaction were both diminished. The level of vigilance seems to be changed. The third examination, after medication had been discontinued, is no real baseline measure because of the preceding pharmacological and psychotherapeutic procedures which altered the initial state in the way we could show with our questionnaire data.

The alpha activity has now reached a higher level again and the beta activity shows a decrease, similar to our first examination.

Discussion of the clinical findings

Longterm therapy with a tranquillizer is open to two principal objections. The first is concerned with the placebo reaction aspect. There is no doubt whatever that there are placebo reactors. The fact that a drug does not produce the effect the doctor expects of it, is not primarily to be imputed to the drug.

Our study shows clearly that diazepam remains 'biologically' effective even after longterm therapy. The fact that a drug acquires another significance in longterm treatment presupposes, as mentioned in the foregoing, a continuous appraisal of the physician–patient relation.

The other objection concerns the abuse potential. In comparison with the classic dependences of the morphine or barbiturate–alcohol type this is low. The discussion in the literature of the dependence potential of benzodiazepines, which is sometimes inaccurately documented and emotionally loaded, possibly derives from the fact that a symptom like 'anxiety', which is at first treated successfully, reappears in an intensified form after discontinuation. Because of the innate need to find a causal connection, this symptom may then be interpreted as a 'withdrawal' symptom. We feel that only when other significant withdrawal symptoms are present can there be any suggestion of a genuine dependence. Apart from sleep disturbances this was not the case in our clinical findings. We have to interpret this symptomatology as a rebound effect. It might be considered that in 5 of 10 patients no reaction to discontinuation could be detected. After discontinuance in 2 of 10 patients a combination therapy was carried on with a neuroleptic and diazepam; in 2 other patients it was necessary to switch to an anxiolytic–antidepressant medication because of a change in symptoms.

References

1. Bond, A. J., James, D. C. and Lader, M. H. (1974). Physiological and psychological measures in anxious patients. *Psychol. Med.*, **4,** 364
2. Bond, A. J., James, D. C. and Lader, M. H. (1974). Sedative effects on physiological and psychological measures in anxious patients. *Psychol. Med.*, **4,** 374
3. Fahrenberg, J., Selg, H. and Hampel, R. (1973). *Das Freiburger Persönlichkeitsinventar, FPI.* (Göttingen: Hogrefe)
4. Feldhege, F. J. and Krauthan, G. (1979). *Verhaltenstrainingsprogramm zum Aufbau sozialer Kompetenz.* (Berlin, Heidelberg, New York: Springer)
5. Fink, M. (1974). EEG profiles and bioavailability measures of psychoactive drugs. *Mod. Probl. Pharmacopsychol.*, Vol. 8, pp. 76–98. (Basel: Karger)
6. Fink, M. and Irwin, P. (1975). EEG and blood level correlations for psychoactive drugs. In Matejcek, M. and Schenk, G. K. (eds.), *Quantitative Analysis of the EEG. Proc. 2nd Symposium of Study Group for EEG-Methodology*, Jongny sur Vevey, pp. 119–126. (Konstanz: AEG-Telefunken)
7. Itil, T. M. (1974). Quantitative pharmaco-electroencephalography. *Mod. Probl. Pharmacopsychol.*, Vol. 8, pp. 43–75. (Basel: Karger)
8. Kielholz, P. (1968). Gesamtschweizerische Enquête über die Häufigkeit des Medikamentenmissbrauchs. *Schweiz. Aerzte-Ztg.*, **49,** 1077
9. Ladewig, D. (1973). Gesamtschweizerische Enquête über die Häufigkeit des Medikamenten- und Drogenmissbrauchs. *Schweiz. Aerzte-Ztg.*, **54,** 971
10. Marjerrison, G. (1974). Effects of minor tranquilizers on the EEG. *Mod. Probl. Pharmacopsychol.*, Vol. 8, pp. 149–157. (Basel: Karger)
11. Marks, J. (1978). *The Benzodiazepines.* (Lancaster: MTP Press)
12. Martinius, J., Schwarz, E., Mayer, F. X. and Clarke, A. (1975). Spectral EEG analysis in neuropsychological experimentation in school age children. In Matejcek, M. and Schenk, G. K. (eds.), *Quantitative analysis of the EEG. Proc. 2nd Symposium of Study Group for EEG-Methodology*, Jongny sur Vevey. pp. 783–793. (Konstanz: AEG-Telefunken)
13. Matejcek, M. (1979). Pharmaco-electroencephalography: The value of quantified EEG in psychopharmacology. *Pharmakopsychiatrie*, **12,** 126
14. Rogers, C. R. (1978). Die klientenzentrierte Gesprächspsychotherapie. (München: Kindler)
15. Saletu, B., Matejcek, M., Knor, K., Ferner, U. and Schneewind, U. (1976). Assessing the psychoactivity of cloxazolam (MT 14-411) by quantitative EEG and psychological studies. *Curr. Ther. Res.*, **20,** 510
16. Schwarz, E., Kielholz, P., Hobi, V., Goldberg, L., Gilsdorf, U., Hofstetter, M., Ladewig, D., Miest, P.-Chr., Reggiani, G. and Richter, R. (1980). Alcohol-induced biphasic background and stimulus-elicited EEG changes in relation to blood alcohol levels. *Int. J. Clin. Pharmacol.* (in press)
17. Siciliani, O., Schiavon, M. and Tansella, M. (1975). Anxiety and EEG alpha activity in neurotic patients. *Acta Psychiatr. Scand.*, **52,** 116

19

Psychosocial Aspects of Mental Health Care in Developing Countries – The Role of the Benzodiazepines

E. D. Busnello

Introduction

The World Health Organization has been involved since 1975 in seeking answers to some of the basic questions related to the possibility of treatment of severe mental disorders prevalent in the developing countries*[1]. A WHO Joint Study on Strategies for Extension of Mental Health Services is being carried out for the purpose of developing and evaluating alternative and low-cost methods for mental health work, including training of personnel, in such countries. This study is scheduled for completion in 1981, but some findings are already available, such as the magnitude of mental health problems in communities and particularly in the services that provide primary health care; reactions of the community to mental diseases; how to select priorities and train health workers for definite tasks; drugs than can be used and the ways in which communities manage to identify and take care of persons with mental disorders.

Four countries were at first involved in the study: Columbia, India, Senegal and Sudan. Later three more countries, Egypt, Philippines and Brazil, joined.

This paper is based on the initial results of this Joint Study and some

* Working material used in the 4th Meeting of the Investigators of the WHO Collaborative Study on Strategies for Extending of Mental Health Care, which took place from June 5th to 12th, 1979, in Dakar, Senegal, under the auspices of the Mental Health Division of the World Health Organization.

observations from the preparatory studies and working documents are also presented. Observations related to the prevalence of mental health problems, reactions of the community to mental disease and the availability of some of these methods of intervention are discussed.

Significance of mental health problems

Epidemiological studies have shown that serious mental diseases are as prevalent in developing countries as in developed ones, with those due to organic–cerebral problems being more frequent. Another WHO report estimates that 20% of the serious disabling diseases in world derive from mental disorders[7, 8]. The WHO Joint Study has confirmed these findings. The percentage of mental disease varies between 10.5 and 17% among adults of the areas studied. For children the levels are higher, between 11 and 29%. Among adults, the majority presented neuroses, while among children, the most common were behaviour disorders and mental retardation. Most complaints of adults were about physical symptoms: the larger the number of physical complaints (generally more than three in each person) the greater the possibility that they were due to underlying mental disorders.

Reaction of the community to the mental diseases

At this stage of the study, we can already say with some certainty that mental diseases are perceived as a very serious problem by the community. It is recognized that mental diseases constitute a significant health problem that leads to serious disability and causes important social problems. Recourse to traditional religious aid is very common because this is often the only source of help. Once modern health services are available, however, people respond to them with enthusiasm and there is active community involvement in the treatment of patients. People show an interest in seeking help for both physical and mental problems from services that use methods of treatment derived from modern medicine. It has become increasingly evident that, once informed, people make use of local health services and wish to keep patients in the community thus avoiding the expense and inconvenience of sending them to hospitals; and that it is possible to work in collaboration with traditional sources of help, such as witch-doctors and religion. Modern treatment is viewed as complementary to and compatible with the beliefs held by a given population.

Selection of priorities, definition of tasks

These findings demonstrate that it is a matter of some urgency to select mental health priorities, which is done according to criteria of prevalence, serious consequences for the individual and society, concern of the community, and availability of methods of treatment that are simple, efficient and inexpensive[3, 6].

The teams that are investigating the extension of health services in the seven countries have chosen as their first priority psychiatric emergencies, epilepsy and chronic psychosis. Some countries also chose the care of retarded children, depressions and alcoholism.

Once the priorities have been defined, the means of dealing with them are selected, together with the methods for training the personnel who will put them into effect.

Availability of methods of intervention

In the developing countries, the majority of mental health services are concentrated in hospitals the custodial function of which is well known. Most patients receive no help or only traditional care which, although often beneficial, sometimes deprives them of the advantages of modern psychopharmacological and social treatment.

The community health worker

Although the material and human resources in the health services of the developing countries are limited, some progress has been made, such as introduction of mental care in General Health Services. Primary health workers or the community health workers chosen by the community, after a short period of training, can give general health care.

The purpose of the WHO study is to determine whether these workers are also able to include mental health care among their activities.

The answer to this question depends on the answers to some specific points:

(1) Are problems of mental health prevalent in the community, and do they have consequences sufficiently serious to cause concern to the communities?
(2) Can the methods of diagnosis and treatment be made simple and safe enough so that the community health worker could be trained to give mental health care?
(3) What steps are needed to implement mental health care in the communities and what is their relation to the already existing services and training program?

At this stage of the research, we can already confidently reply that mental diseases are perceived as very serious problems by the communities, that it is possible to train already existing health staffs to enable them to give basic mental health care, that patients come to consultation regularly, and that it is possible to involve the community in the care of patients.

Dealing with chronic psychosomatic illness

Giel and Workneh†, in a working paper aimed at the training of health workers, suggest the need to attend to chronically complaining persons because of their great number. They constitute about 1% among the 20% of persons with mental disorders who call the Out-Patient Health Services in Ethiopia, and their complaints are partially or wholly of emotional origin[2,4]. These patients result in additional expenditure for the health services; they repeat consultations, and generally are poorly dealt with by health workers and services.

There is a tendency to subject this type of patient to a series of examinations which, on the one hand, increases the patient's belief that his complaints are of a physical nature and, on the other hand, follows the natural tendency of modern medical services to direct their efforts mainly to the diagnosis of physical health problems.

There is no great difference in the approach to adult patients, mostly neurotics, who require primary health care in regional services and present mental disorders.

Treatment to relieve basic physical complaints, when justified by the basic cause, must be supplemented by attending to the underlying psychological and social factors, which are as important as the physical, or even more so. The physiological support given to the patient, both by means of explanation of the psychosocial nature of his symptoms, and by helping him bear the psychological problems he is experiencing, is of maximum importance.

In achieving this objective, the use of a suitable tranquillizer or a placebo is plainly justified, since the deep psychological analysis of the symptomatology presented becomes difficult in the context of a health service that offers primary care to a broad population and must tend a great number of patients.

The use of psychotropic agents, especially the benzodiazepines, in developing countries

Another approach to the problem has been made by Harding and Chrusciel[5], who state that health workers are easily trained to administer psychotropics in a safe and effective manner. These drugs can be used by non-specialized staff.

† Giel, R. and Workneh, F. Coping with patients who cannot cope: Management of persistent complainers in an African country. Working paper presented at Fourth Meeting of Investigators, Dakar, June 5th to 12th, 1979, WHO Collaborative Study on Strategies for Extending Mental Health Care.

Provision of medication is an important part of the intervention phase. In recognition of this fact, the World Health Organization has drawn up a list of 15 essential drugs[9].

The introduction of medication in dealing with these patients is recommended and, in the case of neurotic patients and those presenting chronic complaints basically of a emotional nature, the benzodiazepines figure as a powerful aid in health problems of populations in developing countries on account of their ease of management, safety, efficacy and efficiency. It should not be forgotten, however, that the possibility exists that these drugs can result in dependence or in increasing use, a danger which should be adequately controlled by the community health worker.

In extending mental health care, the use of benzodiazepines in the treatment of acute crises of anxiety and in epilepsy has also been recommended[5]. In this case again, non-specialists can be trained to use this type of drug and a large proportion of all patients who are in need of this type of medication can be safely treated. The use of benzodiazepines in the context of extending mental health services to the community, and their introduction into primary health care, thus deserves mention in this connection.

Concluding remarks

It is my opinion that all those who, like myself, are concerned with the social aspects of psychiatry and work for the development of mental health care within the community should take into consideration the abovementioned data when planning how to deal with multiple health problems in the context of primary health care in developing countries. It is possible that this experience, primarily directed to problems of health in underdeveloped countries, may result in the organization of health services which are not very different from those designed for the developed countries.

This statement derives from the magnitude of the mental health problems within the framework of the health problems of populations of both poor and rich countries, and leads naturally to the development of this line of thought.

Summary

This paper presents some of the initial results of a WHO Joint Study on Strategies for Extension of Mental Health Services with the objective of developing alternative and low-cost methods for mental health work in developing countries. Observations related to the prevalence of mental health problems, reactions of the community to mental diseases and the availability of some of the methods of intervention are presented. Preliminary findings from the working documents indicate that serious mental diseases are as prevalent in developing countries as in developed ones and that the community is extremely concerned about them. Psychotropic drugs, particularly benzodiazepines, can be used in a safe and effective manner by non-specialized health workers who can be easily trained to deal with them.

References

1. Diop, B., Collignon, R. and Guéye, M. (1976). Présentation de l'étude concertée de l'OMS sur les stratégies pour l'extension de soins de santé mentale. *Psychopathol. Africaine*, **XII**, 173
2. Dormaar, M., Giel, R. and Van Luijk, J. N. (1977). Psychiatric illness in two contrasting Ethiopian populations. *Soc. Psychiatry*, **9**, 155
3. Giel, R. and Harding, T. W. (1976). Psychiatric priorities in developing countries. *J. Psychiatry*, **128**, 513
4. Giel, R. and Van Luijk, J. N. (1969). Psychiatric morbidity in a small Ethiopian town. *Br. J. Psychiatry*, **115**, 149
5. Harding, T. W. and Chrusciel, T. L. (1975). The use of psychotropic drugs in developing countries. *Bull. WHO*, **52**, 359
6. Morley, D. (1973). *Paediatric Priorities in the Developing World.* (London: Butterworths)
7. World Health Organization (1975). Organization of mental health services in developing countries. Sixteenth report of the Expert Committee on Mental Health. *Tech. Rep. Ser.*, **564**, (Geneva)
8. World Health Organization (1976). Reports on specific technical matters: disability prevention and rehabilitation. WHO document A29/INF. DOC/1.
9. World Health Organization (1976). Report of a consultation in drug therapy for neuropsychiatric disorders in developing countries. Offset document, Geneva

20

Longterm Treatment with Anxiolytic Drugs: Possibilities of Pharmacodependence

J. R. Bueno

All 'pills' are equal; but some 'pills' are more equal than others.

Adapted from George Orwell

Introduction

Since the introduction of meprobamate as an anxiolytic or ataraxic substance, the possibility of drug dependence has been discussed. The reason is that these substances, both meprobamate and benzodiazepines, could be included in the broad classification of sedatives, since the prototype of sedatives is still the barbiturate group.

This article presents a more or less critical analysis of this problem, comparing our data with those in the literature.

Patients and methods

The Out-Patient Clinic of the Post-Graduate Course at the Institute of Psychiatry has, since 1972, determined in patients with anxiety states the possibility of drug dependence induced by anxiolytics. Furthermore, it was also of interest to compare the therapeutic efficacy of various anxiolytics. Patients who were pregnant or concomitantly presented neurological disorders, glaucoma and/or prostatic disorders were excluded from the study. On this basis, 600 patients (65.8% women) participated in several double-blind studies. All previously treated patients went on a 10-day washout programme. The selected patient was then randomly put into either the treated or the placebo group. In comparative studies, they were randomly put in one or the other drug (anxiolytic) group. Therapeutic efficacy was evaluated by the scale of Hamilton. The average duration of treatment was 28 days.

Over a period of 6 years, 420 patients completed studies in which the following anxiolytic agents were evaluated: chlordiazepoxide, diazepam, clobazam, lorazepam, bromazepam, dipotassium chlorazepate and trazodone (a non-benzodiazepine).

Results

In general, there was no detectable difference between the treated and placebo group during the first week of treatment. Both groups showed improvement, thus demonstrating a very high degree of placebo effect. From the 14th day on, however, while the placebo group began to deteriorate, the drug group continued to show improvement which was maintained during the remaining period of the study. In comparative studies, the efficacy of all the benzodiazepines were indistinguishable from each other after 28 days of treatment.

Since the data has not been completely analysed, we can only give you our clinical impression at the moment. It seems that there is a risk of dependence when anxiolytics are administered for long periods, favouring the appearance of signs of tolerance and progressive increase of dose, and it seems also that there is some relation between the type of anxiolytic drug and the appearance of dependence. However, since symptoms (exacerbation of anxiety, insomnia, motor agitation, tremor and increase in somatic complaints) associated with the termination of treatment are similar to those which brought the patients to the clinic, assessment of drug dependence is very difficult. In addition, some patients presented ataxia, gastro-intestinal cramps and dysphoria which did not respond to placebo during the post-treatment phase. These 'withdrawal symptoms' seem to be inversely related to duration of action of the anxiolytic drugs, i.e. the shorter the duration of their action, the higher the frequency of these symptoms.

Conclusion

Two factors may contribute to the abuse of anxiolytics.

(1) Since benzodiazepines are therapeutically very effective and have not only minor but also a very low incidence of side-effects, physicians in general have the tendency of prescribing them without making a proper diagnosis and to continue prescribing without first ascertaining whether or not the patients still need such a treatment.

(2) The majority of the patients treated are not informed of their illness. Neither are they being told of the nature of the treatment they receive. The consequence is that the patient believes that his well-being is solely dependent on the availability of the treatment.

I, therefore, feel that most of the dependence associated with benzodiazepines is iatrogenic in nature! However, I do not deny the possibility of real drug dependence induced by the anxiolytics.

In a survey of the literature, the most common statement found was the following: 'The risk of pharmacodependence with benzodiazepines has been largely exaggerated'. I have found this idea under varied constructions in papers by Leo Hollister[2], John Marks[3], or in those by Greenblatt and Shader[1]. We believe that there is indeed a certain exaggeration when the risk of drug dependence with benzodiazepines is discussed.

In an attempt to reduce or prevent real benzodiazepine-induced dependence via our Service, no patient is treated longer than 90 days on one specific anxiolytic agent. If, at the end of this period, it is established that the patient still needs medication, an anxiolytic of a different class (an antidepressant, a neuroleptic or an antihistaminic) is then prescribed.

References

1. Greenblatt, D.J. and Shader, R.I. (1978). Dependence, tolerance, and addiction to benzodiazepines: Clinical and pharmacokinetic considerations. *Drug Metab. Rev.*, **8,** 13
2. Hollister, L.E. (1973). *Clinical Use of Psychotherapeutic Drugs.* (Springfield: Charles C. Thomas)
3. Marks, J. (1978). *The Benzodiazepines.* (Lancaster: MTP Press)

21

Comparative Study of the Use of Benzodiazepines in a University Psychiatric Clinic and in Public and Private Services

O. Bastos, M.C.C.A. Martins, J. Lemos and M.A.S.L. Santos

Introduction

The aim of this study was to compare the use of benzodiazepines in different types of psychiatric services: university clinic, private practice, public service and private enterprises. Twenty practitioners from each professional group were surveyed about their attitudes towards and prescribing habits of benzodiazepines by means of a questionnaire containing 22 questions. The hypothesis was that there would be variations in the ways in which benzodiazepines are used and in the therapeutic results obtained according to the type of psychiatric services and patients' socio-economic level.

Material and methods

A questionnaire containing 22 questions was distributed to a cross-section of doctors working in this field. The answers were given in free form. Seventy-seven of the returned questionnaires were considered in the analysis, and 19 of the questions and answers are considered in the following report.

The individual questions, together with a tabular presentation of the responses, are given in the following section. In Brazil, it is usual for medical doctors to have more than one professional appointment and, in our study, all respondents held at least two different positions. The most common combination was of public and private service. Classification was according to the more permanent occupation and main activity in one of the following groups:

Group A: university clinical medical personnel: $N = 17$

Group B: psychiatrists engaged mainly in private practice: $N = 20$

Group C: medical doctors working in public health services: $N = 20$

Group D: psychiatrists working for private enterprises: $N = 20$

Group A consisted mainly of young professionals, probably on account of the presence of residents. The majority of those in group B were doctors of longer professional activity (11 to 20 years), while group C had a large number of younger specialists, although most had between 11 and 20 years' experience in the field. Group D was made up mainly of younger doctors who would tend to discontinue work in this position in the course of time (Table 21.1). All doctors interviewed are regularly in direct contact with patients.

Table 21.1 Number of years active in this specialist branch of medicine

Activity in the medical speciality	*Group A* ($N = 17$) %	*Group B* ($N = 20$) %	*Group C* ($N = 20$) %	*Group D* ($N = 20$) %	*Total* ($N = 77$) %
Up to 10 years	53	35	55	85	57
11–20 years	23.5	45	45	5	30
More than 20 years	23.5	20	0	10	13

Results

Socio-economic status of patients and time spent attending them

Group B practitioners primarily treat patients of middle or high socio-economic status, while groups A, C and D care exclusively for patients of low socio-economic level (Table 21.2). Those of group B spend significantly more time with their patients (maximum: 2 patients per hour), while group A and particularly group C and D doctors see 4 or more patients in an hour. One of those interviewed in group D acknowledged seeing about 12 patients every 60 minutes. Social problems are more frequently encountered in patients treated by groups A, C and D, and sometimes food would be more important than medical care.

Table 21.2 Socio-economic status of the patients treated by the different medical groups

Socio-economic level of patients	*Treated by*				
	Group A ($N = 17$) %	*Group B* ($N = 20$) %	*Group C* ($N = 20$) %	*Group D* ($N = 20$) %	*Total* ($N = 77$) %
Low	88	5	90	100	70
Middle + high	0	65	0	0	17
Variable	6	30	0	0	9
Not specified	6	0	10	0	4

'*What remarks would you like to make on the use of benzodiazepines with regard to the particular needs of the patients in your practice*?'

A large number of different answers to this question was received from all groups. The most frequent response (22% of those surveyed) mentioned the use of benzodiazepines to cope with social problems or insufficient support and assistance. In group B, in contrast to the other groups, this aspect was mentioned only once ($p < 0.01$). The incidence of the other answers was not related to group classification.

Benzodiazepines are indicated in pictures of anxiety, alcoholism and behavioural problems but not in psychotic patients with organic and intellectual deficiency problems (stated by 21% of those surveyed).

Benzodiazepines find approval because of their excellent anxiolytic action, good tolerance, low price and free distribution (mentioned by 10%).

Benzodiazepines influence the psychodynamic behaviour of the patient (17%).

Benzodiazepines are widely used and frequently requested (13%).

Benzodiazepines are not accepted by some patients (8%).

Conditions in which benzodiazepines are of most use

All groups agreed that anxiety, whether alone or associated with insomnia or convulsions, is the condition for which benzodiazepine therapy is most useful. Neuroses and alcoholism were mentioned by neither group A doctors, whose patients were mainly women, nor by group B doctors, whose practices had a lower incidence of alcoholism and who had a more pronounced tendency to treat anxiety symptoms and not neurotic disease with benzodiazepines (Table 21.3).

Table 21.3 Conditions in which benzodiazepines are of most use

	Group A ($N = 17$) %	*Group B* ($N = 20$) %	*Group C* ($N = 20$) %	*Group D* ($N = 20$) %	*Total* ($N = 77$) %
In cases of anxiety	70	80	65	75	73
Alone	64	70	55	55	61
With insomnia	6	5	0	15	7
With convulsive fits	0	5	10	5	5
In neurotics and alcoholics	0	0	5	20	6
Others	12	10	0	5	6
When physician deems necessary	12	0	5	0	4
When there is no possibility for systematic psychotherapy	6	0	5	0	3
No answer	0	0	5	0	1

Some answers deserve special attention: 'when the anxiety level is high and hinders psychotherapy, or in cases of initial insomnia'; 'when there is no possibility of regular psychotherapy'; 'in patients with neurotic anxiety, without severe social problems'; 'in the initial phase of treatment for crisis'; 'as symptomatic medication'; etc.

Type of patient who benefits most from benzodiazepine therapy

This question was frequently misunderstood and confused with the previous question. It was answered correctly by only 16% of those surveyed, who saw those most likely to benefit from benzodiazepine therapy as having a high IQ, being motivated to seek treatment or being young people with the possibility of psychotherapy.

Conditions in which benzodiazepines are of less use

Of those interviewed, 40% mentioned patients with psychopathological conditions, such as psychosis, intellectual deficiency, drug addiction, while 16% criticized prescription of benzodiazepines for psychoneurosis, preferring psychotherapy. Group C and D doctors strongly emphasized the inapplicability of psychotropic agents in conditions in which social problems are of primary importance. Group B doctors, on the other hand, referred only in exceptional cases to such problems. This difference may reflect the different socio-economic levels of the patients being treated by

Table 21.4 Conditions in which benzodiazepines are of less use

	Group A (N = 17) %	*Group B* (N = 20) %	*Group C* (N = 20) %	*Group D* (N = 20) %	*Total* (N = 77) %
In psychotic patients psychopaths, intellectual deficiency and drug addiction	47	40	30	45	40
In psychoneurotic patients	12	30	15	5	16
In face of social problems	6	0	30	20	14
In old age	12	5	0	15	8
Do not use	0	10	15	0	6
During psychotherapy	6	5	0	0	3
Others	18	10	10	15	13

the various groups (see Table 21.4). A smaller number of those interviewed (8 %) commented that the benzodiazepines are of little use in the elderly.

Situations in which the use of benzodiazepines is considered prejudicial

The use of benzodiazepines in dependent personalities, drug addicts, persons at risk of drug dependence or in cases where they could hinder psychotherapy was most frequently considered prejudicial by groups A and B. Groups C and D referred more often to the disadvantages of prescribing these drugs when socio-economic problems were present (Table 21.5).

Some answers were as follows: 'when they hinder psychotherapy or there is risk of psychic or physical dependence'; 'when I feel I am deceiving the patient by prescribing diazepam instead of the food he needs'; 'when the psychopathological picture is caused by hunger or poverty'; 'when it is used as a certificate of illness'; 'in addiction-prone personalities'; 'in patients who develop tolerance and change the dosage on their own initiative'.

Role of the benzodiazepines in the doctor–patient relationship

The great majority of all those interviewed were convinced of the important and positive role of the benzodiazepines in the doctor–patient relationship (66 % positive response). A much smaller percentage (10 %) attributed to them an insignificant, unnecessary, minimal function, and some found them to be either beneficial or detrimental, according to the circumstances in which they were used.

Table 21.5 Situations in which the use of benzodiazepines is considered prejudicial

	Group A (*N* = 17) %	*Group B* (*N* = 20) %	*Group C* (*N* = 20) %	*Group D* (*N* = 20) %	*Total* (*N* = 77) %
In dependent personalities, drug addicts, when there is risk of drug dependence or detriment to psychotherapy	47	55	10	30	35
'When there is no indication and/or there are formal contra-indications'	18	20	20	15	18
When there are socio-economic problems	12	5	30	15	16
In aged and psychotic patients	0	5	10	25	10
Never	12	10	5	10	9
Others	12	0	10	5	6
Do not use	0	5	15	0	5

Some answers could be noted: 'very important, most patients only come to get drugs'; 'as a means of dealing with both the patients' needs and expectations and the physician's own anxiety'; 'the drug is the sufferer's ever-present requirement: it satisfies both the doctor's need to do something for and give something to the patient, and the latter's expectation of receiving something from the doctor'; 'they jeopardize the relationship seriously'; 'the effects ascribed to the drug are in fact due to the doctor–patient relationship itself'; 'they make things easy, prescribing is an act of giving attention' (Table 21.6).

The usefulness of benzodiazepines in association with systematic psychotherapy

Most members of the 4 groups (71 %) considered the use of benzodiazepines simultaneously with systematic psychotherapy as being useful or significant, particularly in crisis conditions or in the initial phase of treatment.

Table 21.6 Role of benzodiazepines in the doctor–patient relationship

	Group A ($N = 17$) %	*Group B* ($N = 20$) %	*Group C* ($N = 20$) %	*Group D* ($N = 20$) %	*Total* ($N = 77$) %
Excellent, very important, necessary, positive, useful, easing relationship	71	45	60	70	61
As an aid in initial phase	12	5	0	0	4
Alleviation of anxiety	12	5	0	5	5
'Armed psychotherapy'	0	0	0	10	3
Subtotal: Benzodiazepines make easier doctor–patient relationship	95	55	60	85	73
Sometimes useful, sometimes prejudicial	6	15	0	0	5
Indifferent, unnecessary, minimal etc.	0	20	10	10	10
Prejudicial	0	5	5	5	4
Subtotal: Benzodiazepines are of little or no use in doctor–patient relationship	6	40	15	15	19
Left blank, or others (don't know, difficult etc.)	0	5	25	0	8

A smaller proportion (10 %) found them to be 'sometimes useful, sometimes prejudicial' (Table 21.7).

Use of benzodiazepines in the absence of systematic psychotherapy

In all groups, the great majority (70 %) of the psychiatrists were of the opinion that benzodiazepines are useful or are even the only alternative when it is not possible to conduct systematic psychotherapy, that they are necessary in the initial phases of treatment or in minimal doses for a short period, during crises or as 'armed psychotherapy' (Table 21.8). Some of those in groups A and C (30 %) referred to their symptomatic effect, while 20 % of those in groups B and C considered benzodiazepines administered under these conditions to be inefficient and palliative medicine,

Table 21.7 The usefulness of benzodiazepines in association with systematic psychotherapy

	Group A (*N* = 17) %	*Group B* (*N* = 20) %	*Group C* (*N* = 20) %	*Group D* (*N* = 20) %	*Total* (*N* = 77) %
Exceptional, essential, etc.	6	0	10	5	5
Important, useful, auxiliary, etc.	41	30	50	65	47
Useful in crisis conditions	29	15	0	0	10
Useful in the beginning of the treatment	0	25	5	5	9
Subtotal: Benzodiazepines useful combined with psychotherapy	76	70	65	75	71
Sometimes useful, sometimes prejudicial	6	25	0	10	10
Unnecessary, dispensable, etc.	12	0	5	5	5
Prejudicial	0	5	0	0	1
Subtotal: Benzodiazepines not useful combined with psychotherapy or of little use	18	30	5	15	16
Left blank or does not conduct systematic psychotherapy	6	0	30	10	12

claiming that 'there is always possibility for a psychotherapeutic approach or assistance', and pointing to the risk of dependence.

'*How do you view the prospects of treatment by means of exclusive use of benzodiazepines?*'

The majority of the doctors interviewed (61 %) viewed the prospects of exclusive use of benzodiazepines in a negative light, pointing to the risks of iatrogenesis and the development of dependence and chronic habits of

Table 21.8 Use of benzodiazepines in the absence of systematic psychotherapy

	Group A (*N* = 17) %	*Group B* (*N* = 20) %	*Group C* (*N* = 20) %	*Group D* (*N* = 20) %	*Total* (*N* = 77) %
The only alternative, compulsory, of fundamental importance, helpful, good results, etc.	18	65	25	65	44
Reference to symptomatic effect	35	0	25	0	14
Reference to usefulness in initial phase of treatment or in minimal doses for a short period	0	0	20	5	6
Reference to usefulness in crisis	12	0	0	0	3
Reference to 'armed psychotherapy'	12	0	5	0	4
Subtotal: favourable	77	65	75	70	71
Inefficient, palliative medicine, etc.	0	15	0	25	10
Reference to risk of dependence	0	10	0	0	3
Subtotal: unfavourable	0	25	0	25	13
Assertion that there is always a possibility of psychotherapeutic attitude or 'I do regular psychotherapy'	17	10	5	0	8
Blank	6	0	20	5	8

use. A less significant percentage (24%) considered exclusive benzodiazepine therapy as useful, especially in 'cases of crises'.

However, a significant number of group B and C psychiatrists stated their opposition to this practice, group B mentioning that they do not use drugs exclusively. Some comments were 'it is far from being what one might wish'; 'treatment exclusively with drugs is the same as iatrogenesis'; 'treatment tends to consist exclusively of drug therapy on account of the instability of socio-economic conditions'; 'it is not feasible'; 'drugs are always used simultaneously with psychotherapy' (Table 21.9).

Table 21.9 The prospects of treatment by means of exclusive use of benzodiazepines

	Group A ($N = 17$) %	*Group B* ($N = 20$) %	*Group C* ($N = 20$) %	*Group D* ($N = 20$) %	*Total* ($N = 77$) %
Very good, good, useful, etc.	18	10	5	30	16
Called for in case of crisis	12	10	5	5	8
Subtotal	30	20	10	35	24
Poor, unpredictable, inefficient, very poor, chaotic	29	40	70	50	48
With risk of iatrogenesis	12	0	5	0	4
With risk of dependence	12	5	5	5	6
With risk of chronic use	0	0	5	5	3
Subtotal	53	45	85	60	61
'I do not use drugs' or 'I do not use drugs exclusively' etc.	17	35	5	5	15

Drugs most usefully administered in combination with benzodiazepines

The great majority (74%) of those surveyed favour combination of benzodiazepines with antidepressants, and a relatively small group (13–17%) stated anticonvulsants, hypnotics and neuroleptics to be the most useful drugs for combination with benzodiazepines (Table 21.10).

Particular benzodiazepines preferred for therapy

Diazepam, as a single prescription or in conjunction with chlordiazepoxide, lorazepam or bromazepam, was the first preference amongst the surveyed population. Group A (university clinic) and group C (public health services) referred to the free distribution of diazepam by CEME*. Group B preferred bromazepam to a degree which was statistically significant. A

* Central Drug Institute

Table 21.10 Drugs most usefully administered in combination with benzodiazepines (more than one answer possible)

Advantageous combinations: Benzodiazepines with	*Group A* ($N = 17$) %	*Group B* ($N = 20$) %	*Group C* ($N = 20$) %	*Group D* ($N = 20$) %	*Total* ($N = 77$) %
Antidepressants	76	75	60	85	74
Anticonvulsants	12	10	20	15	14
Hypnotics	6	5	5	35	13
Neuroleptics	6	20	25	15	17
Others or blank	6	10	15	0	8
Do not use combinations	12	0	5	5	5

Table 21.11 Particular benzodiazepines preferred for therapy (2 answers possible)

	Group A ($N = 17$) %	*Group B* ($N = 20$) %	*Group C* ($N = 20$) %	*Group D* ($N = 20$) %	*Total* ($N = 77$) %
Diazepam	65	20	35	25	35
Bromazepam	0	25	5	5	9
Lorazepam	12	5	10	10	9
Chlordiazepoxide	12	0	0	5	4
Non-existent	18	35	20	55	32
Others	6	5	10	10	8
Blank, not specified	6	15	25	0	11

relatively large group (32%) had no particular preference for any benzodiazepine derivative (Table 21.11).

Use and results with hypnotic benzodiazepines

Most of those participating in the survey (68%) mentioned that they prescribed hypnotic benzodiazepines. Forty-five per cent did not comment on results, 13% commented positively on their effects and 9% viewed them as being only moderately effective.

Personal observation of psychic or physical dependence or increasing tolerance to benzodiazepines

In regard to this question, most of those interviewed (73%) reported some experience with such effects, but 21% did not specify the type of phenomenon observed. Twenty-one per cent emphasized psychic dependence,

17% mentioned psychic dependence with increased tolerance, 9% referred to psychic and physical dependence with increased tolerance and 5% mentioned only increasing tolerance. More psychiatrists in groups C and D reported psychic dependence and increased tolerance than in groups A and B (Table 21.12).

Table 21.12 Personal observation of psychic or physical dependence, or increasing tolerance to benzodiazepine

		Group A ($N = 17$) %	*Group B* ($N = 20$) %	*Group C* ($N = 20$) %	*Group D* ($N = 20$) %	*Total* ($N = 77$) %
YES	Without specification of type	18	10	25	30	21
	Psychic dependence	29	35	10	10	21
	Psychic dependence and development of tolerance	6	5	20	35	17
	Psychic and physical dependence and development of tolerance	6	15	5	10	9
	Development of tolerance	0	10	10	0	5
	Subtotal	59	75	70	85	73
NO		29	15	15	15	18
Nil		0	10	15	0	6
No experience		12	0	0	0	3

Physicians' reaction to signs of psychic or physical dependence, or increasing tolerance to benzodiazepines

When faced with psychic or physical dependence or increasing tolerance to benzodiazepines, 38% of those asked mentioned the following measures: suspension, reduction or replacement of the benzodiazepine, with greater emphasis on psychotherapy. On the other hand, 34% stated that they would suspend or replace the drug without referring to alternative therapeutic measures, while 10% proposed lower doses of neuroleptics to replace benzodiazepines (Table 21.13).

Table 21.13 Physicians' reaction to signs of psychic or physical dependence, or increasing tolerance of benzodiazepines

Measures taken	*Group A* (*N* = 17) %	*Group B* (*N* = 20) %	*Group C* (*N* = 20) %	*Group D* (*N* = 20) %	*Total* (*N* = 77) %
Suspension, reduction or replacement of drug with emphasis on psychotherapy	53	55	15	30	38
Suspension, replacement without mention of other solutions tried	18	25	45	45	34
Replacement by low doses of neuroleptics	12	0	20	10	10
Others or blank	18	20	20	15	18

Level of demand for, acceptance of, or resistance to prescription of benzodiazepines

In this regard, most of those interviewed (57%) answered 'high demand, total acceptance and rare resistance'. A much smaller proportion (17%) emphasized acceptance without mentioning demand or resistance, while an even smaller percentage placed emphasis on resistance. Group B psychiatrists, however, clearly and emphatically expressed the resistance

Table 21.14 Level of demand for, acceptance of, or resistance to prescription of benzodiazepines

	Group A (*N* = 17) %	*Group B* (*N* = 20) %	*Group C* (*N* = 20) %	*Group D* (*N* = 20) %	*Total* (*N* = 77) %
High demand, total acceptance and rare resistance	71	30	60	70	57
Emphasis on acceptance without reference to demand resistance	18	10	10	30	17
Emphasis on resistance	0	50	5	0	14
Others or blank	12	10	25	0	12

of their patients to the prescription of benzodiazepines. This attitude differed to a statistically significant degree from those held by patients treated by the other groups (Table 21.14).

Some answers: 'high demand, good level of acceptance and rare resistance'; 'resistance as a result of publicity in the lay press'; 'resistance in cases of psychotherapy'; 'wide acceptance, with minimal resistance'; 'good acceptance but fear of becoming addicted'; 'small demand, with resistance, particularly in persons of higher social level'.

Alternatives to benzodiazepines therapy

Presented with the hypothetical situation that benzodiazepines had been withdrawn from the market, 40% of those surveyed answered that they would substitute neuroleptics in low doses. Others (14%) would replace them with some other form of medication with psychotherapy, 9% would use some other medication alone and a further 9% would substitute psychotherapy alone. Some of those asked regarded such a hypothetical situation as being unlikely to occur in real life while others (5%) stated that they would revert to using pre-benzodiazepine tranquillizers (Table 21.15).

The answers to this question varied widely: 'This possibility seems remote to me'; 'neuroleptics in low dosages'; 'by placebo and vitamins'; 'by sweetness and affection'; 'there was a time when they did not exist and physicians prescribed other formulae'; 'I would not know how to replace

Table 21.15 Alternatives to benzodiazepine therapy

	Group A ($N = 17$) %	*Group B* ($N = 20$) %	*Group C* ($N = 20$) %	*Group D* ($N = 20$) %	*Total* ($N = 77$) %
Neuroleptics in low doses	35	35	40	50	40
Other medication and psychotherapy	24	20	10	5	14
Other medication (not specified)	12	0	10	15	9
Psychotherapy	6	15	10	5	9
Pre-benzodiazepine tranquillizers	6	10	5	0	5
Considers the need for alternatives unlikely	6	5	5	5	5
No substitute	0	5	5	10	5
Blank or other	12	10	15	10	12

them, but the psychiatrist should compensate for this lack with better human assistance'; 'by the same means as present, but without benzodiazepines' (psychotherapist); 'if they were withdrawn from the market, a new drug would be developed for the same purpose'; 'by means of a psychotherapeutic approach'; 'I can find no substitute at the same level'; 'I would have difficulties'; 'I don't know'.

The place of benzodiazepines relative to other psychotropic agents

Most of those interviewed in all groups (58 %) gave a definite first place to benzodiazepines, ahead of all other psychotropic agents, with favourable remarks. A rather lower percentage (10 %) classified them in second or third place after neuroleptics and/or antidepressants and 6 % of psychiatrists criticized the action of benzodiazepines, considering them as symptomatic therapy, supportive, complementary, panacea etc. An even smaller number (4 %) also placed them in second or third position with regard to therapeutic results, while classifying them in first place in terms of prescription volume (Table 21.16).

Table 21.16 The place of benzodiazepines relative to other psychotropic agents

The future of the benzodiazepines

With regard to the future of the benzodiazepines, most psychiatrists of the 4 groups predicted an increase in their use, with criticism of society, psychiatric practice and the pharmaceutical industry's advertising (45%). Others believed that things would continue as at present (21%), while only 13% foresaw a decrease in the use of the benzodiazepines under the improved conditions of the future, with its better social development and improved psychiatric training and practice. A small number referred to future progress and the improvement of chemical aspects, favouring better psychopharmacology.

Those interviewed answered in general terms, making no reference to such specific aspects of the question as the future of benzodiazepines in psychiatry, internal medicine and surgery (Table 21.17).

Table 21.17 Future of the benzodiazepines

	Group A ($N = 17$) %	*Group B* ($N = 20$) %	*Group C* ($N = 20$) %	*Group D* ($N = 20$) %	*Total* ($N = 77$) %
Increase in use with criticism of society, psychiatrists and advertising	41	45	50	45	45
Same as present situation	24	20	10	30	21
Decrease in use in a better future (from the social point of view, with improved psychiatric training and practice)	12	10	20	10	13
I don't know, no answer, vague answers	18	20	10	5	13
Reference to improvement in chemical processes	6	5	10	10	8

Discussion and conclusions

We stated in our working hypothesis that there would be variations in the ways in which benzodiazepines are used and in the therapeutic results obtained, according to the type of psychiatric service and patients' socio-economic level. Comparing the answers provided by the four groups (university clinic: A; private practice: B; public health services: C; private enterprises: D), we found a high degree of conformity, the number of those in disagreement with general opinion being relatively small.

Differences in the socio-economic status of patients, their particular characteristics, types of conflicts and specific needs have some influence on the results obtained with benzodiazepines.

The 4 groups agreed upon the following aspects:

(1) Benzodiazepines are indicated in anxiety states, alcoholism and behavioural disorders.

(2) The benzodiazepines are very useful for treating anxiety, either alone or associated with insomnia and convulsions.

(3) Benzodiazepines are less useful in certain psychopathological conditions: psychosis, intellectual deficiency, drug addiction.

(4) Benzodiazepines are useful in the doctor–patient relationship, favouring the success of therapy, facilitating the initial phase of treatment and alleviating anxiety of both parties.

(5) Benzodiazepines are useful and important during systematic psychotherapy, particularly in crisis situations at the beginning of treatment.

(6) These drugs are needed as adjuvant, symptomatic therapy in the initial phase of treatment or in low doses for short periods at times of crisis, and as 'armed psychotherapy' when there is no possibility of applying systematic psychotherapeutic methods.

(7) There was disapproval of the exclusive use of benzodiazepines, and mention was made of the risks of iatrogenesis, dependence and the development of habits of chronic use.

(8) There was a tendency to combine benzodiazepine therapy with administration of antidepressants or also with anticonvulsants, neuroleptics and hypnotics.

(9) Diazepam was most frequently considered the most effective benzodiazepine.

(10) Doctors stated that psychic or physical dependence or increased tolerance have occurred. They saw the latter two effects as being secondary to psychic dependence.

(11) When faced with patients presenting psychic or physical dependence or rising threshold of tolerance to the drug, the doctors adopt the following methods: suspension, reduction or replacement of the drug with emphasis on psychotherapy; suspending or replacing the drug, but no mention of a substitute therapy; replacement by low doses of neuroleptics.

(12) It was stated that the level of demand for benzodiazepines amongst patients is high; they are wholly accepted and rarely resisted by those for whom they are prescribed.

(13) Presented with the hypothetical case that benzodiazepines had been

withdrawn from the market, those interviewed stated that, in the case of their absence, they would substitute neuroleptics in reduced dosage or a combination of another drug and psychotherapy.

(14) The benzodiazepines were, in general, preferred to other psychotropic agents available.

(15) For the above-mentioned reasons, it was anticipated that benzodiazepine use would increase, although criticism was made of psychiatric practice and pharmaceutical industry advertising.

There was a marked discrepancy between the responses furnished by psychiatrists in private practice and those from practitioners in public service or employed by private enterprises, a variance attributable mainly to the difference in socio-economic level of the patients who attended:

Those working in the public health service (C) or for private enterprises (D) strongly emphasized the inability of the benzodiazepines to help in cases where the problems are of social origin.

Groups A (university clinic) and B (private practice) pointed to the detrimental effect of benzodiazepine use in certain clinical pictures and specific therapeutic situations such as in dependent personalities, drug addicts, personalities at risk of developing drug dependence, or when prescription of these drugs may be prejudicial to systematic psychotherapy.

With regard to the question of exclusive use of benzodiazepines, those in private practice (B) tended to oppose such a practice, stating that they 'do not make exclusive use of drugs'.

With regard to preference for a particular benzodiazepine, groups A (university clinic) and C (public health service) stated that they prescribed diazepam exclusively as it was distributed free by the CEME (Central Drug Institute). Those in private practice preferred to prescribe bromazepam.

With regard to the appearance of psychic dependence and raising of the therapeutic threshold, these phenomena were reported to have been observed by more psychiatrists in groups C (public health services) and D (private enterprises) than in the other 2 groups.

As to the question regarding level of demand for, acceptance of or resistance to benzodiazepines, group B (private practice) clearly and emphatically expressed their patients' resistance, a fact not observed in the other groups.

From the analysis of the data presented, we may conclude that the private practice group maintains its autonomy and independence from the other groups, while the groups from private health services and private enterprises are largely similar. The university clinic group most closely resembles the latter 2 groups, while having some aspects in common with the private practice group. The differences observed are related mainly to the various socio-economic levels represented among the patients of the groups studied, and the conditions under which they are treated. This fact fully confirms our hypothesis that such conditions significantly influence the behaviour of the groups studied.

22

A Brazilian Contribution to Benzodiazepine Psychopharmacology: Research on Anticonvulsant Therapeutics and the Dependence Problem

J.C. Madalena

Introduction

In 1962, a small book of 150 pages came to my attention: *Psychochemotherapy* (*The Physician's Manual*), by E. Remmen, S. Cohen, K. S. Ditman and J. R. Frantz[11]. On page 94, reference was made to a substance that was synthesized by Dr. Leo H. Sternbach, who is today honouring Brazilian Psychopharmacology with his presence. It was the first agent of a new class of psychotherapeutic compounds which could be applied in a wide area of psychopathology.

As Chairman of this Section of the Symposium on 'Contributions of Brazilian Clinical Research', I have dedicated it to the Medical Scientific Department of F. Hoffmann–La Roche & Co. and its brilliant researcher, Dr Leo H. Sternbach.

Benzodiazepines as anticonvulsants[1,2]

In 1960, I. N. Rosenstein[12] discovered the anticonvulsive action of chlordiazepoxide while studying a case of GM (grand mal). All over the world,

Table 22.1 Controlled substances: Use and effect (Justice Department of USA)

	Drugs	*Scale**	*Trade names*	*Medical use*	*Dependence potential*	
					Physical	*Psychic*
Narcotics	Opium	II	Dover's Powder Paregoric Elixir	Analgesic Antidiarrhoeal	High	High
	Morphine	II	Morphine	Analgesic	"	"
	Codeine	II, III, V	Codeine	Analgesic Antitussive	Moderate	Moderate
	Heroin	I	None	None	High	High
	Meperidine	II	Demerol	Analgesic	"	"
	Methadone	II	Methadone	Analgesic Substitute heroin	"	"
	Other narcotics	I, II, III V	Dilaudid	Analgesic Antidiarrhoeal Antitussive	"	"
Depressives	Chloral hydrate	IV	Chloralat	Hypnotic	Moderate	Moderate
	Barbiturates	II, III, V	Amytal Nembutal Phenobarbital	Anaesthetic Anticonvulsive, Sedation, Sleep	High	High
	Glutethimide	III	Doriden	Sedation, Sleep	"	"
	Methaqualone	II	Mandrax Mequelon	Sedation, Sleep	"	"
	Tranquillizers	IV	Equanil Librium, Miltown Valium	Anti-anxiety Muscle relaxant Sedation	Moderate	Moderate
	Other depressives	III, IV	Noludar	Anti-anxiety Sedative Somniferous Hypnotic	Possible	Possible
Stimulants	Cocaine**	II	Cocaine	Local anaesthetic	"	High
	Amphetamines	II, III	Benzedrine Dexedrine	Hypercathesia Narcolepsy Anorexiant	"	"
	Phenmetrazine	II	Preludin	Weight control	"	"
	Methylphenidate	II	Ritalin	Hypercinesia	"	"
	Other stimulants	III, IV	—	Weight control	"	Possible
Hallucinogens	LSD	I	None	None	None	Unknown degree
	Mescaline	I	"	"	"	"
	Psilocybin	I	"	"	"	"
	MDA	I	"	"	"	"
	PCP***	III	"	Veterinary Anaesthetic	"	"
	Other hallucinogens	I	"	None	"	"
Cannabis	Hashish Hashish oil Marihuana	I	"	"	Unknown degree	Moderate

* *Scale* Classifications vary for each drug because the controlled substances are often sold in combination with other medicinal ingredients

** *Cocaine* Classified as narcotic by 'Controlled Substances' Act

*** RGB Classified as denressive by the same law

Tolerance	*Duration of effects (h)*	*Administration route*	*Possible effects*	*Hyperdosage effects*	*Abstinence syndrome*
Yes	3–6	Oral – Smoked			
			Sleepiness	Slow and superficial	Lachrymose eyes
			Euphoria	respiration	Rhinorrhoea
,,	,,	Injection –	Respiratory	Viscous skin	Yawning
		Smoked	depression	Coma	Anorexia
,,	,,	Oral –	Myosis	Convulsions	Irritability
		Injection			
,,	,,	Injection	Nausea	Possible death	Tremors
		Inhalation			Panic
,,	,,	Oral – Injection			Shivers
,,	12–24	,, ,,			Perspiration
					Cramps
,,	3–6	,, ,,			Nausea
Probable	5–8	Oral			
Yes	1–16	Oral – Injection			
			Senseless talk	Superficial	Anxiety
,,	4–8	Oral	Disorientation	respiration	Insomnia
,,	,,	,,	Ebrious behaviour	Cold and viscous	Tremors
			without smell of	skin	Delirium
,,	,,	,,	alcohol	Dilated pupils	Convulsions
				Weak and rapid	Possible death
				pulse	
				Coma and possible	
Yes	4–8	Oral		death	
,,	2	Injection –	Increased	Agitation	Apathy
		Aspiration	vigilance	Hyperthermia	Long periods
,,	2–4	Oral – Injection	Excitement	Hallucinations	of sleep
			Euphoria	Convulsions	Irritability
			Mydriasis	Possible death	Depression
,,	,,	Oral	Tachysphygmia		Disorientation
,,	,,	,,	Hypertension		
,,	,,	,,	Insomnia		
			Anorexia		
,,	Variable	,,			
,,	,,	Oral – Injection	Delusions and	Longer and more	Abstinence
,,	,,	Oral	hallucinations	extensive trips	syndrome not
,,	,,	Oral – Injection	(except MDA)	Psychosis	mentioned
		Aspiration	Disorientation in	Possible death	
,,	,,	Oral – Injection	time and space		
		Smoked			
,,	,,	Oral – Injection			
		Aspiration			
			Euphoria	Tiredness	Insomnia
,,	2–4	Oral – Smoked	Increased appetite	Delirium	Hyperactivity
			Bewildered	Possible psychosis	Decreased
			behaviour		appetite in few
			Unrestraint		patients

Table 22.2 Controlled substances: Use and effect (Justice Department of USA)
Table modified by Dr. J. Caruso Madalena, Head of the Programming and Technical Norms of the National Menta Health Division of the Health Ministry, Brazil

*Degree of dependence risk-factor (Kielholz)****	*Group*	*Substances*	*Scale**	*Trade names*	*Medical use*
0.2	Tranquillizers	Tranquillizers (Benzodiazepines) Meprobamate	—	Librium Valium Equanil	Anti-anxiety Muscle relaxant Anticonvulsive
2.7	Hypnotics	Methaqualone	II	Mandrax Mequelon	Sedation Sleep
		Chloral hydrate	IV	Chloralat	Hypnotic
		Barbiturates	II, III, IV	Amytal Nembutal Phenobarbital Seconal	Anticonvulsive Sedative Anaesthetic
		Glutethimide	III	Doriden	Sedative Sleep
n.d.		Cocaine**	II	Cocaine	Local anaesthetic
3.8	Stimulants	Amphetamines	II, III	Benzedrine Dexedrine	Hypercathesia Narcolepsy
		Phenmetrazine	II	Preludine	Weight control
		Methylphenidate	II	Ritalin	Hypercinesia
		Other stimulants	III, IV	,,	Weight control
n.d.	Narcotics	Opium	II	Dover's Powder Paregoric Elixir	Analgesic Anti-diarrhoeal
		Morphine	II	Morphine	Analgesic
		Codeine	II, III, IV	Codeine	Analgesic Antitussive
		Heroin	I	None	None
		Meperidine	II	Demerol	Analgesic
		Methadone	II	Methadone	Substitute for heroin

* *Scale* Classifications vary for each drug as controlled substances are often sold in combination with other medic ingredients
** *Cocaine* Classified as narcotic by 'Controlled Substances' Act
*** Dependence risk factors for drug groups[3] (Risk factor for Analgetica = 1)
n.d. = not determined

many studies followed with chlordiazepoxide[4] and other benzodiazepines, particularly the benzodiazepine-2-one group, as anticonvulsant substances[5–9].

At the May 24, 1963, session of the Centro de Estudos of the Instituto de Psiquiatria at the Federal University of Rio de Janeiro, I presented the results of my clinical–therapeutic and electroencephalographic investigations of epilepsy with Ro 5-0690 (chlordiazepoxide) and Ro 5-2807 (diazepam). The results were compared with those presented by A. Creso and G. R. Hernandez at the Second Latin American Congress on Psychiatry, Mexico, November 11–17, 1962.

Dependence potential		*Tolerance*	*Duration of effects (h)*	*Administration route*	*Possible effects*	*Hyperdosage effects*	*Abstinence syndrome*
Physical	*Psychic*						
Not confirmed	Not confirmed	Not confirmed	4–8	Oral	Sleepiness Asthenia	Sleepiness Asthenia	Not confirmed
Moderate	Moderate	Yes	4–8	Oral	,,	,,	Anxiety Insomnia
Moderate	Moderate	Probable	5–8	Oral	Ebrious behaviour Dysarthria Disorientation	Superficial respiration Cold skin Dilated pupils Weak and rapid pulse Coma Death	Anxiety Insomnia Tremors Delirium Convulsions Death
High	High	Yes	1–16	Oral – Injection			
,,	,,	,,	4–8	Oral			
Possible	,,	,,	2	Injection Aspiration	Increased vigilance Excitement Euphoria Mydriasis Tachysphygmia Hypertension Insomnia Anorexia	Agitation Hyperthermia Hallucinations Convulsions and possible death	Apathy Long periods of sleep Irritability Depression Disorientation
,,	,,	,,	2–4	Oral – Injection			
,,	,,	,,	,,	Oral			
,,	,,	,,	,,	,,			
,,	Possible	,,	,,	,,			
High	High	,,	3–6	Oral (smoked)	Sleepiness Euphoria Respiratory depression Myosis Nausea	Slow and superficial respiration Viscous skin Convulsions Coma Possible death	Lachrymose eyes Rhinorrhea Yawning Anorexia Irritability Tremors Panic Shivers Nausea Cramps
,,	,,	,,	,,	Injection Smoked			
Moderate	Moderate	,,	,,	Oral – Injection			
High	High	,,	,,	Injection Inhalation			
,,	,,	,,	,,	Oral – Injection			
,,	,,	,,	12–24	Oral – Injection			

For the first time in Brazil, benzodiazepines were used systematically as a new class of anticonvulsant substances.

Use of clonazepam

My experience with benzodiazepines as anti-epileptic drugs is extensive, beginning in 1961 with the use of chlordiazepoxide as a substitute for earlier anti-epileptic agents (particularly barbiturates and hydantoins) and later on in studies comparing chlordiazepoxide, diazepam and clonazepam with post-benzodiazepine anti-epileptic agents (such as sulthiame carbamazepine). In clinical practice clonazepam has proved superior to the two other benzodiazepines. However, in the rare cases when clonazepam has failed, better results have been achieved with the classic chlordiazepoxide.

In my opinion, clonazepam has the following advantages compared with chlordiazepoxide and diazepam:

(1) Much lower dosage with impressive efficacy in GM;

(2) Completely safe, with excellent tolerance even in chronic use;

(3) Almost complete absence of side-effects;

(4) Better euhypnic effect in epileptic patients;

(5) Clearly better effects on behavioural disorders associated with epilepsy;

(6) Selective favourable effect on PM (petit mal) crises, which does not occur with chlordiazepoxide and diazepam.

According to my experience since 1961, I can confirm today that the benzodiazepines are the best anticonvulsant drugs on account of their efficacy, safety and absence of dependence risk.

The dependence problem[10]

With regard to the controversy surrounding benzodiazepine dependence, I report the following Brazilian contribution I made as Head of the Programming and Technical Norms Service of the National Mental Health Division of the Health Ministry. I modified the official US Justice Department Table of Controlled Substances (Use and Effect), which can be seen in Table 22.1. The modified version is presented in Table 22.2. As can be seen, I have replaced 'drugs' by 'substances' in the first column because I was dealing with a table of substances. I classified the groups of psychotherapeutic substances according to the degrees of dependence ('risk-factor'), after the classification of Kielholz[3], which appears best adapted to the current clinical situation. I removed from the table substances with no specific medical indication. I separated the barbiturate group from that of the benzodiazepines, since in neuro-anatomical, pharmacodynamic and clinical aspects and dependence risk, they represent two very distinct sectors.

References

1. Audisio, M. and Picat, J. Le traitement des épilepsies. In Laffont, A. and Durieux, F. *Encyclopédie Médico-Chirurgicale*, 37250, A 20, p. 1. (Paris: Editions Techniques)

2. Garattini, S., Mussini, E., Randall, L. O. (eds.), (1973). *The Benzodiazepines*. (New York: Raven Press)
3. Kielholz, P. (1968). Gesamtschweizerische Enquête über die Häufigkeit des Medikamentenmissbrauches. *Schweiz. Aerzteztg.*, **49**, 1077
4. Madalena, J. C. (1962). O clordiazepóxido como medicamento antiepiléptico. *J. Bras. Psiq.*, **11**, 211
5. Madalena, J. C. (1963). Ro 4-8180 – Novo benzodiazepínico. Seu ensaio na neurose e na epilepsia. *J. Bras. Psiq.*, **12**, 323
6. Madalena, J. C. (1963). As benzodiazepinas: nova classe de substâncias anticonvulsivantes. Primeiras comparações. *J. Bras. Psiq.*, **12**, 313
7. Madalena, J. C. (1967). A situação atual da medicação anti-epiléptica sob o enfoque psicofarmocológico. Nossa experiência. *Rev. Bras. Psiq.*, **1**, 241
8. Madalena, J. C. (1972). Observações clínicas preliminares com o clonazepam (Ro 5-4023) na epilepsia. *Rev. Bras. Clín. Terap.*, **1**, 357
9. Madalena, J. C. (1973). As benzodiazepinas no tratamento dos distúrbios epilépticos. *Folha Méd.*, **67**, 685
10. Marks, J. (1978). *The Benzodiazepines. – Use, Overuse, Misuse, Abuse.* (Lancaster: MTP Press Limited)
11. Remmen, E., Cohen, S., Ditman, K. S. and Frantz, J. R. (1962). *Psychochemotherapy. – The Physician's Manual.* (Los Angeles: Western Medical Publications)
12. Rosenstein, I. N. (1960). A new psychosedative (Librium) as an anticonvulsant in grand mal type convulsive seizures. *Dis. Nerv. Syst.*, **21**, (suppl.) 57

23

Flurazepam in Insomnia

A. J. M. de Paula

Introduction

Sleep disturbances are, next to pain of various origins, the most commonly encountered complaints in man, judging by the number and type of drugs used in their treatment.

For patients and physicians, the most important form of sleep disturbances is insomnia. This most prevalent of sleep disorders has been called 'the great underground ailment of modern society'*. Difficulties with sleeping arise for many reasons and physicians should, in treating their patients, take into account all factors that can provoke insomnia. If hypnotic drugs are necessary, they should be effective, safe, well-tolerated and appropriate to the different types of insomnia.

The successful management of insomnia will depend on the choice of the hypnotic and its acceptability to the patient. The benzodiazepines appear to possess interesting pharmacological properties and have an established efficacy in a number of diverse neuropsychiatric conditions. They are useful in a wide variety of clinical situations ranging from the treatment of anxiety to the management of insomnia.

Benzodiazepines probably exert their pharmacological and clinical effects through interaction with specific benzodiazepine receptors in the central nervous system.

The management of insomnia – flurazepam

Basic information

Flurazepam – a cyclic and fluorated benzodiazepine derivative – has been

* *J. Am. Med. Assoc.* (1978). **23**, 25

widely studied and used in the treatment of insomnia. Its chemical denomination is: 7-chloro-1-[2-(diethylamino)ethyl]-5-(*o*-fluorophenyl)-1,3-dihydro-2H-1,4-benzodiazepin-2-one mono- or dihydrochloride, and it has the following structural formula:

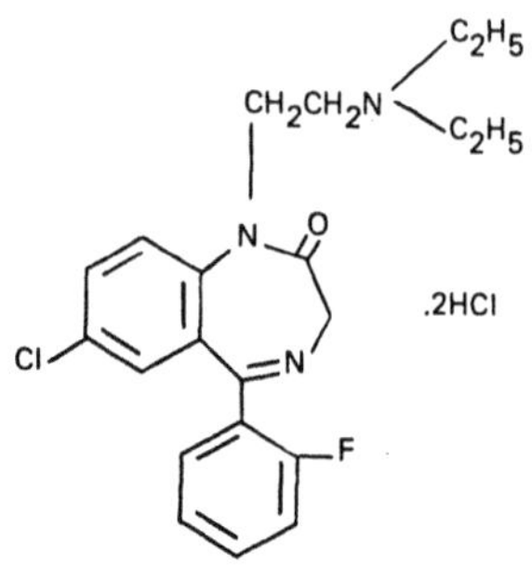

In experiments on animals it has been demonstrated that it possesses all the well-known pharmacological properties of benzodiazepines, e.g.: anxiolytic, sedative, anticonvulsant and muscle-relaxant. In humans, flurazepam is readily absorbed and rapidly metabolized. The pathways of the flurazepam biotransformation in man and dog are given in Figure 23.1[19].

Clinical evidence

Flurazepam was the first hypnotic to be extensively studied in sleep laboratories, in volunteers as well as in insomniac patients. In these studies, during the night continuous electroencephalographic (EEG), electromyographic and electro-oculographic (EOG) recordings were made.

Subjective ratings of sleep quality and duration were also recorded. Short-, medium- and longterm studies were performed in order to demonstrate efficacy after single and repeated administration for several weeks.

In most of these studies, it was possible to demonstrate that flurazepam in appropriate dosage (30 mg or 15 mg)

Reduces the time needed for sleep induction, that is, the period between going to bed and first signs of sleep ('detachment from the external world'). In the mean, sleep latency was reduced to 50% of that without flurazepam and was approximately 15 minutes;

Reduces the mean time awake after initial sleep onset. The typical outcome was a decrease from more than 30 minutes without flurazepam to less than 15 minutes during the flurazepam period;

Increases the total sleep time by a mean of between 30 and 60 minutes;

Decreases the number of awakenings during the night.

In contrast to other hypnotics, Dalmadorm continued to exercise a satisfactory therapeutic effect at the end of a treatment period of 3 weeks without any need to increase the dosage.

Dalmadorm was superior to placebo in all parameters measured and, overall, more effective than other hypnotics[10, 15]. Dement *et al.*[9] found that although the drug reduces slow-wave sleep significantly, it does not strongly suppress REM sleep, as is the case with other hypnotics.

It seems that, in parallel to the accumulation of the active metabolite,

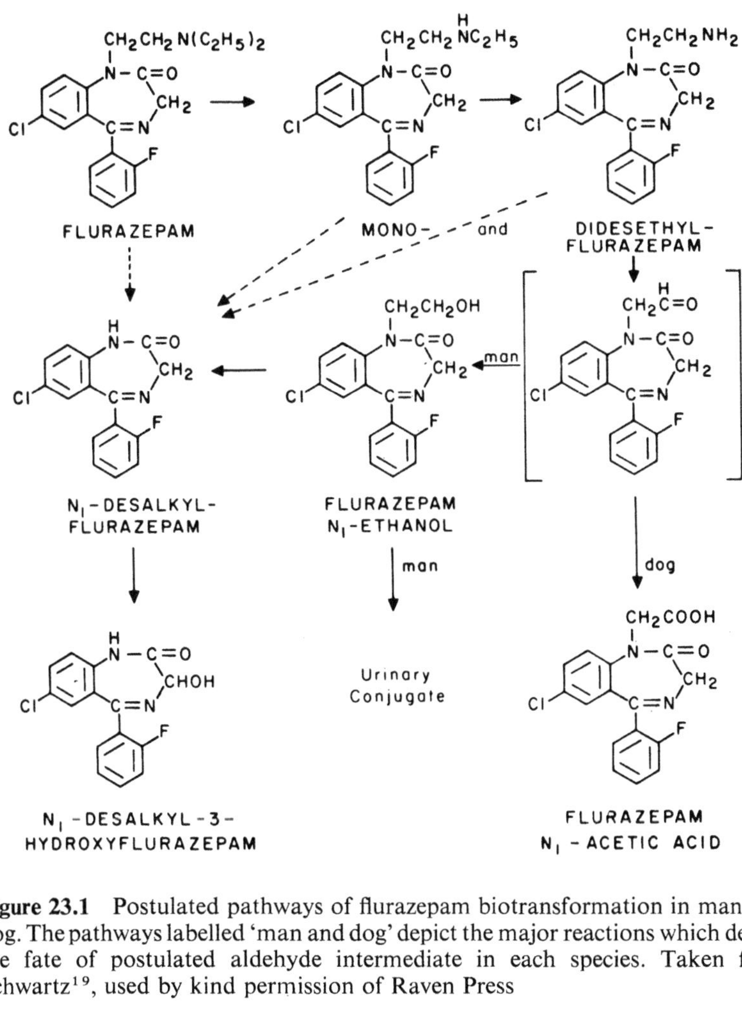

Figure 23.1 Postulated pathways of flurazepam biotransformation in man and dog. The pathways labelled 'man and dog' depict the major reactions which decide the fate of postulated aldehyde intermediate in each species. Taken from Schwartz[19], used by kind permission of Raven Press

desalkyl flurazepam, there is a better effect on the second night than on the first night.

Sleep laboratory studies are important since they provide objective proof of the effectiveness of an hypnotic agent. On the other hand, these studies can be carried out in only a relatively small number of subjects and in a highly sophisticated technical environment.

Therefore, well-controlled clinical trials to assess tolerance and efficacy are for clinicians even more important than electrophysiological studies.

In open longterm tolerance studies carried out with 271 patients[8] doses of 15mg to 120mg of flurazepam were administered during 90 nights. Side-effects such as dizziness, sleepiness, tottering gait and ataxia were dose-dependent and disappeared within a few days as the treatment continued, without reduction or discontinuation of the administration of the drug. The low toxicity of flurazepam was conclusively confirmed by double-blind studies involving more than 2000 patients. Side-effects such as dizziness and sleepiness appeared chiefly in aged and debilitated patients.

No interference with cardiac and respiratory functions was noted: patients given up to 200mg of flurazepam in multiple doses, or single doses of up to 120mg, did not present any functional change in the circulatory and respiratory systems. In usual dosage (15–30 mg), hangover was only seldom present.

Today there is extensive literature[1–7, 11–14, 16–18, 20–23] on the subject of performance the day after drug intake. Even after multiple doses, flurazepam 15mg did not affect performance in tests in any study. However, impaired performance in some tests after 30mg flurazepam has been mentioned by a few authors.

In double-blind clinical studies (cross-over or parallel groups) conducted to determine the effectiveness of Dalmadorm compared with placebo or usual hypnotics like glutethimide, chloral hydrate or methaqualone, Dalmadorm was preferred by patients and was more effective in reducing the time taken to fall asleep and in maintaining sleep. More than 2000 patients, including psychiatric cases, participated in these clinical trials.

Conclusions

On the basis of open and comparative studies carried out with flurazepam and other hypnotic agents and sleep induction agents, it can be concluded that flurazepam is clearly superior to other drugs for the treatment of insomnia and sleep disturbances, because it induces physiological sleep without altering phases and cycles. It is characterized by good tolerance and awakenings without hangover, and does not interact with other drugs or cause tachyphylaxis. Finally, and above all, flurazepam is effective in all dimensions of insomnia, whatever the cause, type or severity, and whoever the patient.

References

1. Bixler, E. O., Kales, A., Tan, T.-L. and Kales, J. D. (1973). The effect of hypnotic drugs on performance. *Curr. Ther. Res.*, **15,** 13
2. Bixler, E. O., Scharf, M. B., Leo, L. A. and Kales, A. (1975). Hypnotic drugs and performance: a review of theoretical and methodological considerations. In Kagan, F., Harwook, T., Rickels, K., *et al.* (eds.), *Hypnotics: Methods of Development and Evaluation*, pp. 175–196. (New York: Spectrum)
3. Bocci, U., Inga, E. F., Mariani, L., Pigani, G., Resele, L. F. and Senini, G. (1977). The residual effects of some sleep-inducing benzodiazepines and pentobarbital on some performance tests. *Drugs Exp. Clin. Res.*, **1,** 341
4. Bond, A. J. and Lader, M. H. (1973). The residual effects of flurazepam. *Psychopharmacologia (Berlin)* **32,** 223
5. Borland, R. G. and Nicholson, A. N. (1975). Comparison of the residual effects of two benzodiazepines (nitrazepam and flurazepam hydrochloride) and pentobarbitone sodium on human performance. *Br. J. Clin. Pharmacol.*, **2,** 9
6. Broadhurst, A. D. and Arenillas, L. (1975). A clinical and psychometric evaluation of flurazepam as a hypnotic in psychiatric patients. *Curr. Med. Res. Opin.*, **3,** 413
7. Church, M. V. and Johnson, L. C. (1979). Mood and performance of poor sleepers during repeated use of flurazepam. *Psychopharmacology*, **61,** 309
8. Data on file, Medical Department, Hoffmann–La Roche Inc. Nutley, N. J.
9. Dement, E. C., Carskadon, M. A., Mitler, M. M., Phillips, R. L. and Zarcone, V. P. (1978). Prolonged use of flurazepam. – A sleep laboratory study. *Behav. Med.*, 5, 10, 25
10. Frost, J. D., Carrie, J. R. G., Borda, R. P. and Kellaway, P. (1973). The effects of Dalmane (flurazepam hydrochloride) on human EEG characteristics. *Electroencephalogr. Clin. Neurophysiol.*, **34,** 171
11. Grunberger, J., Saletu, B., Linzmayer, L., Kalk, A. and Berner, P. (1978). Pharmacodynamic investigations with WE 941, a new triazolodiazepine, by means of psychometric analyses. *Curr. Ther. Res.*, **24,** 427
12. Hablitz, J. J. and Borda, R. P. (1973). The effects of Dalmane (flurazepam hydrochloride) on the contingent negative variation. *Electroencephalogr. Clin. Neurophysiol.*, (*Suppl.* 33), 317
13. Harper, C. R. and Kidera, G. S. (1972). Aviator performance and the use of hypnotic drugs. *Aerosp. Med.*, **43,** 197
14. Hindmarch, I. (1977). A repeated dose comparison of three benzodiazepine derivatives (nitrazepam, flurazepam and flunitrazepam) on subjective appraisals of sleep and measures of psychomotor performance the morning following night-time medication. *Acta Psychiat. Scand.*, **56,** 373
15. Kales, A., Bixler, E. O., Scharf, M. and Kales, J. D. (1976). Sleep laboratory studies of flurazepam. – A model for evaluating hypnotic drugs: *Clin. Pharmacol. Ther.*, **19,** 576
16. Linnoila, M. and Erwin, C. W. *J. Clin. Pharmacol.* (In Press)
17. Saario, I. and Linnoila, M. (1976). Effect of subacute treatment with hypnotics, alone or in combination with alcohol, on psychomotor skills related to driving. *Acta Pharmacol. Toxicol.*, **38,** 382
18. Salkind, M. R. and Silverstone, T. (1975). A clinical and psychometric evaluation of flurazepam. *Br. J. Clin. Pharmacol.*, **2,** 223

19. Schwartz, M. A. (1973). Pathways of metabolism of the benzodiazepines. In Garattini, S., Mussini, E. and Randall, L. O. (eds.). *The Benzodiazepines*, pp. 53–73. (New York: Raven Press)
20. Siegler, P. W., Winston, D. and Nodine, J. H. (1966). Common hypnotics and a psychomotor performance task. *Curr. Ther. Res.*, **8,** 215
21. Veldkamp, W., Straw, R. N., Metzler, C. M. and DeMissianos, H. V. (1974). Efficacy and residual effect evaluation of a new hypnotic triazolam. *J. Clin. Pharmacol.*, **14,** 102
22. Viukari, M., Linnoila, M. and Aalto, U. (1978). Efficacy and side effects of flurazepam, fosazepam and nitrazepam as sleeping aids in psychogeriatric patients. *Acta Psychiat. Scand.*, **57,** 27
23. Vogel, G. W., Barker, K., Gibbons, P. and Thurmond, A. (1976). A comparison of the effects of flurazepam 30mg and triazolam 0.5mg on the sleep of insomniacs. *Psychopharmacol.*, **47,** 81

Bibliography

Flurazepam

Anonymous (1972). A clinical evaluation of flurazepam. *J. Clin. Pharmacol.*, **12,** 217

Adachi, K. and Muranaka, A. (1973). Clinical experience of flurazepam in gynecology. *Basic Pharmacol. Ther.*, **1,** 238

Allen, C., Scharf, M. B. and Kales, A. (1971). The effect of flurazepam (Dalmane) administration and withdrawal on REM density. *Psychophysiol.*, **9,** 92

Andreani, G., Martelli, G. and Mascellani, A. (1973). Valutazione clinica dell'azione ipnotica del flurazepam nel trattamento dell'insonnia. *Neuropsichiatria* **29,** 251

Autera, C. (1974). Un preparato a base di flurazepam. Studio di tollerabilità e di efficacia. *Minerva Ginec.*, **26,** 657

Azuma, Y., Yasui, M., Asai, T., Kawasaki, G., Momotani, Y. and Tsuda, T. (1973). Therapeutic experience of flurazepam, a new sleep inducer. *Basic Pharmacol. Ther.*, **1,** 97

Azuma, Y., Yasui, M., Asai, T., Kawasaki, G., Momotani, Y. and Tsuda, T. (1973). Experimental therapy of flurazepam, new sleep inducer. *J. Pharmacol. Ther.*, **1,** 471

Babbini, M., Torrielli, M. V., Strumia, E., Gaiardi, M., Bartoletti, M. and De Marchi, F. (1975). Sedative-hypnotic properties of a new benzodiazepine in comparison with flurazepam. Pharmacological and clinical findings. *Arzneim. Forsch.*, **25,** 1294

Bussone, G., Boiardi, A. and Lazzaroni, M. (1975). Sperimentazione clinica controllata di una nuova benzodiazepina (Ro 5-6901) attiva sui disturbi del sonno. *Clin. Ter.*, **73,** 561

Cernibori, A. (1974). Osservazioni cliniche e rilievi elettroencefalografici di un nuovo preparato benzodiazepinico ad azione ipnotica – il flurazepam. *Gazz. Med. Ital.*, **133,** 513

Cirignotta, F., Rasi, F., Sacquegna, T., Forti, A. and Lugaresi, E. (1975). Effects on sleep of the drug Ro 5-6901 (flurazepam). A polygraphic study. In Levin, P.

and Koella, W. P. (eds.). *Sleep 1974, Proceedings of the 2nd European Congress on Sleep Research*, Apr. 1974, Rome, pp. 491–495. (Basel: Karger)

Dement, W. C., Phillips, R. L., Mitler, M., Billard, M. and Zarcone, V. (1975). Long-term effectiveness of flurazepam 30 mg h.s. on chronic insomniacs. In Chase, M. H., Stern, W. C. and Walter, P. L. (eds.). *2nd International Congress of Sleep Research* held in Edinburgh, June 30–July 4. *Sleep Research* Vol. 4, p. 94. (Los Angeles: Brain Inf. Serv.)

Di Perri, R. and Meduri, M. (1975). Polygraphic findings on the influence of flurazepam on nocturnal sleep. Preliminary report. In Levin, P. and Koella, W. P. (eds.). *Sleep 1974, Proceedings of the 2nd European Congress on Sleep Research*, Apr. 1974, Rome, pp. 496–499. (Basel: Karger)

Fujii, K., Takahashi, R. and Yamada, H. (1975). Clinical experience of flurazepam to insomnia in the field of psychiatry. *Basic Pharmacol. Ther.*, **3,** 1353

Gaillard, J. M. and Tissot, R. (1975). EEG sleep studies of insomniacs under flunitrazepam treatment. *Int. Pharmacopsychiatry*, **10,** 199

Gancedo, R., Wolfenson, M., Martín, N. E., Paz, J. M. and Hettinger, C. H. (1978). Evaluación clínica del flunitrazepam en el tratamiento del insomnio. *El Día Méd.*, **50,** 81, 84, 86, 88

Gerli, G. C. (1974). Contributo allo studio dell'effetto ipnoinduttivo di flurazepam in pazienti ricoverati in un reparto medico. *Gazz. Med. Ital.*, **133,** 100

Grattarola, F. R. and Marone, A. (1974). Studio clinico in doppio cieco del flurazepam. Presented at the *Symposium sulle Insonnie*, May 14, Bologna.

Greenblatt, D. J., Shader, R. I. and Koch-Weser, J. (1975). Flurazepam hydrochloride. *Clin. Pharmacol. Ther.*, **17,** 1

Hara, T. (1975). Comparison of drug effect between flurazepam (F) and nitrazepam (N) on occasional insomnia. *Jpn. J. Clin. Psychiatry*, **4,** 97

Hirai, S. and Morimatsu, M. (1973). Clinical study of flurazepam in senile insomniac subjects. *J. Pharmacol. Ther.*, **1,** 118

Ishihara, O., Fukushima, H., Nishitani, S., Fujimatsu, K. and Nakada, C. (1973). The effects of flurazepam as a sleep inducer in clinical electroencephalography. *Basic Pharmacol. Ther.*, **1,** 88

Kales, A., Kales, J. D., Bixler, E. O. and Scharf, M. B. (1975). Effectiveness of hypnotic drugs with prolonged use. – Flurazepam and pentobarbital. *Clin. Pharmacol. Ther.*, **18,** 356

Kales, A., Bixler, E. O., Leo, L. A., Starkey, K. and Kales, J. (1975). Flurazepam (Dalmane). – A composite of short and intermediate term studies. In Chase, M. H., Stern, W. C. and Walter, P. L. (eds.). *2nd Intern. Congress of Sleep Research* held in Edinburgh, June 30–July 4, *Sleep Research*, Vol. 4, p. 101. (Los Angeles: Brain Inf. Serv.)

Kales, A., Bixler, E. O., Scharf, M. B., Kales, J. D. and Franchini, E. (1976). Clinical implications of the sleep laboratory and pharmacological profile of flurazepam (Dalmane). In Chase, M. H., Mitler, M. M. and Walter, P. L. (eds.). *Sleep Research* Vol. 5, with Abstr. *16th Annu. Meet. Assoc. Psychophysiol. Study of Sleep*, Cincinnati, Jun. 1976, p. 68. (Los Angeles: Brain Inf. Serv.)

Kan, K., Katsube, S., Andoh, H., Yasuoka, K., Kikichi, S., Sugita, F., Endoh, H., and Kobayashi, H. (1974). Clinical experience of new sleep-inducer, flurazepam, in the field of internal medicine. *Basic Pharmacol. Ther.*, **2,** 1729

Kawai, S., Uemura, S., Hijiyama, T. and Sagara, M. (1973). Clinical experience of flurazepam in surgery. *Basic Pharmacol. Ther.*, **1,** 245

Keston, M. and Brocklehurst, J.C. (1974). Flurazepam and meprobamate. – A clinical trial. *Age Ageing*, **3**, 54
Kim, C.W. and Shin, Y.K. (1975). Clinical trial with flurazepam. *Yonsei J. Med. Sci.*, **8**, 88
Kimura, M., Ohno, Y., Suematsu, K., Kawano, T., Takayama, T., Matsumoto, K.I., Takeya, T., Mori, S., Moronaga, M., Inaba, Y., Itoh, H. (1974). Clinical pharmacological study on sleep inducer. Comparison of drug effect between nitrazepam and flurazepam of new sleeping drug by double-blind test. *Igaku No Ayumi*, **89**, 111
Kitamura, K. (1973). Investigation of hypnotic effect of flurazepam. *J. Pharmacol. Ther.*, **1**, 127
Kojo, J., Kawaike, K., Tsuru, N., Matsushita, K., Kuniyoshi, M., Kawano, K. *et al.* (1976). Clinical investigation of hypnotic effect of flurazepam by double-blind method. *Jpn. J. Clin. Exp. Med.*, **53**, 237
Kotorii, K., Oshima, M., Mizuki, Y., Matsuki, T., Ueda, S., Hasuzawa, H., Imasato, K. *et al.* (1977). Comparison of flurazepam free base with nitrazepam by the double-blind method of cross-over design. *Basic Pharmacol. Ther.*, **5**, 1059
Kubota, I., Fujiki, T., Sato, T., Tahira, H. and Harada, K. (1976). Clinical experience with flurazepam free base, a benzodiazepine derivative and new hypnotic. *J. New Remedies Clin.*, **25**, 413
Leickert, K.H. (1976). Estudio clínico experimental de un hipnótico eficaz – flurazepam. *Invest. Med. Intern.*, **3**, 18
Lynch, T. and Greene, V.T. (1975). Double-blind crossover trial of flurazepam (Dalmane) and nitrazepam (Mogadon) in the treatment of insomnia in psychiatric patients. *J. Ir. Coll. Physic. Surg.*, **4**, 87
Matta, B., Franco, A.E., Le Zotte, L.A., Rudzik, A.D. and Veldkamp, W. (1974). Comparison of triazolam, flurazepam and placebo as hypnotic agents in presurgical patients. *Curr. Ther. Res.*, **16**, 958
Mattioli, G. and Amati, A. (1974). Studio clinico del flurazepam. *Riv. Neurol.*, **44**, 1
Mattioli, G. and Amati, A. (1974). Studio clinico del flurazepam. *Riv. Neurol.*, **44**, 205
Melo de Paula, A.J. (1976). Ensaio duplo-cégo entre flurazepam (Dalmadorm) e metaqualona no tratamento de insónias médias e graves. *Folha Méd.*, **72**, 185
Meyer, J.A. and Kurland, K.Z. (1973). Controlled evaluation of flurazepam hydrochloride, a new nonbarbiturate hypnotic. *Milit. Med.*, **138**, 471
Muñoz Tarrero, J.L., Guillen Llera, F., Lavin Cobo, A. and Martín Alvarez, M. (1974). Ensayo del preparado Ro 5-6901 (Dormodor) en geriatría. *Panmin. Med.*, **4**, 258
Murata, T. (1973). Clinical investigation of flurazepam in neuropsychiatry. *J. Pharmacol. Ther.*, **1**, 67
Murata, T., Ito, K., Miura, K., Morita, A., Kato, T., Ishijima, G., Okajima, K., Onodera, I., Yamashita, I. and Jakahashi, S. (1973). Clinical experiment of flurazepam in the psychoneurotic field. *Basic Pharmacol. Ther.*, **1**, 441
Nagahama, T. (1976). Clinical experience of sedative hypnotics flurazepam. *Jpn. J. Clin. Exp. Med.*, **53**, 1483
Nagai, H., Nishikawa, Y., Nakayama, E. and Kuroki, K. (1973). Clinical study of flurazepam. *J. Pharmacol. Ther.*, **1**, 78

Nagao, K. (1974). Clinical experience of flurazepam in the patients with sleeping disturbance. *Basic Pharmacol. Ther.*, **2,** 1706

Nakanishi, M. (1976). Clinical study of flurazepam free base in out-patients of psychiatry. *Med. Cons. New Remedies*, **13,** 831

Nomura, J. and Hatotori, N. (1976). Clinical effect of flurazepam, a sleep-inducer, in comparison with nitrazepam by double-blind method. *Jpn. J. Clin. Psychiatry*, **5,** 917

Ogawa, H. and Nanba, M. (1973). Clinical evaluation of flurazepam hydrochloride (Ro 5-6901) as a preanesthetic medicament. *Basic Pharmacol. Ther.*, **1,** 180

Panaccio, L. and Tetreault, L. (1972). A comparative investigation of the hypnotic properties of flurazepam (30 mg) secobarbital (100 mg) and placebo in psychotic patients presenting four types of insomnia. In McClure, D. J. (ed.), *First Canadian Intern. Symposium on Sleep* April, pp. 51–64. (Montreal: Roche)

Pines, A., Rooney, J. F. and Arenillas, L. (1976). Flurazepam (Dalmane) in the treatment of insomnia in patients with respiratory disorders. *Practitioner*, **217,** 281

Reyes, B., Puertollano, A. S. and Puertollano, R. A. (1975). Flurazepam as a hypnotic in insomnia cases. – An open trial. *Philipp. J. Intern. Med.*, **13,** 131

Riemann, D. (1975). Ergebnisse mit Flurazepam. Prüfung eines neuen barbituratfreien Schlafmittels. *Aerztl. Prax.*, **27,** 1469, 1473

Rooke, K. C. (1976). The use of flurazepam (Dalmane) as a substitute for barbiturates and methaqualone (diphenhydramine) (Mandrax) in general practice. *J. Intern. Med. Res.*, **4,** 355

Rovati, V. and Galeone, M. (1972). Flurazepam. – Nuovo ipnotico di tipo fisiologico. Studio clinico. *Riv. Sper. Freniat.*, **96,** 1579

Sakamoto, F. and Yoshimura, M. (1973). Medical treatment for insomnia. – Special reference to the effects of flurazepam. *Med. Cons. New Remedies*, **10,** 841

Sakamoto, F., Koga, S., Mizuguchi, K. and Azuma, K. (1973). On effects of a hypnotic agent, flurazepam on sleeping disturbance. *Basic Pharmacol. Ther.*, **1,** 169

Sato, Y., Kato, N., Ukita, G. and Murase, T. (1973). Clinical experiment of a new sleep-inducer, flurazepam. *Basic Pharmacol. Ther.*, **1,** 478

Shoji, S. (1973). Clinical report of a hypnotic agent, flurazepam. *Basic Pharmacol. Ther.*, **1,** 157

Silverstone, T. and Salkind, M. (1974). A clinical and psychometric valuation of flurazepam (Dalmane). *J. Pharmacol.*, **5,** (Suppl. 2), Abstr. No. CV2, 92

Singer, K., Lo, C. W. and Tam, Y. K. (1978). Comparative evaluation of hypnotic efficacy of flunitrazepam in psychiatric in-patients. *Acta Psychiatr. Scand.*, **57,** 382

Suzuki, Y. and Okamoto, H. (1976). Clinical experience of flurazepam free base. *Clin. Rep.*, **10,** 541

Takeuchi, H., Kaji, S., Izumi, T., Tsukada, K., Hasegawa, S., Itoh, H., Nishida, M. *et al.* (1976). Effect of flurazepam monohydrochloride (Dalmate) on insomnia – specially on neuropathic insomnia. *J. New Remedies Clin.*, **25,** 1427

Taws, E. R., Brunning, J. and Arenillas, L. (1975). A clinical evaluation of flurazepam (Dalmane) as a hypnotic in psychiatric patients. *J. Intern. Med. Res.*, **3,** 417

Vogel, G. W., Hickman, J., Thurmond, A., Barrowclough, B. and Giesler, D.

(1972). The effect of Dalmane (flurazepam) on the sleep cycle of good and poor sleepers. *Psychophysiology*, **9**, 96

Yamada, S., Ohmi, S., Asao, Y. and Tanaka, Y. (1974). Clinical experience of new sleep-inducer, Ro 5-6901 (flurazepam). *Basic Pharmacol. Ther.*, **2**, 1721

Yamagata, M., Miura, K. and Mita, M. (1974). Clinical study of flurazepam, a sleep inducer. *J. New Remedies Clin.*, **23**, 397

Yokoyama, S., Kubo, S., Inai, K. and Watanabe, M. (1976). Clinical experiment of a new sleep inducer flurazepam free base in comparison with nitrazepam. *Med. Treat.*, **9**, 971

24

The Use of a Combination of β-Blockers and Benzodiazepines in Anxiety

I.G. Karniol, A.E. Piedrabuena, E.G. Matos, W.A. Vilela and M.J.F. Moreira

The use of benzodiazepines as anti-anxiety agents is one of the most important breakthroughs in modern psychopharmacology. Their efficacy and safety is undoubtedly greater than that of other anxiolytics available at the beginning of the fifties, but their widespread use has brought some problems.

In Brazil we are already facing what British investigators have termed the 'benzodiazepine bonanza'. There is a proliferation of fiercely competitive products among which carefully controlled studies demonstrate differences in overall clinical action which may be quite subtle and sometimes relevant only to selected groups of patients.

As of January 1978, eleven benzodiazepine agents were available for clinical use in Brazil. Those eleven drugs corresponded to 32 brand names. There were also available 38 pre-packed anti-distonic preparations in which benzodiazepines are combined with other drugs such as anticholinergics.

Although such combinations can be useful in some selected groups of patients, there is no scientific evidence that they are better than benzodiazepines alone in treating anxiety states. Probably economic and not medical factors are important here.[6]

It is very difficult to understand why there is a strict control on benzodiazepines when sold alone and not when combined with others in the antidistonic preparations. In the second case no medical prescription is required and the tendency to self-medication can increase.

This can lead to strict measures of control and difficulties in prescribing benzodiazepines in the future to patients who really need these drugs.

One of the recommendations in modern clinical psychopharmacology is not to use combinations of drugs when the same results can be obtained using only one of them, in which case one has to take into account the pharmacodynamic and pharmacokinetic properties of the drug and adjust accordingly the schedule of administration and dosage.

As an example, much evidence suggests that a single bedtime administration of a benzodiazepine in suitable dosage can serve a double function, initially inducing an hypnotic effect and, the following day, continuing to exert an anxiolytic influence.

According to our clinical experience, however, psychomotor and intellectual impairment occur when, as a result of such an approach, higher doses of benzodiazepines are necessary. The same side-effects appear when the total daily dose is divided into two or three administrations or when benzodiazepines of shorter halflife are used. Even with small doses of benzodiazepines some patients experience disabling side-effects.

To avoid such side-effects while relieving the symptoms of anxiety can be a difficult task. If we conclude that a benzodiazepine alone will not suffice, then β-blockers may be a rational adjunct.

It is known that some of the most disabling manifestations of anxiety are peripheral symptoms mediated by β-adrenergic sympathetic activity. Among these symptoms, tachycardia, palpitations, hyperventilation and tremulousness are frequently found. Such symptoms can be self-reinforcing, making the patient more anxious. β-Blockers, owing to their ability to block such manifestations, were prominent. However, studies to date have not definitively confirmed the superiority of this class of drug over benzodiazepines, or sometimes even over placebo[1,3,7,10].

Let us localize in Lader's model[8] of anxiety the probable site of action of benzodiazepines and β-blockers (Figure 24.1). In this formulation, external stimuli impinge on the organism. They can be physical, social or psychosocial. Internal stimuli are also important and consist of thoughts, needs, aspirations, and so on (so-called 'drives'). External and internal stimuli are appraised for possible threats to the organism or individual: genetic endowment and past experience, nature and nurture, which interact to modify the internal stimuli.

The conscious or unconscious appraisal of threat is followed by two processes. First, the activity of certain parts of the central nervous system increases, constituting arousal. Second, an affect is experienced: the benzodiazepines act at this site, at 'A' in Figure 24.1. The CNS arousal is accompanied by widespread physiological changes, which are relayed back to the CNS by proprioceptive pathways but can also be consciously perceived by the subject. These may reinforce the emotion by acting as internal stimuli, thereby constituting a positive feedback loop. 'B' is the site of action of the β-blockers. In the combination of β-blockers and benzodiazepines we thought that lower doses of the latter could be used.

We are now going to present the results of an investigation in which the combination of 10 mg diazepam or its corresponding placebo with a slow-release 80 mg oxprenolol dose or placebo were administered in a single bedtime dose to neurotic anxious outpatients in a crossover double-blind design in which each patient in a random order was to receive all the treatments.

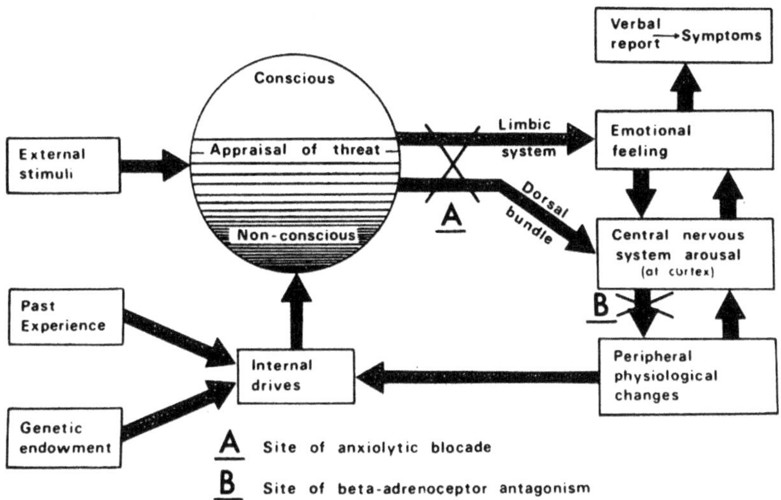

Figure 24.1 A model of anxiety (reprinted from Lipton, M. A., DiMascio, A. and Killam, K. F. (eds), *Psychopharmacology: A Generation of Progress* (New York: Raven Press))

The patients chosen had experienced continuous symptoms for at least two months. Patients with cardiac disease and asthma were excluded and there was a one-week washout period before starting the treatments. A period of two weeks' treatment with each of the four possible combinations of drugs was thought to be enough to decrease the residual effects of the drugs.

Of the eighteen patients who started the trial, to date only ten have received all the treatments and have been evaluated. Although the Latin Square experimental design planned to assess the effects of the order of treatments has not been completed, a non-parametric analysis using the Kruskal–Wallis test indicates that this order probably has not had any influence on the results[5, 9].

The degree of anxiety was rated in each patient before the trial and after each treatment according to a modified Hamilton Rating Scale [2, 4, 11, 12] in which 100 mm linear scores were used instead of categorical ones. The severity of illness was rated on the same occasions using the first item of the Clinical Global Impression (CGI). In that scale, seven possibilities are allowed from 0 (not assessed), 1 (normal, not at all ill) to 7 (among the most extremely ill patients). There was a high and statistically significant correlation between the CGI ratings and the Hamilton Scale ratings.

There was a greater tendency toward improvement when both drugs were used together in combination than when each drug was combined with the placebo of the other, at least when the CGI scale was considered.

One point that has to be considered is that β-blockers have the ability to reduce hepatic blood flow and, as a consequence, they could impair the hepatic clearance of drugs. In that case, the apparently good results obtained with the combination could be attributed to an increase in the plasma levels of active benzodiazepines. The possible importance of such a mechanism will have to be studied before claiming any advantages for the use of a combination of β-blockers and benzodiazepines.

References

1. Burrows, G. D., Davies, B., Fail, L., Poynton, C. and Stevenson, H. (1976). A placebo controlled trial of diazepam and oxprenolol for anxiety. *Psychopharmacology*, **50**, 177
2. ECDEU (1976). *Assessment Manual for Psychopharmacology*. Guy, W. (ed.) (US Department of Health, Education, and Welfare)
3. Greenblatt, D. J. and Shader, R. I. (1978). Pharmacotherapy of anxiety with benzodiazepines and beta-adrenergic blockers. In Lipton, M. A., DiMascio, A. and Killam, K. F. (eds.) *Psychopharmacology: a Generation of Progress*, pp. 1381–1390. (New York: Raven Press)
4. Hamilton, M. (1959). The assessment of anxiety states by rating. *Br. J. Med. Psychol.*, **32**, 50
5. Hoel, P. G. (1968). *Estadística Elementar*. (Rio de Janeiro: Fundo de Cultura)
6. Hollister, L.E. (1978). Antianxiety drugs. In Hollister, L. E. (ed.) *Clinical Pharmacology of Psychotherapeutic Drugs*, pp. 12–49. (New York: Churchill Livingstone)
7. Johnson, G., Singh, B. and Leeman, M. (1976). Controlled evaluation of the adrenoceptor blocking drug oxprenolol in anxiety. *Med. J. Aust.*, **1**, 908
8. Lader, M. (1978). Current psychophysiological theories of anxiety. In Lipton, M. A., DiMascio, A. and Killam, K. F. (eds.). *Psychopharmacology: a Generation of Progress*, pp. 1375–1380. (New York: Raven Press)
9. Lehman, E. L. (1974). *Nonparametrics Methods Based on Ranks*. (New York: McGraw Hill)
10. Moreira, M. J. C., Karniol, I. G. and Knobel, M. (1979). Some considerations on the use of anxiolytics in our community. *Rev. Assoc. Bras. Psiq.*, **1**, 10
11. Tyrer, P. J. and Lader, M. H. (1974). Response to propranolol and diazepam in somatic and psychic anxiety. *Br. Med. J.*, **1**, 14
12. Williams, F. J. (1949) Experimental design balanced for the estimation of residual effects of treatments. *Aust. J. Sci. Res. Series B*, **2**, 149

Bibliography

Benzodiazepines and β-blockers

Marmo, E., Rossi, F., Lampa, E., Pedone, P., Rosatti, F. and del Vecchio, F. (1977). Analisi sperimentale delle interazioni tra un beta-adrenolitico, la D (−) inpea, e un tranquillante minore, il diazepam. *Clin. Ter.*, **82**, 425

Sellers, E. M. (1976). Chlordiazepoxide and popranolol in the treatment of alcoholic withdrawal. Presented at *The Canadian Society for Clinical Investigation Meeting*, January 20, Quebec City.

Sellers, E. M., Zilm, D.H. and Degani, N. C. (1977). Comparative efficacy of propranolol and chlordiazepoxide in alcohol withdrawal. *J. Stud. Alc.*, **38**, 2096

Sellers, E. M., Zilm, D. H., MacLeod, S. M., Degani, H. and Giles, H. G. (1975). Chlordiazepoxide and propranolol treatment of alcoholic withdrawal. *Clin. Res.*, **23**, 610A

Winters, W. D. and Kott, K. S. (1976). Neuropharmacological interaction between ketamine, and physostigmine, diazepam or propranolol. *Proc. West. Pharmacol.*, **19**, 232

Ziegler, A. (1971). Beitrag zur Behandlung der Hyperthyreose mit Propranolol und Diazepam. *Z. Ges. Inn. Med. Grenzgeb.*, **26**, 622

25

Clinical Evaluation of the Sulpiride–Bromazepam Combination, Ro 10-7122, for Patients with a Depressive–Anxious Syndrome

M. S. Moreira and F. J. Braga de Almeida

Introduction

It is common knowledge that the clinical expression of diseases changes according to the context in which they occur, as was demonstrated by Alves Garcia in two of his excellent studies.

According to Alves Garcia, 'Man is the only being that has to adapt itself to the geographical, historical and cultural environment in which it lives, both in health and in sickness. One should not expect to see at the end of the 20th century the neuroses and psychoses of the demonological age, nor even the cases described by the last century's psychiatrists. Today, the Salpêtrière hysteria is merely something that belongs to the files of historical pathology.'

As far as manic-depressive psychosis is concerned, one does not see so often nowadays the crises of excitation and melancholia that were major symptoms in the past. More benign and shorter-lived forms are more usual and are mainly the result of rapid changes in social and cultural structures. The same is true of schizophrenia. The deliria of the past, with their greater mystical and religious cast, have been today replaced by space and astronautical deliria; for instance, hypochondriac delirium is often accompanied by coenaesthesic hallucinations.

This kind of clinical picture naturally makes these patients seek medical and surgical outpatients' clinics for vague and imprecise complaints which puzzle doctors who are not specialized in mental disease care. After exhaustive laboratory examinations, when nothing has been found in support of the patients' complaints, they are labelled 'nervous patients' and a tranquillizer is usually prescribed.

This does not really solve the problem, because their aetiopathogenic basis lies elsewhere, being not related to disorders of the limbic system, but rather to deeper, diencephalic changes.

The major usefulness of the bromazepam–sulpiride combination, in our opinion, is the treatment of such syndromes. Bromazepam, because of its well-known anxiety-relieving characteristics, and the neuroleptic–antidepressant sulpiride, with its polyvalent effect, in combination constitute a powerful delirolytic and hallucinolytic medication acting mainly on the hypothalamus. The combination also has an effective thymoanaleptic action without central sedative effect or diminished attentiveness.

Due to these special features, therefore, the bromazepam–sulpiride combination seems to be a useful product for the general practitioner for the treatment of dysthymic, chronically complaining and stressed patients, particularly when repeated laboratory tests show nothing to justify the symptoms of which they complain.

For the reasons described above, we think this is the therapeutic combination of choice for use in clinical practice. Psychiatrists will find it helpful in cases of moderately severe depressive–anxious syndromes.

Materials and methods

A total of 43 patients (14 males and 29 females with ages ranging from 10 to 68 years) participated in an open study to examine the anxiety-relieving and antidepressant effects of the bromazepam–sulpiride combination, at the Psychiatric Clinic of the Gaffrée-e-Guinle Hospital of the School of Medicine and Surgery of Rio de Janeiro (Table 25.1).

Table 25.1 Age (y) distribution of patients

Age group	*Number of cases*
10–19	4
20–29	5
30–39	12
40–49	10
50–59	7
over 60	5
TOTAL	43

Our aim was to observe the clinical response of the following symptoms: anxiety, tension, depressive mood, lack of initiative, insomnia, delirium, hallucinations, restlessness, nervousness, phobias, irritability, aggressiveness, impotence, obsessive rituals, rumination, tiredness, memory disturbances, tachycardia, dizziness.

As regards treatment, 40 were outpatients and 3 were hospitalized. Case distribution is shown in Table 25.2. Lexpiride (1 mg bromazepam + 25 mg sulpiride; Ro 10-7122) was administered in a dosage of 3 capsules daily in nearly all cases. In only one case did we use five capsules daily, and six capsules daily were used in three other cases (see Table 25.3).

Table 25.2 Clinical status of patients

Diagnosis	*Number of cases*
Neurosis (several clinical forms)	32
Manic–depressive psychosis	4
Paraphrenia	1
Reactive depression	4
Neurasthenic syndrome	1
Schizophrenic psychosis	1
TOTAL	43

The concomitant use of other psychotropic drugs was avoided as far as possible, and occurred only in a few patients in whom another product was already being used for treatment of other symptoms, or whenever, during treatment, it became absolutely necessary to prescribe a new drug to treat symptoms other than those being treated with the trial product. The final results, therefore, were not influenced by the concomitant medication. The average duration of treatment was 42 days.

Evaluation was carried out on a weekly basis by filling out a standard record sheet of signs and symptoms supplied by the Medical Department of the Company Produtos Roche Químicos e Farmaceuticos S.A.

The therapeutic efficacy was assessed using two rating scales, one for psychic and another for somatic symptoms.

Results

Besides the psychiatric symptomatology for which Ro 10-7122 was prescribed, epilepsy was also present in two patients. The clinical condition of one of these patients worsened in spite of concomitant diphenyl-hydantoin use. Ro 10-7122 was therefore stopped. In the other patient Ro 10-7122 was well tolerated and the therapeutical outcome excellent. In this case, clonazepam was used concomitantly.

In the four cases diagnosed as manic–depressive psychosis, there were one excellent, one good and one moderate result. In the remaining case, the psychiatric condition worsened.

In four cases, medication had to be suspended. In three cases, this was due to deterioration of the patient's condition, which was independent of the trial conditions. In the fourth case, suspension was due to the strong side-effects observed. Two further patients refused to continue with the treatment for irrelevant reasons and another gave it up soon after having begun.

The initial dose was individually adapted to each case according to severity of the symptoms (Table 25.3).

Table 25.3 Initial dose

Capsules per day	*Number of cases*
3	39
5	1
6	3
TOTAL	43

Table 25.4 Maintenance dose

Capsules per day	*Number of cases*
2	4
3	15
4	3
5	1
6	7
9	1
TOTAL	31

Table 25.5 Therapeutic response to Lexpiride (Ro 10-7122)

	Evaluation	
Result	*By patient*	*By doctor*
Excellent	24	23
Good	6	8
Average	1	1
No change	7	7
Worse	4	2
No evaluation	1	2
TOTAL	43	43

Table 25.4 presents the maintenance dosage for patients who completed 4 weeks of treatment.

There was slight difference in physician's and patients' efficacy assessment (excellent and good results: according to physician 72%, according to patients 70%) (Table 25.5).

Table 25.6 Tolerance

	Evaluation	
Tolerance	*By patient*	*By doctor*
Good	37	37
Average	1	1
Bad	1	1
No evaluation	4	4
TOTAL	43	43

Tolerance was good in 86% of the cases, as can be seen from Table 25.6. The side-effects were slight and occurred only in seven cases (16%). The effects were such as epigastralgia, sleepiness, anorexia, dysuria, dizziness and dryness of the mouth, as shown in Table 25.7.

Table 25.7 Side-effects

Side-effects	*Number of cases*
Epigastralgia	2
Sleepiness	1
Anorexia	1
Dysuria	1
Dizziness	1
Dryness of mouth	1
TOTAL	7

Discussion and conclusion

A fixed combination of bromazepam (1 mg) with sulpiride (25 mg), Ro 10-7122, is effective in most cases of mild depressive–anxiety syndromes whatever their aetiology (72% of results from excellent to good).

Accelerated evolution of the social and cultural environment modified the clinical expression of mental diseases. The polyvalent action of this combination makes it useful for the management of this changing symptomatology. Mild, incomplete manic–depressive or schizophrenic syndromes could therefore benefit from therapy with Ro 10-7122.

Summary

Lexpiride (Ro 10-7122), a combination of 1 mg bromazepam with 25 mg sulpiride, was investigated in a group of 43 patients whose ages ranged from 10 to 68. The medication was administered for an average period of 42 days. The patients were controlled on a weekly basis by means of physical examinations and by filling out a standard record form for signs and symptoms, developed by the Medical Department of the Roche Laboratory. The results were considered as excellent or good in 72% of the cases.

The preparation was generally well tolerated. Seven patients complained of slight unwanted effects, as follows: heartburn (2 patients), sleepiness, anorexia, dysuria, dizziness and dryness of the mouth (one patient for each symptom).

We believe that this combination is the best and most convenient preparation for the treatment of the vague and imprecise complaints of mildly depressed and anxious patients.

Bibliography

Lexpiride

Alpanez, E. O., Bernat, A. C., Campos, A. L., Eucinas, J. R., Giner, R. C., Girona, J. J., Herrero, F. J. *et al.* (1976). Ensaio multicentrico com o Ro 10-7122. *Folha Méd.*, **73,** 409

Alpanez, E. O., Bernat, A. C., Campos, A. L., Girona, J. J., Eucinas, J. R., Giner, R. C., Herrero, F. J. *et al.* (1976). Emprego do Ro 10-7122 em pacientes de medicina psicossomatica. Estudo multicentrico. *Folha Méd.*, **73,** 515

Andrade Gomide, C. H. (1978). Avaliação clínica F/D-1-25 (sulpiride-bromazepam) em cardiologia em pacientes portadores de ansiedade e depressão. *Folha Méd.*, **77,** 131

Couderc, L., Martin, M., Dufour, H. and Poisson, D. (1970). Le sulpiride dans la thérapeutique et le pronostic des psychoses. *Gaz. Méd. Fr.*, **77,** 3137

Cumin, R. (1976). Ação do bromazepam, do sulpiride e da combinação bromazepam/sulpiride (1-25) em ratos, avaliada pelo 'flash-light–waterlicking conflict test'. *Folha Méd.*, **73,** 277

de Barros, D. S., Machado, N. S., de Barros, C. C. and Warszawski, E. (1977). Ensaio com a associação bromazepam–sulpiride (Ro 10-7122) no tratamento de distúrbios de conduta e de personalidade em crianças e adolescentes. *Folha Méd.*, **74,** 611

Ganança, M., Albernaz, P. L. and Lanzellotti, W. P. (1977). Atividade antivertiginosa da associação bromazepam e sulpride. *Rev. Bras. Clin. Ter.*, **6,** 487

Kawano, M., Nozoe, S. I., Yamanaka, T., Nagata, Y., Takayama, I., Kawa, A., Kanehisa, T., Yoshimuta, T., Okubo, N. and Sonoda, J. I. (1975). Study on the effectiveness of sulpride for neurosis and psychosomatic diseases by the double-blind method. *Jpn. J. Clin. Exp. Med.*, **52,** 636

Lastra, L., Alsasua, A. and De Andres, F. (1976). Avaliação farmacólogica do Ro 10-7122. Pharmacological appraisal of Ro 10-7122. *Folha Méd.*, **73,** 273

Lins, F. E., Zalmon, I. and Teixeira, I. V. (1978). Estudo clínico do novo produto F/D-1-25 sulpan (associação sulpiride–bromazepam) no tratamento dos sintomas psicossomáticos do climaterio. *J. Bras. Ginecologia*, **85**, 37

Muzio, M., Giberti, F., Cichetti, V. and Gabrielli, F. (1975). Sulpiride versus diazépam et sulpiride plus diazépam dans le traitement en ambulatoire des névroses. *Psychol. Méd.*, **7**, 1645

Ordonez Alpanez, E., Luguero Campos, F. and Martinez Lopes, F. (1976). Ensaio sobre o emprego do Ro 10-7122 (Lexpiride) em gastrenterologia. *Folha Méd.*, **73**, 397

Penteado, J. F., Barbosa de Medeiros, R., Mauro de Magalhães, J. and Bonio, M. F. (1977). Avaliação clínica do F/D-1-25 sulpan (sulpiride–bromazepam) em gastrenterologia em pacientes portadores de ansiedade e depressão. *Folha Méd.*, **75**, 727

Santos Moreira, M. and Braga de Almeida, F. J. (1978). Avaliação clínica da associação sulpride–bromazepam, Ro 10-7122, em pacientes com sindrome depressivo-ansiosa. *Folha Méd.*, **76**, 45

Toru, M., Moriya, H., Yamamoto, K., Shimazono, Y., Ishiguro, T., Sugano, K. *et al.* (1976). A double-blind comparison of sulpiride with chlordiazepoxide in neurosis. *Fol. Psychiat. Neurol. Jpn.*, **30**, 153

Workshop A:

Benzodiazepines Today and Tomorrow, from a Pharmacological Point of View

Coordinated by **W.E. Haefely** (Switzerland) and **V. Gentil Filho** (Brazil)

Participants: **R. Amrein** (Switzerland), **L.H. Sternbach** (USA) **W.G. Crouthamel** (USA) and **L.M. Lessa** (Brazil)

The workshop 'Benzodiazepines today and tomorrow from a pharmacological point of view' consisted of very lively discussions on various aspects which could be grossly divided into problems related to molecular, synaptic and behavioural pharmacology as well as to the pharmacokinetics and metabolism of benzodiazepines.

Molecular pharmacology

The basis of the pharmacological effects of benzodiazepines is the existence in the central nervous system of benzodiazepine receptors; these are protein molecules with a very high affinity for benzodiazepine derivatives and a high specificity for this chemical class. Benzodiazepine receptors are characterized by a relative affinity for derivatives which corresponds to their clinical potency and are only present in the central nervous system;

some peripheral tissues contain benzodiazepine binding sites, however, with a low affinity and a specificity unrelated to central activity. The benzodiazepine receptor is a relatively late acquisition in phylogenetic development and does not occur in animal species with a very primitive nervous system, e.g. in crustaceans, although their nervous system contains most or all of the neurotransmitters which are also present in the mammalian brain. The question of whether the benzodiazepine receptors represent a homogeneous group of identical molecules or whether several populations of benzodiazepine receptors exist is not yet clear. Preliminary results seem to indicate the existence of at least two populations of benzodiazepine receptors which differ slightly in their affinity for drugs. Whether different receptors are responsible for the various effects of the benzodiazepines is still an open question.

In analogy to the situation with opiate receptors, many investigators are searching for brain constituents that could act as endogenous ligands of the benzodiazepine receptors. Theoretically, an endogenous ligand could physiologically stimulate the receptor and thereby prevent overstimulation of the central nervous system (acting as an 'endogenous anti-anxiety compound') or it could be lacking under pathological conditions and then be replaced by therapy with benzodiazepines. Alternatively, an endogenous ligand could occur only under pathological conditions and benzodiazepines could act as antagonists of such a hypothetical 'anxiogenic substance'. It is also possible that there does not exist any physiological or pathological endogenous ligand with either of these two activities.

Brain constituents have been found which displace benzodiazepines from their receptors. In the Roche laboratories three low molecular weight compounds were found: the two purine derivatives, inosine and hypoxanthine, as well as nicotinamide. The affinity of these compounds for the benzodiazepine receptors is extremely low in comparison to the benzodiazepines. Of the three compounds, nicotinamide possesses some pharmacological properties in common with benzodiazepines, although very high doses are required. Also high molecular weight substances in the brain as well as indole derivatives from the urine have been reported to interfere with the binding of benzodiazepines to their receptors. The significance of these findings is at present completely unknown.

Knowing that benzodiazepines interact specifically with GABAergic transmission and that specific molecules exist in the central nervous system to which benzodiazepines have to bind to in order to produce their effects, raises the question of how benzodiazepine receptors are coupled to GABAergic synapses.

Although it has recently been possible in the Roche laboratories to locate the benzodiazepine receptor at GABAergic synapses with the aid of photo-affinity-labelling and EM autoradiography, we do not yet know whether the benzodiazepine receptor is located presynaptically, i.e. on the GABA neurons, or postsynaptically near the GABA receptor on the subsynaptic membrane. Some experimental evidence has been presented for the location of benzodiazepine receptors on the GABAergic neuron itself. Theoretically, GABAergic interneurons might become hyperexcitable under the effect of benzodiazepines. This means that they fire a greater number of action potentials in response to one input to the cells and, therefore, that more GABA is released at the GABAergic endings. There is also some evidence that benzodiazepines could act at the nerve terminals of GABAergic neurons and may improve excitation–secretion coupling, thus increasing the amount of GABA which is released at the ending in response to an action potential.

Most work so far, however, has been done on postsynaptic location of the benzodiazepine receptors and it is Costa's group at the NIH which claims the existence of a supra-molecular complex consisting of the GABA-receptor, a GABA-modulating protein ('gabamodulin'), the benzodiazepine receptor and the chloride channel. The work of this group of investigators suggest that benzodiazepines interact with an endogenous protein which physiologically reduces the affinity of the GABA-receptor to GABA, thereby increasing the effectiveness of GABA. This work, albeit highly interesting and able to explain most of the electrophysiological findings, has not yet been reproduced in other laboratories.

Synaptic pharmacology

How can one benzodiazepine receptor, assuming that there is only one population, explain the different effects of the benzodiazepines? In other words, how is it possible that benzodiazepines differ in their pharmacological profile, although they seem to interact at an identical receptor molecule? An answer to this question cannot be given at the moment. It is possible that different affinities of the various receptors and different pharmacokinetic conditions, such as distribution in the central nervous system, may explain the different pharmacological activities.

It is obvious also to raise the question of whether GABA-mimetics could replace benzodiazepines. This question has been studied intensively in the past few years mainly with the help of muscimol, a GABA-mimetic compound which enters the brain and is a potent stimulant of GABA-receptors. The results obtained seem to indicate that GABA-mimetics are not a useful approach to therapy. This is probably due to the fact that GABA-receptors are present on all neurons and that the stimulation of these receptors throughout the central nervous system does not result in a specific effect. The difference between the GABA-mimetic compounds and the benzodiazepines seems to be that the benzodiazepines enhance GABA-receptor activity only at those sites where GABAergic neurons are present and active.

Behavioural pharmacology

A question raised at the workshop was whether benzodiazepines induced an amnesic effect and how this could be explained. It seems that all benzodiazepines, like many other central depressant agents, are able in principle to produce anterograde amnesia. This anterograde amnesia depends on the dose and, probably more important, on the rapidity with which the drug reaches the central nervous system. This anterograde amnesia is a welcome effect of benzodiazepines, e.g. in anaesthesiology, but is, of course, an unwanted effect in other indications.

Clinical studies indicate that the amnesic effect does not occur with the usual therapeutic doses for the treatment of anxiety or insomnia. Surprisingly, even an improvement of memory has been found with benzodiazepines in a clinical study; it was discussed whether this improvement of memory could be related to the enhancing effect of benzodiazepines on presynaptic inhibition, which would lead to a more effective filtering of the input to the brain, e.g. a better separation between incoming relevant and irrelevant information.

Another problem which was discussed was whether it is possible to predict addiction liability of a drug from animal experiments. This question is of great importance since most health authorities are requesting animal experiments on addiction liability. It is highly questionable whether animal experiments are able to predict the liability of a compound to induce psychic dependence in man. The way these experiments are usually carried out is to make animals physically dependent on a drug, which is, of course, quite different from the question of whether a drug would have a primary reinforcing effect in man. There is no doubt that some physical dependence can be produced with benzodiazepines in animals when very high doses are given over a long period of time. Rare cases of physical dependence in man are reported in the literature.

Another question which was raised was whether the animal tests used today in the screening of new compounds were able to detect new interesting psychotropic activities, or, in other words, whether animal tests were relevant in predicting drug activity in human disease. It was explained that in fact all animal tests in use today were devised after the discovery of new groups of psychotropic agents and that the only possibility for the experimental pharmacologists to find useful compounds with new profiles of activity was to consider all behavioural, neurochemical and electrophysiological effects produced in animals.

Pharmacokinetics and metabolism

We have to realize that we do not know at present the relationships between the concentration of psychotropic drugs, and, hence, also of benzodiazepines, in the plasma and the number of specific receptors occupied in the central nervous system. This problem can be solved in the near future in animal experiments using the receptor binding assay. It is important to keep in mind that the kinetics of a drug in the blood gives useful information on the overall fate of a drug in the body but that the brain is a very special inhomogeneous organ, in which pharmacologically inert structures for the same drug molecules are present together with specific receptors. The situation is further complicated by the fact that receptor occupancy by a drug at a given moment may not be the only decisive factor for a pharmacological activity because the brain is certainly able to adapt to an altered activity of its neurons.

A question which was raised many times is whether it would be possible to devise new molecules with an anti-anxiety effect but without sedative side-effects. Most participants agreed on the fact that anxiety could not be regarded simply as an excessive arousal state. It was mentioned that observations in the clinic showed that drug-induced sedation could occur without reduction of anxiety and therefore, that, the anti-anxiety effect was in principle separable from a sedative effect. However, in the group of benzodiazepines and in all drugs known at present a complete separation has not been achieved.

It is clear that treatment of insomnia, epilepsy and anxiety requires different kinetic properties of a benzodiazepine. Although most of the benzodiazepines produce essentially the same pharmacological effects, it is not possible to have one drug which would be equally useful for all indications. The particular value of a given benzodiazepine in a given clinical situation can only be assessed in clinical trials relying on pharmacokinetic properties and pharmacological profiles because the animal experiment is not discriminative enough to predict such fine differences in clinical use. The continuous cooperation of clinical and experimental pharmacologists is the prerequisite for the development of optimal drugs.

Workshop B:

Benzodiazepines Today and in the Future

Coordinated by **R.G.Priest** (Great Britain) and **J. Paprocki** (Brazil)

Participants: **W. Pöldinger** (Switzerland), **J.R. Bueno** (Brazil) and **D. Kelly** (Great Britain)

The short-term efficacy of benzodiazepines has clearly been demonstrated but we still know very little about the longterm effects. In addition to this it would be desirable to know more about the sub-groups of patients who respond to different drugs. We also considered the links between the relief of anxiety and the production of drowsiness and Dr Paprocki emphasized that ideally we should like to be closer to the position that we are in when treating schizophrenic patients with neuroleptics in an attempt to normalize the patients' psychological state. We would like to do the same with the benzodiazepines in treating emotional reactions. Even so, in spite of these opening statements, Dr Paprocki endorsed the conclusion of the symposium. In addition to developing new drugs we do need a better understanding of the drugs we have today at our disposal.

Dr Pöldinger pointed out an interesting paradox. From animals we are familiar with the anti-aggressive effects of benzodiazepines. And yet, what happens today in clinical practice? We treat aggressive patients with neuroleptic drugs. Maybe we can in the future produce a new benzodiazepine that is thoroughly anti-aggressive in humans.

Dr Pöldinger also considered antidepressant effects. To establish that a drug is antidepressant we have to establish that it does elevate the mood. Does this really happen at present with benzodiazepines or is what we are seeing an indirect effect produced by the relief of anxiety?

Dr Kelly pointed out another unsolved problem, that of panic attacks. Panic attacks are very common in psychiatric outpatients. But, although benzodiazepines are very useful for sustained anxiety, they are less useful for blocking these panic attacks. These can be blocked with antidepressants but it would be an advantage if we could find some way of using anti-anxiety drugs to block panic attacks, because if we can do that we can enable our patients to overcome the feared situation that at present produces the panic.

Reverting to the topic of producing relief of anxiety without producing drowsiness, Dr Kelly pointed out that this is possible at present with a different group of drugs, the β-blockers. These block anxiety without producing drowsiness. However, they are good only for somatic features of anxiety, such as palpitations and possibly tremor. What we need now is a drug which relieves the psychic anxiety without producing drowsiness.

Dr Bueno addressed himself to the social issues that we meet with the use of benzodiazepines and to the need to try to avoid the problem of dependence on anti-anxiety drugs. It may be that we can do this by developing longer-acting benzodiazepines: possibly, by developing drugs which are free from a hangover effect. However Dr Bueno thought that we should not ignore the very pressing need for fundamental research into the neurophysiology of anxiety so that we might come up with new ideas from a logical approach.

Dr Paprocki addressed further questions to the members of the panel and he asked Dr Pöldinger: to what extent does biochemical individuality affect the response to benzodiazepines? Dr Pöldinger thought it is possible that there are biochemical differences in human beings that affect their response, and he drew the analogy with depression. We know that we have different types of depression, endogenous depression, reactive depression and so forth, where there seems to be a biochemical difference between them. He thought that it would be worth looking for differences within the different clinical groups of anxiety states, to investigate the possibility of a different biochemical basis.

Dr Kelly was asked for how long should benzodiazepines be administered. Again there was an analogy with antidepressant drugs where even after six months on the drug it can be demonstrated that the placebos are poorer than the active compound in preventing relapse. Would the same be true for benzodiazepines? We know there are many cases in which it does not seem to be important for the patient to receive benzodiazepines regularly.

Dr Kelly was quite sure that there were many situations where it was important. The whole adaptation to life of some patients had been altered by the administration of benzodiazepines where repeated attempts to take the patient off benzodiazepines led to relapse and where it seemed likely that the patient would need to continue with drugs for many years, if not indefinitely.

Professor Bueno asked Dr Pöldinger whether it was legitimate to give benzodiazepines together with other psychotropic drugs. Dr Pöldinger thought that this was proper and that certainly combination with neuroleptic drugs and with antidepressants was in order. He went on to emphasize that it is not just a simultaneous administration of drugs that is important. Sometimes it is important they should be in the same tablet or in the same capsule. For instance, patients being treated to depression with a combination tablet of benzodiazepine and tricyclic antidepressant would take the tablet because they felt in the first place it helped them, they got immediate subjective relief, and they were favourably disposed towards the medication. If you separated the two, the patient may say to himself, 'well, in the second tablet I find I get unpleasant side-effects, I get lots of dry mouth and constipation', and the patient may in fact stop the antidepressant and may then relapse into a suicidal state of depression and this could be very dangerous. Thus there was a definite place for combined preparations under these circumstances.

I would like to end by thanking Dr Paprocki, who did so much to make this workshop successful with his careful preparation and his skilled coordination.

Workshop C:

Psychopharmacotherapy with Benzodiazepines

Coordinated by **W. Pöldinger** (Switzerland) and **Á. Rubim de Pinho** (Brazil)

Participants: **J.A. Costa e Silva** (Brazil), **T.R. Browne** (USA) and **R.G. Priest** (Great Britain)

In Workshop C we were discussing three topics. The discussion started with the problem of correlating psychopharmacotherapy with psychotherapy. It was pointed out that there has been a change in opinion. In former times, the dominating opinion was that administration of drugs has an antagonistic effect to psychotherapy. For example, it was mentioned that in former times some therapists believed that by reducing the anxiety of a patient the latter will be less willing to go to psychotherapy. Now this opinion has changed. In more recent times we can see an increasing instance of combining psychopharmacotherapy with psychotherapy. For instance, the reduction of anxiety, especially of severe anxiety, is necessary to be able to speak with the patient and to discuss his problems. There may be also an influence on this new aspect in the opinion about neurosis and how a neurosis can be treated. In former days, it was pointed out that pharmacotherapy, especially with benzodiazepines, is a so-called symptomatic therapy while psychotherapy is a real basic therapy. Unfortunately, there are only a few follow-up studies in neurosis but those studies show the difficulty of curing a neurosis by psychotherapy. It seems to be that we need another concept of neurosis to be able to see during a neurotic development phases of decompensation and phases of compensation. This is because we know that many neurotic persons can live for a longer time without severe problems and then a phase of decompensation can start again.

In some neurotic problems psychotherapy alone is advisable, and in another decompensation, for instance with a severe neurotic depression, we combine antidepressive therapy with psychotherapy.

The second topic was the problem of abuse, overuse and dependence development in the field of pharmacotherapy with minor tranquillizers. First of all it was pointed out that in the case of treatment with neuroleptics in psychosis we can administer those for a long time. If we administer the minor tranquillizers, especially benzodiazepines, in psychogenic states, we have to be aware of dependence development. Therefore we should administer them for shorter periods than the neuroleptics in psychosis. Then it was pointed out that the problem of misuse of drugs is not only a problem of pharmacokinetics of the drug. The development of dependence can be seen as an interaction between the personality, the social environment and the drug pharmacokinetics. It seems to play an important role whether the drug is socially accepted or not.

The third topic of our workshop was the problem of the treatment of alcoholics, especially of the meta-alcoholic psychoses like delirium tremens and withdrawal symptoms. It was pointed out in our discussion that chlordiazepoxide is a very successful medicament for treating delirium tremens. Benzodiazepines in general are also very useful for the treatment of other withdrawal symptoms. The general opinion of our group was that the benzodiazepines can be used very successfully if their administration is for a limited period.

Workshop D:

Social Aspects of Benzodiazepines Therapy

Coordinated by **D. Ladewig** (Switzerland) and **M. Levy, Jr.** (Brazil)

Participants: **E.D. Busnello** (Brazil), **S.C. Kaim** (USA) and **M.A. Albuquerque** (Brazil)

It is a paradox that the usefulness as well as the availability of psychotropic drugs today has produced an ambivalent approach by society. We see on the one hand an increasing tolerance towards mental illness, which is more or less accepted, but in the meantime we are confronted with hostility towards behavioural disorders caused by drugs themselves.

The medical question on treating people with states of anxiety is: at what state does anxiety need treatment, and what kind of treatment? Anxiety is a normal emotion and might be seen as a valuable function inducing beneficial adaptive change. The intervention of treatment merely to suppress anxiety will prevent or retard the appropriate adaptation and sometimes may do more harm than good. Every anxiolytic treatment should be based on a clear medical diagnosis and should be integrated in a broader concept of a total therapy which means an integration in psychosocial and even religious resources of a society.

Using the drug only as *one* part – and clearly the most inexpensive one – of the therapeutic armamentarium and prescribing it for the minimum period necessary to achieve a therapeutic effect is the best way of reducing the risk of abuse or dependence, which is generally very low in benzodiazepines. This has been demonstrated many times.

Dr Kaim discussed the risks of benzodiazepines utilization: those that abuse them are already tendentious because of their personality structure and, in general, combine other drugs or have a history of multiple drug abuse before using benzodiazepines. He even considered harmful the promotion contrary to their use, as patients who really need them may be led to abandon the therapy.

Dr Busnello, after taking into consideration some aspects of mental health, referred to the advantages of a suitable tranquillizer – like the benzodiazepines – of easy and safe usage, there being even the possibility of their use by beginners in mental health. Their utilization not only relates to anxiety and epilepsy crises but also to the fact that psychiatrists must consider social problems related to mental health in general. Worrying with other persons involved in mental health treatment about social problems, the psychiatrist has to stress the importance of adequate treatment procedures.

Finally Dr Albuquerque said that the drug must not be an isolated therapeutic agent; it must be completely appropriate for the patient and not be used just to tranquillize the doctor. He called attention to considering the country as a big organism, avoiding a 'collective dependence' on psychotropic drugs without motivation and energies to be applied to general health problems such as basic cleanliness, habitation, welfare etc. In addition to medical treatment it was generally considered that education in an appropriate way must be directed to all kinds of mental and physical hygiene to *reduce* the increasing incidence of psychosocial stress in order to *prevent* a worsening of psychosomatic disturbances and to *change* attitudes and prejudices regarding psychosomatic disturbances.

Closing Speech

U. Vianna Filho

I believe that man has a natural horror of endings. This is a psychological characteristic of the human being who is the only creature in the zoological scale to have the notion of finiteness; this idea of finiteness is really given or actually imposed by medicine which makes us turn our thoughts to the idea of the end.

It is very difficult to analyse correctly the facts reported here because they always lead us to more profound reflections. Possibly, it is not opportune to report here on the background of these reflections, yet I believe that one of the merits of these congresses is to provide us with many problems to meditate upon. This stimulating effect is, in my opinion, one of the great values of meetings such as this one.

I also believe such reflection to be of tremendous importance and that thorough comprehension requires a longer time. I hope that all those present will be sensitive to the problems raised here; we know that, although to present a problem is not to solve it, the mere fact of becoming aware of such questions has enriched us all extraordinarily.

With reference to the sessions, which were well coordinated, there is one aspect raised by our esteemed co-president, Professor Sternbach, which led to extremely important considerations – I refer to the film that was shown here. I commented to him that it might give more force to the anti-psychiatry arguments when we see that, through the use of drugs, we may be altering the inborn characteristics of the human being. Everything leads us to believe that man is the perfect end-product in the history of living beings on this planet and that the human being possesses really special characteristics which do not permit comparison with the findings of animal experimentation.

The research being done in the pharmacokinetic field (revealed in one magnificent session on 'Benzodiazepines today and tomorrow, from a pharmacological point of view' (Workshop A)) demonstrates perfectly the importance of these pharmacological, physiological and biochemical aspects within the pharmacological context of the use of such a drug. The insight provided by progress in neurophysiology and all the instruments with which research technology provides us, can and does shed light on the various questions presented.

It is evident that the progress made in these last 10 years has been great and that the majority of the questions posed have not yet found a solution in technology. Yet this is the destiny of the sciences, of activity, of reflection, of epistemology, of neurophysiological knowledge. This is a question which only time and more research can answer.

Following the film, we had the splendid papers by Professor Priest on clinical reviews. The psychophysiological effects were well dealt with by Dr V. Gentil Filho.

The application of benzodiazepines in psychosomatic illness was also discussed, just at a time when we are beginning to achieve new insights into such disorders through interpreting the endogenous factors within the group of depressant equivalents. Our new understanding of psychosomatic illness and related aspects, together with the research on anxiety, has opened up a very fertile field of possibilities for the use of associated medications.

The next session, again, mainly covered work on other clinical aspects of the benzodiazepines, including the work by Brown on the neurological aspects and the specific problem of the use of these medications in the treatment of epilepsy.

The tendency of the later reports was to point out an intimate relationship between the psychological and the psychotherapeutic approach. This is very important because there is no basic conflict between these methods and the utilization of medicinal agents: we have passed the age of omnipotency and the progress of medicine depends on a multidisciplinary outlook, dealing with all aspects of the problems.

Concern was also expressed by Dr S. Kaim at the treatment of alcoholism, and Dr Ladewig examined the utilization of anxiety-reducing drugs and the possibilities of pharmacodependence.

Finally, we dealt with Brazilian research. Problems that involved social factors were presented, highlighted by Professor Othon Bastos' paper on the use of benzodiazepines in a university clinic and in the public service. Perhaps the invited speakers will have realized the importance which these matters acquire in our country; they are social problems, involving the generalization and, perhaps, even mass action in the treatment of the ill. I have the impression that it is not a specific problem but that it is a function of the degree of development which our country has reached, being tied to its level of economic development and the social and economic disparities which prevail in a country labelled 'a developing nation'.

This preoccupation of the Brazilian speakers with the social element, is, perhaps, to compensate for the fact that we have not been able to achieve sufficient technological development to do the research which our guests have reported, with all the sophistication of today's scientific technology. Evidently, we have not yet reached a state of development that allows a contribution of this nature but I also believe that our country should be given credit for its interest in the human and social dimensions of problems.

Perhaps there has been some antagonism between the purely pharmacological, the purely biochemical, the purely neurophysiological and even the physiopathological approach and psychological and socio-economic methods.

In this connection, we are tempted into the dualistic way of thinking with which our occidental civilization is strongly stigmatized. I believe the time has come for us to think of man as an integral whole, not as a fragmented being functioning on several disparate levels broken up into his biological, social and genetic components. Consideration must be given to the peculiar nature of the human manner of living, concentrating on the special conditions prevailing today.

Another point to which almost all the speakers referred was the need to provide for the future of this man, living in constantly changing conditions in which the mechanisms of adaptation are unpredictable.

Another important subject that was discussed and was, perhaps, the preoccupation of all the commentators and many of the speakers, was the possibility of the use of the benzodiazepines in combination with other drugs. I refer, for example, to the work of Karniol and of his experience in São Paulo with the combined use of β-blockers and benzodiazepines.

One of the thoughts that has come to me during this symposium concerns the separation that could have emerged between our guest speakers and our Brazilian speakers in the absence of any local Brazilian research technology and in view of the socio-economic and psychological concerns that guide Brazilian psychiatry at the present time.

I did feel that during the first sessions there was, perhaps, a certain communication difficulty between our internationally well-known guests and our Brazilian speakers. The workshops, however, permitted more immediate human contact between the two facets of the works presented: on the one hand, the pharmacological and clinical research aspects, and on the other, the greater concern of the Brazilian work with another facet of the philosophy of psychiatry.

Finally, I believe that the Symposium has brought us much material for thought and that the implications of the problems raised are very far-reaching. I hope that at a later date the knowledge imparted here concerning these problems, and the manner in which they were dealt with, will have repercussions on Brazilian psychiatric thinking. For this we are extremely grateful to all our guest speakers who brought us their knowledge and came to raise philosophical, human and socio-economic questions relating to this great problem, perhaps the most serious problem faced by mankind today.

I also want to say that looking at the problem of the benzodiazepines from a futuristic point of view is like the mediaeval preoccupation with the quest for the philosophical touchstone. We are here searching for the ideal drug, the drug that does not bring about dependence, the drug that has no unwanted additional effects, the omnipotent drug, the ideal drug. This is, perhaps, just a brief reflection on certain themes inspired by this modern-day quest for the philosophical touchstone, the search for the ideal drug which may serve to relieve the problem of contemporary man.

Index of Participants

Subject Index

GPSR Compliance

The European Union's (EU) General Product Safety Regulation (GPSR) is a set of rules that requires consumer products to be safe and our obligations to ensure this.

If you have any concerns about our products, you can contact us on ProductSafety@springernature.com

In case Publisher is established outside the EU, the EU authorized representative is:

Springer Nature Customer Service Center GmbH
Europaplatz 3
69115 Heidelberg, Germany

Batch number: 10583998

Printed by Printforce, the Netherlands